Overview

D1484674

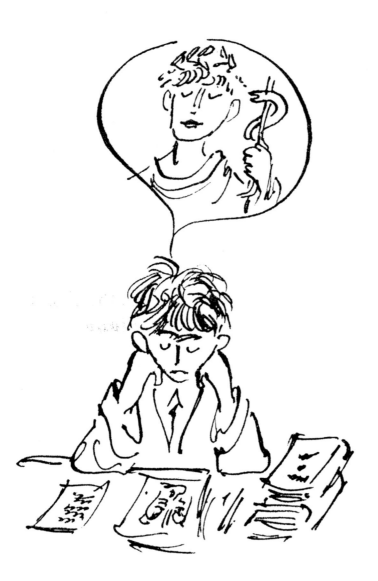

Illustration by Robert Wyss

Fundamentals of Neurology
An Illustrated Guide

Mark Mumenthaler, M.D.

Professor Emeritus of Neurology
Former Head of the Department
of Neurology
Berne University
Inselspital Berne
Switzerland

Heinrich Mattle, M.D.

Professor of Neurology
Berne University
Inselspital Berne
Switzerland

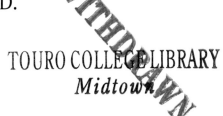

Translated and adapted by Ethan Taub, M.D.

396 illustrations

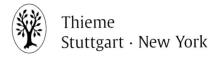

Thieme
Stuttgart · New York

Library of Congress Cataloging-in-Publication Data
Mumenthaler, Marco, 1925-
  [Grundkurs Neurologie. English]
  Neurology : an illustrated guide / Mark Mumenthaler,
  Heinrich Mattle ; translated by Ethan Taub.
    p. ; cm.
  Includes index.
  "Revised translation of the German edition ... Grund-
kurs Neurologie. Illustriertes Basiswissen für das Stu-
dium" – T.p. verso.
    ISBN 1-58890-450-4 (GTV : alk. paper) –
    ISBN 3-13-136451-3 (TNY : alk. paper)
    1. Neurology—Outlines, syllabi, etc. I. Mattle, Heinrich.
II. Title. [DNLM: 1. Nervous System Diseases—Hand-
books. WL 39 M962g 2006a]
RC357.M8613 2006
616.8–dc22   2005032828

This book is an authorized and revised translation of the
German edition published and copyrighted 2002 by
Georg Thieme Verlag, Stuttgart, Germany. Title of the
German edition: Grundkurs Neurologie. Illustriertes
Basiswissen für das Studium

Translator: Ethan Taub, M.D., Klinik im Park, Zurich,
Switzerland

Illustrators: Malgorzata and Piotr Gusta,
Champigny sur Marne, France

Important note: Medicine is an ever-changing science undergoing continual development. Research and clinical experience are continually expanding our knowledge, in particular our knowledge of proper treatment and drug therapy. Insofar as this book mentions any dosage or application, readers may rest assured that the authors, editors, and publishers have made every effort to ensure that such references are in accordance with **the state of knowledge at the time of production of the book.**

Nevertheless, this does not involve, imply, or express any guarantee or responsibility on the part of the publishers in respect to any dosage instructions and forms of applications stated in the book. **Every user is requested to examine carefully** the manufacturers' leaflets accompanying each drug and to check, if necessary in consultation with a physician or specialist, whether the dosage schedules mentioned therein or the contraindications stated by the manufacturers differ from the statements made in the present book. Such examination is particularly important with drugs that are either rarely used or have been newly released on the market. Every dosage schedule or every form of application used is entirely at the user's own risk and responsibility. The authors and publishers request every user to report to the publishers any discrepancies or inaccuracies noticed. If errors in this work are found after publication, errata will be posted at www.thieme.com on the product description page.

© 2006 Georg Thieme Verlag,
Rüdigerstrasse 14, 70469 Stuttgart, Germany
http://www.thieme.de
Thieme New York, 333 Seventh Avenue,
New York, NY 10001 USA
http://www.thieme.com

Typesetting by primustype Hurler GmbH, Notzingen
Printed in Germany by Appl, Wemding

ISBN 3–13–136451–3 (GTV)
ISBN 1–58890–450–4 (TNY)   1 2 3 4 5 6

12/19/08

Preface

This textbook of neurology, a translation and revision of the original book in German, was written for students of medicine. Persons starting their careers in the other health professions may also find it useful.

We the authors are two Swiss academic neurologists with our own narrow subspecialties in the broad field of neurology. In writing this book, we have set our personal interests aside, presenting in detail only what seemed to us to be most important for the student. The book begins with a brief review of fundamentals, then deals with the syndromes affecting each major component of the nervous system. It also includes chapters on the clinical neurological examination and on common ancillary tests, with explanations of their underlying principles.

The main emphasis of the book is on clinical disease states. Most of its chapters are thus devoted to the diseases affecting a particular part of the nervous system.

Despite enormous progress in our understanding of pathogenesis, especially in microbiology and molecular genetics, and despite advances in neuroimaging and electrophysiology, diagnostic evaluation in neurology still crucially depends on the meticulous analysis of clinical information, i. e., the findings of the clinical history and neurological examination. The book includes many illustrations of abnormalities that can be seen either in radiological images or directly on examination of the patient.

The information in the book, and the degree of detail in which each item is discussed, reflect the subjective and, sometimes, arbitrary choices of the authors. In choosing what to include, we have tried to answer the questions that our students have asked us most often over the years. We hope that the book will also meet the needs of readers of this English edition.

An English translation of a European book for medical students in America, Britain, and elsewhere might seem superfluous. Yet, having both lived, studied, and worked in the United States for many years, we have happily discovered that, in the interconnected world of medicine, all national and linguistic borders tend to lose their significance.

Finally, we offer thanks in advance to any readers who care to give us their criticism, thoughts, or suggestions for future editions.

Mark Mumenthaler
Heinrich Mattle

Translator's Note

"The tongue of the wise brings healing" (Proverbs 12:18). Once again, it has been my privilege to translate and revise an important work by Professors Mumenthaler and Mattle. The fourth English edition of their comprehensive text, *Neurology*, was published by Thieme in 2004 and has met with an appreciative audience. This shorter but still highly informative book is a teaching text intended to give the medical student a plentiful fund of knowledge in this wide-ranging and challenging field. May it enjoy a similar success.

Ethan Taub

Contents

1 Fundamentals

Microscopic Anatomy of the Nervous System

Neurons are the structural and functional building blocks of the nervous system. This type of cell is specialized for the **reception**, **integration**, and **transmission of electrical impulses**.

Neurons. The cell body (**soma**) of the neuron is enclosed by the cell membrane and contains the cell nucleus, mitochondria, endoplasmic reticulum, neurotubules, and neurofilaments (Fig. 1.1). Dendrites are short, more or less extensively branched, cellular processes that conduct *afferent* impulses toward the cell body. They provide the cell with a much larger surface area than the cell body alone, thereby increasing the area available for intercellular contact and for the deployment of cell membrane receptors. Different types of neurons have different characteristic morphological types of dendrites; those of the cerebellar Purkinje cells, for example, resemble a deer's antlers (Fig. 1.2). The **axon** is a single cell process, usually longer than a dendrite, which emerges from the cell body at the axon hillock. It conducts *efferent* impulses away from the cell body to another neuron or an effector organ.

Generally speaking, every neuron has a soma, an axon, and one or more dendrites. The structure and configuration of the nerve cell processes (especially the dendrites) vary depending on the function of the neuron. Thus, neurons can be classified into a number of morphological subtypes (Fig. 1.3).

Fig. 1.**1 Fine structure of a neuron** (after Wilkinson, J.L.: *Neuroanatomy for Medical Students*, 2nd edn, Butterworth–Heinemann, Oxford 1992).

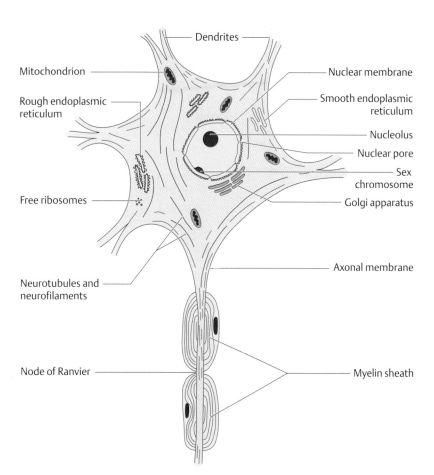

Dendrites

Mitochondrion

Rough endoplasmic reticulum

Free ribosomes

Neurotubules and neurofilaments

Node of Ranvier

Nuclear membrane

Smooth endoplasmic reticulum

Nucleolus

Nuclear pore

Sex chromosome

Golgi apparatus

Axonal membrane

Myelin sheath

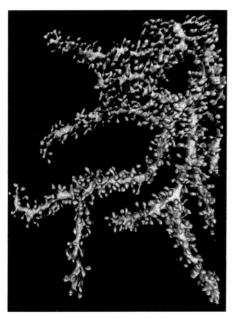

Fig. 1.**2 Cerebellar Purkinje cell** (microphotograph). Note the numerous synapses on the dendrites. (Image obtained by Dr. Marco Vecellio, Histological Institute of the University of Fribourg, Switzerland.)

Neuroglia. The neurons constitute the important functional part of the nervous system; they are surrounded by *supportive cells*, which are collectively called neuroglia. Neuroglial cells of one particular type, the **astrocytes**, have a starlike morphology. They make contact with nonsynaptic sites on the neuronal surface and possess perivascular foot processes that contact 85 % of the capillaries of the nervous system. Astrocytes ensure

an adequate supply of nutrients to the neurons and are an important component of the blood–brain barrier. Other types of supportive cell in the central nervous system include the **oligodendrocytes**, **microglia**, and **ependymal cells**, and the cells of the choroid plexus.

Myelin sheaths. Axons less than 1 μm in diameter are usually unmyelinated, while thicker axons are sheathed in myelin. The **myelin sheath** is generated by the "sinking" of an axon into an oligodendrocyte (or, in the peripheral nervous system, a Schwann cell), forming a *mesaxon*, which consists of a double sheet of cell membrane. The mesaxon wraps around the axon multiple times (Fig. 1.**4c**). Individual segments of myelin, which can be up to 1 mm long, are separated by the intervening **nodes of Ranvier**, which play an important role in the transmission of nerve impulses along the axon (p. 4). The "naked" axonal segments at the nodes of Ranvier, are 1–4 μm wide and are only partly covered by processes of the neighboring Schwann cells. They are thus separated from the surrounding endoneural interstitium only by the neuronal cell membrane (neurilemma or axolemma). The nodal axolemma mainly contains voltage-dependent sodium channels, while the internodal segments mainly contain potassium channels.

Synapse. The sites at which neurons transmit impulses to each other are called synapses. Each synapse is composed of a bulblike expansion of the end of an axon, called an *axon terminal* (or *bouton*); the *synaptic cleft*; and the *postsynaptic membrane* of the receiving neuron or effector organ (Fig. 1.**5**). Myelinated axons lose their myelin sheath just proximal to the axon terminal. A single neuron can receive synaptic input from one or many axons; the impulses it receives can be either exci-

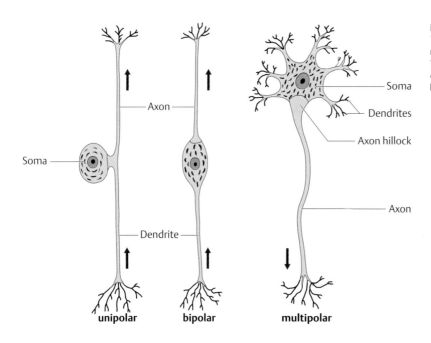

Fig. 1.**3 Three types of neurons.** The arrows indicate the usual direction of impulse conduction (after Wilkinson, J.L.: *Neuroanatomy for Medical Students*, 2nd ed, Butterworth-Heinemann, Oxford 1992).

Soma

Dendrites

Axon hillock

Axon

Axon

Soma

Dendrite

Soma

unipolar   **bipolar**   **multipolar**

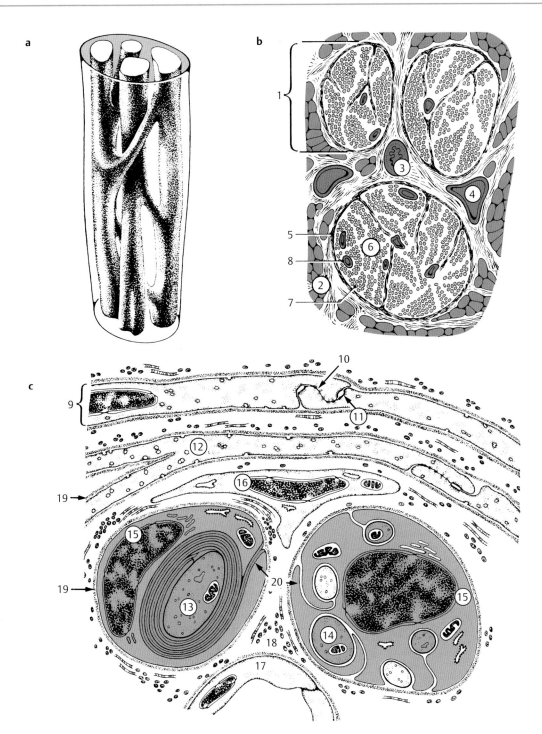

Fig. 1.**4 Peripheral nerve** (schematic drawings). **a** Low magnification reveals the plexuslike structure of the nerve fascicles. **b** The nerve fascicles (**1**) are surrounded by a common epineurium (**2**) composed mainly of fat and connective tissue. Blood vessels (vasa nervorum) lie between the fascicles (**3** = arteries, **4** = veins). The fascicles are subdivided by septa derived from the perineurium (**5**). The endoneurium (**6**) contains myelinated fibers (**7**) and capillaries (**8**). **c** Electron microscopy reveals the flat perineural cells (**9**), which are tightly connected to one another by zonulae occludentes (**10** = tight junctions) and desmosomes (**11**). The perineural cell cytoplasm contains many pinocytotic vesicles (**12**). Within the endoneurium, one can discern myelinated (**13**) and unmyelinated axons (**14**), Schwann cells (**15**), a fibrocyte (**16**), and a capillary (**17** = endothelial cell). The endoneural interstitium contains numerous collagen fibrils (**18**). The perineural, endothelial, and Schwann cells are surrounded by a basal membrane (**19**). A mesaxon (**20**) is formed by the sinking of an axon into a Schwann cell.

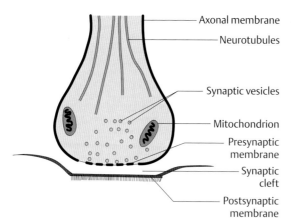

Axonal membrane

Neurotubules

Synaptic vesicles

Mitochondrion

Presynaptic membrane

Synaptic cleft

Postsynaptic membrane

Fig. 1.**5 Fine structure of a synapse** (diagram after Wilkinson, J.L.: *Neuroanatomy for Medical Students*, 2nd edn, Butterworth–Heinemann, Oxford 1992).

tatory or inhibitory. An axon can form a synapse onto a cell body, a dendrite, or another axon. Ongoing processes of structural and functional change at the synaptic contacts between nerve cells provide the nervous system with functional adaptability ("plasticity") even after the individual has reached maturity. Neural impulses are transmitted across synapses by chemical substances called **neurotransmitters**: some of the more important ones in the central nervous system are dopamine, serotonin, acetylcholine, and γ-aminobutyric acid (GABA). Specialized synapses connect the axons of the peripheral nervous system to effector organs such as muscle cells (motor end plates, p. 263) or glandular cells (p. 280).

Elements of Neurophysiology

The resting **membrane potential** of a neuron or muscle cell can undergo a rapid, transient change, called an action potential, in response to an incoming stimulus or impulse. The **action potential** is generated by transient changes of ion permeability across the cell membrane. Action potentials and chemical impulse transmission at the synapses are the specific mechanisms used by the nervous system for information transfer.

Neurons are enclosed by a double-layered **cell membrane** with an inner *phospholipid layer* and an outer *glycoprotein layer*. Specialized protein molecules within the cell membrane form **channels** that are selectively permeable to sodium, potassium, or chloride ions. Some ion channels (e. g., on the postsynaptic membrane) open only when a specific ligand binds to them, e. g., the neurotransmitter molecule that conveys neural impulses from cell to cell. These channels are called **ligand-dependent ion channels. Voltage-dependent ion channels**, on the other hand, are found mainly on the axonal membrane. They open and close depending on the transmembrane electrical potential.

Resting potential. A difference of electrical potential arises across the neuronal membrane because of the unequal concentrations of ions in the intracellular and extracellular spaces (ICS, ECS) combined with the varying electrical conductivity of the membrane to different types of ion. The resting potential is mainly determined by the **ratio of intracellular and extracellular potassium concentration**, because, at rest, the membrane is highly permeable to potassium ions and relatively impermeable to sodium ions. The potassium concentration in the ICS is roughly 35 times higher than in the ECS. Thus, potassium ions tend to diffuse out of the cell. The inner surface of the membrane thereby loses positive charges and becomes negatively charged. As negative charge builds up on the inner surface of the membrane, a differ-

ence of electrical potential is generated, which opposes further outward flow of potassium ions; negative charge continues to build up until the potential difference exactly cancels out the force arising from the difference in potassium ion concentration. The net effect is that there is no further net transfer of potassium ions across the membrane in either direction and a stable, resting membrane potential is generated, with a value ranging from − 60 to − 90 mV.

Action potential. The sodium ion concentration is roughly 20 times higher in the ECS than in the ICS. Therefore, neurotransmitter-induced opening of ligand-sensitive postsynaptic sodium channels is followed by a **rapid influx of sodium ions** into the cell. The inner surface of the cell membrane becomes positively charged and an action potential is generated whose amplitude and time course are independent of the nature and intensity of the depolarizing impulse (this is the **all-or-nothing law** of cellular excitation). The transmembrane potential difference reaches a peak positive value ranging from + 20 to + 50 mV. After a brief delay, the potassium channels of the cell membrane become more permeable than at rest, so that a net outflow of potassium ions results. This compensates for the preceding sodium influx and causes repolarization of the membrane to its resting potential. An active sodium pump also participates in this process. Until repolarization is complete, the membrane is temporarily unable to conduct any further impulses; the initial *absolute refractory period* is followed by a *relative refractory period*.

Impulse conduction. The axon potential begins at the axon hillock and is then conducted forward along the axonal membrane by the successive opening of voltage-dependent sodium channels. This wave of excitation (local depolarization) travels down the axon at a speed that depends on the thickness of the axon and the thickness of its myelin sheath. The nodes of Ranvier play an especially important role in this process: the isolating myelin sheaths lower the capacitance of the axonal membrane and raise its electrical resistance. The action potentials are therefore initiated only at the nodes, "jumping over" the internodal axon segments (so-called **saltatory conduction**). Because of this special mecha-nism, myelinated nerve fibers conduct action potentials much more rapidly than unmyelinated fibers. The nor-mal motor and sensory conduction velocity of periph-eral nerves is 50–60 m/s.

Elements of Neurogenetics

Many neurological diseases are caused by genetic defects or tend to arise in the presence of a genetic predisposition. In this section, we will present the basics of both **"classical" (Mendelian) inheritance** and **molecular genetics**, as a necessary prerequisite for the understanding of these diseases and for the counseling of affected patients and their families.

General Genetics

The physical characteristics (**phenotype**) of an in-dividual are determined both by the totality of that in-dividual's genetic information (the **genotype**) and by environmental influences during gestation and after-ward. Genetic information is contained in DNA molecules in the cell nucleus and mitochondria. A seg-ment of DNA containing the information necessary for the synthesis of a protein molecule is called a **gene** and the totality of the organism's genes is called the **genome**. The nuclear genes of human beings are con-tained in **23 pairs of chromosomes**—22 pairs of **auto-somes** and one pair of **sex chromosomes** (gonosomes), which can be either XX (in females) or XY (in males).

Recombination of genetic material. The growth of the organism requires a large number of cell divisions (**mi-toses**). In each mitosis, the nuclear genetic material doubles in amount (replicates) and is then distributed to the two daughter cells, so that each daughter cell, like the original cell, contains a complete (diploid) set of chromosomes. For the purpose of sexual reproduction, however, a reductive cell division (**meiosis**) occurs, pro-ducing egg or sperm cells that contain only a haploid set of chromosomes—i. e., only one of each chromosome (22 autosomes and one sex chromosome), as opposed to the 23 pairs found in all other cells. The union of an egg cell and a sperm cell restores a full (diploid) comple-ment of chromosomes, half of which are derived from the maternal genome and half from the paternal genome.

According to the rules of Mendelian inheritance, ma-ternally-derived and paternally-derived properties (genes) are assorted randomly and independently to the germ cells, and thereby to the offspring. An important limitation of this random and independent assortment comes from the fact that genes located on the same chromosome are ordinarily transmitted together (be-cause entire chromosomes are passed on to the germ cells). Yet, in a particular phase of meiosis, correspond-ing DNA segments on homologous chromatids can be exchanged with each other (**crossing over**), producing a new arrangement of genes on the chromatids that take part in the transaction (genetic recombination). The greater the distance between two genes on a chromo-some, the more frequently recombination will occur be-tween them.

In addition to these physiological mechanisms lead-ing to change and reassortment of the genetic material (random assortment of maternal and paternal chromo-somes in meiosis and fertilization, recombination of genes on homologous chromosomes), spontaneous changes in the genome, called **mutations**, can also occur. Mutations in the germ line are passed on to the in-dividual's offspring.

Autosomal dominant inheritance. A gene that markedly influences or completely determines the phenotype of the individual in the heterozygous state is called **dominant**. If the father *or* mother is heterozygous for a dominant allele, then their child has a 50% chance of being heterozygous and displaying the corresponding phenotypic trait.

Autosomal recessive inheritance. An autosomal gene that has no effect in the heterozygous state and only manifests itself phenotypically in homozygotes is called **recessive**. If *both* the father *and* the mother are heterozy-gous for a recessive allele, then 75% of their progeny will also possess at least one copy of the allele: 50% will be heterozygous and 25% will be homozygous. Only the ho-mozygous offspring will display the corresponding phenotypic trait (e. g., a recessively inherited genetic dis-ease). The heterozygous offspring ("carriers") will not display the phenotypic trait; neither will the one-quarter of offspring who do not possess the recessive allele.

X-chromosomal inheritance. Males receive an X-chro-mosome from their mother and a Y-chromosome from their father, while females receive an X-chromosome from both parents. Mothers, therefore, will pass on an X-chromosomal gene to half of their offspring, whether male or female (as long as they are themselves heter-ozygous for it), while fathers will pass it on to all of their daughters, but not to their sons. Dominantly inherited X-chromosomal diseases affect both males and females; recessively inherited X-chromosomal diseases mainly affect males, striking only the rare females that are ho-mozygous for the disease, i. e., only those who have in-herited an X-chromosome with the diseased gene from each of their parents. Any affected male is certain to have received the gene from his mother; as long as his female partner is not a carrier of the disease, all of his daughters will be healthy carriers. Female carriers whose male partners do not have the disease will pass on the disease to 50% of their sons; all of their daughters will be healthy, though half will carry the gene for the disease.

Maternal inheritance of the mitochondrial genome.
Mitochondrial DNA is passed on exclusively in the maternal line: mitochondrial genetic diseases are transmitted only by mothers to their children (both male and female), but never by fathers. Mitochondria with mutated DNA can coexist in the same cell with other mitochondria whose DNA is normal. This phenomenon, called **heteroplasmia**, has no counterpart in the nuclear genome, which is the same in every cell of the body. In mitochondrial genetic diseases, the phenotype, i. e., the extent of damage to the involved cells and tissues, depends on the ratio of mutated to normal mitochondrial DNA and on the number of defective mitochondria that are present.

Mutations are necessary for evolution; without them, the human species would not exist. Yet, adverse mutations can also cause genetic defects and diseases. Mutations can be classified into genomic and intragenic types.

Genomic mutations are of two types, designated as numerical and structural chromosomal aberrations. In the former type of mutation, the number of chromosomes is abnormal (e. g., monosomy, trisomy); in the latter type, the structure of a chromosome is abnormal. Structural aberrations include *deletions, translocations,* and *inversions* of chromosomal segments.

Intragenic mutations involve alterations of the DNA. Within each chromosome, DNA is arranged linearly. DNA segments (genes) that code for amino acid sequences (proteins) are called *exons* and are found in alternation with noncoding sequences called *introns.* Exons account for only about 5% of human chromosomal DNA. When the DNA is transcribed into RNA, the primary RNA transcript contains a copy of the introns. These are then spliced out in a second stage of processing, which yields the mature transcript, *messenger RNA* (mRNA).

Each group of three consecutive nucleotides in the mRNA molecule (called a *triplet* or *codon*) codes for an amino in the protein undergoing biosynthesis. "Stop codons" between the exons signal the beginning and end of the gene and thereby determine the length of the protein that is to be synthesized.

Mutations involving the replacement of a DNA nucleotide by a different nucleotide often alter the sense of the codon to which it belongs (**missense** mutations): the wrong amino acid is inserted into the gene product at this point in protein biosynthesis. The ultimate effect this has on protein function is highly variable. If, however, a nucleotide replacement happens to result in the generation or destruction of a stop codon, an incomplete or excessively long protein will be produced (**nonsense** mutations). Other mutations involving the *insertion* of an extra nucleotide into the DNA, or the *deletion* of a nucleotide, alter the rhythm of nucleotide triplets and are therefore called **frame-shift** mutations. These usually cause severe abnormalities of protein structure and function (e. g., Duchenne muscular dystrophy, p. 265).

Expanded repetitive DNA sequences. A further type of mutation of special importance in neurology affects the number of trinucleotides (triplets). Normal human DNA contains a large number of repetitive sequences of trinucleotides, whose presence affects the function and expression of genes. An important group of neurodegenerative diseases is caused by mutations involving abnormally long (expanded) triplet repeat sequences. These diseases are called **trinucleotide** or **triplet repeat** diseases. Where the normal repeat sequence might contain only a few triplets, the diseased sequence contains dozens or hundreds. The longer the expansion, the earlier the age of onset of disease, and the more severe its manifestations. The repeat sequences tend to lengthen from one generation to the next, so that the disease tends to appear earlier and earlier ("anticipation") and to become increasingly severe.

Mutations of mitochondrial DNA impair oxidative metabolism in the mitochondria, causing a number of different types of disease, including **mitochondrial encephalomyopathies** (p. 272).

Neurogenetics

The **triplet diseases** are of special relevance to neurology. The neurodegenerative diseases caused by expanded triplet repeats are listed in Table 1.1; their common features are summarized in Table 1.2. Some of the more common inherited mitochondrial diseases are listed in Table 1.3 (for their clinical manifestations, cf. p. 272).

Ever more genetic defects are being identified as the cause of neurological and other diseases. Large tables and books are available for those seeking up-to-date information. Rapid access to the current state of knowledge is best obtained via the Internet. Two useful sites are "Online Mendelian Inheritance in Man" (http://www3.ncbi.nlm.nih.gov/OMIM/) and Medline (http://www4.ncbi.nlm.nih.gov/entrez/query.fcgi).

Genetic Counseling

Many genetic mutations can be detected directly by DNA analysis. The results are highly specific. Thus, many diseases can be diagnosed even before they become symptomatic, so that a long-term prognosis can be given. Sadly, these diseases are generally untreatable and inexorably progressive.

Before any DNA analysis is performed, the treating physician should:
- perform a meticulous clinical examination,
- obtain a detailed family history and personally examine the patient's relatives, if possible,
- inform the patient and his or her relatives in detail about the suspected disease, and
- explain the consequences of the proposed DNA analysis to them in a readily understandable manner.

A negative DNA analysis can provide relief and free the patient from anxiety. A positive result, on the other hand, may propel the patient into a severe depression, as he or she will then face the certainty of developing an inherited disease, mostly with a grim prognosis, and may not be able to cope with this knowledge. The knowledge of a genetic abnormality may also put a

Tabelle 1.1 **Some neurodegenerative diseases caused by triplet repeat expansions**

Disease	Major clinical manifestations	Triplet	Chromosomal localization
Fragile X-chromosome	diminished intelligence, sometimes facial dysmorphism, connective tissue dysplasia	CGG	Xq27
Myotonic dystrophy	progressive, mainly distal muscular dystrophy and myotonia	CTG	19q13.3
Friedreich ataxia	ataxia, areflexia, pyramidal tract signs, dysarthria	GAA	9q13–q21.1
Spinobulbar muscle atrophy (Kennedy syndrome)	muscle atrophy, dysarthria, fasciculations, gynecomastia	CAG	Xq13–q21
Huntington disease	chorea, rarely spasticity or rigidity, cognitive and behavioral disturbances	CAG	4p16.3
Spinocerebellar ataxia type 1 (SCA1)	cerebellar ataxia, sometimes chorea or dystonia, polyneuropathy, often pyramidal tract signs, sometimes dementia	CAG	6p24
Spinocerebellar ataxia type 2 (SCA2)	cerebellar ataxia, sometimes chorea or dystonia, myoclonus, polyneuropathy, sometimes pyramidal tract signs and dementia	CAG	12
Spinocerebellar ataxia type 3 (SCA3); Machado–Joseph disease	cerebellar ataxia, sometimes chorea or dystonia, polyneuropathy, sometimes pyramidal tract signs and dementia	CAG	14
Spinocerebellar ataxia type 6 (SCA6)	cerebellar ataxia, sometimes polyneuropathy and pyramidal tract signs	CAG	19p13
Spinocerebellar ataxia type 7 (SCA7)	cerebellar ataxia, sometimes chorea or dystonia, retinal degeneration, polyneuropathy, sometimes pyramidal tract signs	CAG	3p
Spinocerebellar ataxia type 8 (SCA8)	cerebellar ataxia, spasticity, impaired vibration sense	CTG	13q21
Dentato-rubro-pallido-luysian atrophy (DRPLA)	ataxia, myoclonus, epilepsy, choreoathetosis, dementia	CAG	12p

severe stress on a marriage or other partnership. Social problems of yet other kinds may arise, because persons with inherited diseases are, unfortunately, often treated like outcasts in our postindustrial society. They may have troubles in the workplace, not least because they are likely to be uninsurable. For all these reasons, genetic testing generally causes fewer problems if it is performed after the disease has become symptomatic. Asymptomatic children should not be subjected to genetic testing even if their parents ask for it. They should be allowed to decide for themselves whether to undergo testing once they are mature enough to do so and have attained legal majority.

Many patients and their relatives decide not to undergo testing after being fully informed about their potential genetic disease and the consequences of DNA analysis. In particular, presymptomatic and asymptomatic persons would often rather not find out whether they would develop the disease at some time in the future. A positive test result would destroy their hopes for good health in later life.

If the patient does decide to undergo DNA analysis and then tests positive, the physician should inform the patient and his or her relatives in a personal discussion, with ample time to consider all of the implications. Test results should never be imparted over the telephone or in written form. Patients who have tested positive often

Table 1.2 **Common features of triplet repeat diseases**

- Autosomal dominant or X-chromosomal inheritance
- Onset usually between the ages of 25 and 45
- Gradual progression of disease
- Symmetrical neuronal loss and gliosis in the brain
- Anticipation
- The number of triplet repeats is correlated with the age of onset and the severity of the disease
- The diagnosis can be established by DNA analysis

Table 1.3 **Mitochondrial encephalomyopathies**

- Progressive external ophthalmopathy (PEO)
- Kearns–Sayre syndrome (KSS)
- Leber hereditary optic neuropathy (LHON)
- Mitochondrial encephalomyopathy with lactic acidosis and stroke (MELAS)
- Leigh disease
- Neuropathy, ataxia, and retinitis pigmentosa syndrome (NARP)
- Myoclonus epilepsy with ragged red fibers (MERRF)

need long-term psychotherapy. Nor does the physician–patient relationship end once the test results are given: many patients with hereditary neurological diseases can be greatly helped by continuing psychological support and symptomatic treatment.

2 The Clinical Interview in Neurology

General Principles of History Taking

> The clinical history is of paramount importance in neurology, perhaps more so than in any other medical specialty. It is indispensable as a **diagnostic instrument**, it serves to establish a **doctor-patient relationship built on trust**, and it is a prerequisite for the success of any treatment that will follow. The history should always be taken with utmost care.

The type of neurological disturbance from which a patient is suffering can usually be determined from a carefully obtained clinical history even before the physical examination or any further tests are performed. In many patients, the history alone permits the assignment of a precise diagnosis, but only if the physician has been listening closely to the patient.

! *"A blind neurologist is better than a deaf neurologist."*

Skillful history taking is the distinguishing mark of a good clinician.

General prerequisites for good history taking. In any branch of clinical medicine, not just in neurology, a good history can be obtained only if the patient has confidence in the physician. Introduce yourself to the patient and take the history in a place offering the necessary privacy and discretion. The patient should be comfortably seated and emotionally at ease, as far as the circumstances allow, and must not feel rushed. If someone else is present during the interview, e. g., a medical student, introduce this person and make sure the patient really has no objection to his or her presence. Persons other than the physician taking the history should behave discreetly and keep themselves somewhat in the background. The history should be detailed and complete and should be taken by, or under the supervision of, an experienced clinician, as far as possible.

General principles of the clinical interview. While interviewing the patient, observe these principles: in the beginning the patient should be doing most of the talking and you should say as little as possible. You do indeed have to elicit all of the important historical data by specific inquiry, but only after the patient has finished describing the problem in his or her own words. The patient's story may be rambling or vague; even so, you should take care not to seem impatient or irritated. Once your turn comes, however, you must amplify and refine this initial information by persistent or even stubborn questioning, until at last you have obtained a clear picture of the present illness. Never reject the patient's own interpretation of his or her symptoms, even if it seems implausible or absurd. You will then come across as a scoffing know-it-all and will have broken your line of communication with the patient.

Your demeanor toward the patient. Every patient has the right to be treated courteously and tactfully and to receive the physician's full attention during an appropriately set period. You should perform a meticulous physical examination only after you have listened carefully to the patient's story and filled it out with further, detailed questioning. The patient has the right to a full explanation of your findings and of what they imply about his or her illness. You should explain these matters truthfully, in language that the patient can understand and with due respect for his or her feelings. You will often find yourself having to steer a difficult course between bluntness and euphemism.

If the patient is accompanied by another person, such as a spouse, parent, other relative, or friend, the patient should remain the focus of your attention, even if he or she is a child or adolescent. You should communicate mainly with the patient. You might have to ask accompanying persons to leave the room for part of the clinical interview or physical examination, but do not neglect their needs, either; the persons nearest to the patient, after all, may have an important role to play later on, during treatment. Courtesy and consideration for the patient as a fellow human being, palpable respect for his or her dignity, and genuine understanding and sympathy are the foundations of a trusting relationship between the patient and the physician and are therefore essential preconditions for successful treatment.

The history and physical examination are two independent and equally important components of clinical diagnostic assessment. They must complement each other and should, to some extent, be performed in parallel. The experienced clinician, while listening to the patient's history, will already be thinking of specific abnormalities to look for on physical examination. If the examination should then reveal other, perhaps unexpected findings, the clinician can amplify the history by asking further, specific questions. Ideally, the clinician will be able to make the diagnosis from the history and physical examination alone.

Special Aspects of History Taking

The Clinical Interview in Neurology

2

> The "classic" history has certain standard components and is meant to provide a complete picture of the patient, including his or her present complaints, past medical history, personality, and life situation.

The present illness. When taking a clinical history, always first give the patient a chance to describe his or her **current complaints** and the **reason for the consultation**. Only afterward should you begin interrogating the patient systematically to make the history complete, in accordance with the principles presented above. Systematic history taking is performed in standard fashion in all branches of clinical medicine; a basic outline is provided in Table 2.**1**. In each specialty, however, there are further important issues that tend to arise regularly and these should be asked about specifically. The important questions to ask in the neurological history are summarized in Table 2.**2**.

Past medical history, family history, and social history. Once you have a clear and complete picture of the patient's current complaints, you can begin to ask about **earlier symptoms and illnesses**, starting with general questions and then proceeding into greater detail. Always ask about problems that might bear a relation to the present illness: a patient suffering from ischemic stroke, for instance, should be asked about hypertension, heart disease, and smoking. Inquire into the health of the patient's blood relatives, particularly with regard to neurological and other hereditary diseases. Finally, ask about the patient's **familial and social setting**: marriage or other partnership, children, occupation, and any potential problems or conflicts in these areas. Ascertain how the patient's current (or earlier) medical problems affect him or her in everyday life, both at home and in the workplace. Broach these matters as unobtrusively as possible, however, because overzealous questioning might make the patient wrongly think that you believe his or her problems to be primarily psychogenic. Of course, if a thorough diagnostic evaluation reveals that a psychogenic mechanism is the likely cause, then this, too, should be discussed openly with the patient.

Table 2.1 Outline of the general clinical history

1 The patient's spontaneous description of his or her current complaints —more precise information can be elicited by direct questioning

2 Systematic analysis of the current complaints (see Table 2.2)

3 Prior illnesses (past medical and surgical history)
- information spontaneously provided by the patient
- specific questioning by the physician, particularly about earlier conditions of potential relevance to the current complaints
- gestational and birth history, when indicated

4 Life Habits
- alcohol and tobacco
- medications
- illicit drugs
- potentially toxic environmental influences

5 Neurovegetative functions
- sleep, digestion, urination, sexual dysfunction

6 Personality and social situation
- the patient's **personal and social setting**: education, occupation, familial/social/financial position, and any current problems or conflicts (information of this type enables the physician to assess all of the factors affecting the patient's ability to deal with his or her medical problems successfully)
- the patient's behavior, manner of speaking, gestures, facial expressions, emotional responses, and reactions to questions, etc., give the examiner an **overall impression of the patient's personality**

7 Family history

Table 2.2 History of the present illness

Major symptom(s)
- The patient's spontaneous description, refined by specific questioning
- How long have the symptoms been present? Where are they located?
- How did they begin? (suddenly, gradually, or after a specific inducing event?)
- How have they developed over time? (constant, increasing, decreasing, fluctuating?)
- What influences the symptoms? (ameliorating/aggravating influences, medications?)
- Effects
  - How severe are the symptoms in terms of their effect on everyday life at home and at work, and on the patient's emotional well-being? Is treatment required?

Current accompanying symptoms
- Here it is particularly important to supplement the patient's spontaneous complaints with specific questioning. An experienced clinician knows what questions to ask even if the patient has provided very little information.

Relevant past medical history
- Did the patient already have **earlier symptoms** or conditions that might be relevant to the current complaints? (e. g., earlier transient ischemic attacks in a patient suffering from acute stroke?)
- Does the patient have any **predisposing factors** for conditions that might account for the current complaints? (e. g., cigarette smoking leading to a Pancoast tumor of the apex of the lung?)

Relevant family history
- This may lend support to a conjectural diagnosis: e. g., similar symptoms in blood relatives of the patient's parents, if a recessively inherited condition is suspected, or hemicranial headaches in the mother of a patient with suspected migraine

A carefully elicited clinical history ought to enable the experienced clinician to formulate a **tentative diagnosis** even before proceeding to the physical examination. With the tentative diagnosis in mind, he or she can then devote particular attention to certain aspects of the examination. Of course, the clinician must not allow his or her findings to be so colored by prior expectations that they are no longer reliable. The tentative diagnosis should inform the physical examination, not convert it into a pointless exercise.

3 The Neurological Examination

Basic Principles of the Neurological Examination

Neurological diseases can often be diagnosed based on a carefully elicited history in combination with the physical examination. In order to ensure completeness, the examining physician should examine all patients according to the same general scheme, making individual variations where required. One may either test the individual components of the nervous system in a particular sequence (**cranial nerves**, **reflexes**, and **motor**, **sensory**, and **autonomic function**), or else orient the examination along topographic lines (**head**, **upper limbs**, **trunk**, **lower limbs**). The presentation in this chapter is topographically organized.

Neurology stands by itself as an independent medical specialty and field of research. Most neurological illnesses affect only the nervous system. Nonetheless, general medical illnesses often manifest themselves with neurological symptoms and signs (cf. p. 120 ff.). The clinical neurological examination must therefore always include a general physical examination.

The practicing neurologist should indeed lay emphasis on the neurological aspects of the physical examination but cannot neglect its general aspects. Some of the basic principles of physical examination are listed below.

The examiner must **talk to the patient**, briefly explaining the purpose of individual steps in the examination where appropriate. This holds for patients of all ages, even more so for children.

In principle, the neurological examination should always be **complete** and should always be performed in the same sequence, though the examiner is free to use whatever sequence he or she prefers. The individual components of the examination are listed in Table 3.1. In certain exceptional situations, a highly experienced clinician may choose to perform only a partial examination. This is generally to be avoided, however, as even the best neurologist can miss something important in this way. In addition, a thorough, methodical examination helps reassure the patient that the physician is competent and attentive.

Patients should be examined **undressed**, after being given clear instructions about which clothes to remove, usually everything but their underwear. The spine cannot be examined if the upper body remains clothed and, if the patient is wearing socks, sensation cannot be tested in the feet, and the Babinski reflex cannot be elicited.

As we have already stressed, the examination should always be **systematic and complete**; yet, the tentative diagnosis (or diagnoses) suggested by the history will direct the clinician to **lay particular attention on certain aspects of the examination**. There is no sense in the mechanical, unthinking performance of a rigidly identical examination on every patient.

As soon as possible after the examination is completed, the examiner should **document the findings in writing**. Global statements such as "Neuro unremarkable" are worthless. The findings can be summarized in an outline such as the one provided in Table 3.1. The main purpose of precise documentation is to enable the clinician to follow the development of a disease process from one examination to the next. It is also obviously indispensable for medicolegal reasons.

Moreover, certain findings should be **quantified or numerically graded**, particularly muscle strength (see Table 3.4, p. 30). Sensory disturbances should be documented precisely in terms of their topography and extent.

Table 3.**1**   **The neurological examination**

Head and cranial nerves
Head freely mobile
Skull not tender to percussion
No supra- or infraorbital point tenderness
Carotid pulsations strong bilaterally, without bruits
Temporal artery pulsations strong bilaterally, without tenderness

No meningismus
No bruits
No occipital point tenderness
Perioral reflexes not exaggerated

I	Coffee correctly identified by smell in both nostrils (spontaneously named/chosen from list)
II	Corrected visual acuity (distance): R L
	Visual fields full to confrontation
	Optic discs normal bilaterally
III, IV, VI	Eye movements full and coordinated
	No pathological nystagmus
	Pupils equal, round, midsized, and symmetrical, with prompt reaction to light and convergence
V	Sensation in the face intact
	Corneal reflex symmetrically elicitable
	Masseter strong bilaterally
VII	Facial expression normal (both voluntary and involuntary movements)
VIII	Hearing subjectively normal
	Whisper heard at a distance of m (R ear), m (L ear)
	Weber not lateralized
IX, X	Palatal veil symmetrical at rest, elevates symmetrically
	Gag reflex intact
	Swallowing subjectively unimpaired
XI	Sternocleidomastoid strength full and symmetrical
XII	Tongue symmetrical, protrudes in the midline, freely mobile

Language Unremarkable

Upper Limbs   right-handed   Left-handed
Bulk normal bilaterally
Tone normal bilaterally
Full mobility throughout
Raw strength normal in all muscle groups
Postural testing normal bilaterally, without sinking
Rapid alternating movements performed well bilaterally
No rebound phenomenon
Finger–nose test accurate bilaterally, no intention tremor
No finger tremor
Reflexes: Biceps reflex symmetrical, of medium strength
                Triceps reflex symmetrical, of medium strength
                Brachioradialis reflex symmetrical, of medium strength
                Mayer reflex elicitable bilat   Hoffmann, Trömner not exaggerated bilat.
Sensation bilaterally intact to touch
Pain sensation bilaterally intact   Two-point discrimination < 5 mm bilat.
Temperature sensation bilaterally intact
Position sense in the fingers bilaterally intact
Vibration sense bilaterally intact
Stereognosis prompt bilaterally   Coin recognition good bilaterally

Trunk
Spine unremarkable, without percussion tenderness anywhere
Sensation on trunk intact   "Saddle" sensation intact
Abdominal skin reflex symmetrically intact   Finger-to-floor distance: .../... cm
Cremaster reflex bilaterally present (males only)   Small Schober .../... cm

Lower limbs
Bulk normal bilaterally
Tone normal bilaterally
Full mobility throughout
Raw strength normal in all muscle groups, incl. plantar flexors
and dorsiflexors
Lasègue negative bilaterally   No nerve trunk tenderness
Postural testing (supine position) normal bilaterally, without sinking
Heel–knee–shin test accurate bilaterally
Reflexes: Quadriceps reflex symmetrical, of medium strength   Oppenheim negative bilaterally
                Achilles' reflex symmetrical, of medium strength
                Babinski negative bilaterally
                Gordon negative bilaterally

Continued →

Table 3.**1**   **The neurological examination** (continued)

Sensation bilaterally intact to touch
Pain sensation bilaterally intact
Temperature sensation bilaterally intact
Position sense in the toes bilaterally intact
Vibration sense bilaterally intact
Graphesthesia (number recognition) good on both legs

Stance and gait
Romberg negative (in various positions of the head)
Normal gait with normal accessory movements
Walks well on heels bilaterally   Walks well on tiptoes bilaterally
No unsteadiness in heel-to-toe walk

Mental status grossly unremarkable without further testing   **General physical examination:** blood pressure, pulse, heart, lungs, abdomen, lymph nodes, peripheral pulses

(Only those items marked with a check ✓ or plus sign + have been examined)

Stance and Gait

General remarks. Though stance and gait are listed at the bottom of Table 3.**1**, we in fact recommend testing these functions as the first step in the examination of the undressed patient. Mere **observation** of the patient in a standing position can reveal evidence of a disease process, e. g., muscle atrophy, spinal deformities, and winging of the scapula. The patient's **posture at rest** may be abnormal, e. g., the exaggerated lumbar lordosis of muscular dystrophy (cf. Fig. 14.**3**, p. 266) or the stooped, rigid posture of the patient with Parkinson disease (cf. Fig. 6.**33**, p. 128). Stance and gait are best examined with the patient barefoot; meaningful findings can be obtained only if the patient has enough room to walk in. The testing of **stance and gait** often provides important clues to the type of disease process that is present. The sequence of tests is shown in Fig. 3.**1a–g**. The most important features of gait are whether the patient can walk at normal speed and without limping. If the patient limps, then the pathological side is the side that bears weight for the *shorter* time. The examiner should note the length of the patient's steps, the manner in which the feet are planted on and rolled off the ground, and the accompanying swinging of the arms. Some characteristic disturbances of gait are described in Table 3.**2**.

Walking on tiptoe and walking on the heels (Figs. 3.**1b, c**) let the clinician judge the strength of the calf muscles and the foot and toe extensors. If the plantar flexors are only mildly weak, the patient will still be able to walk on tiptoe, but will not be able to raise himself or herself on tiptoe while standing on one leg, or hop repeatedly on one foot (10 times in succession).

The "tightrope walk" (heel-to-toe walk) (Fig. 3.**1d**) is a very sensitive test of equilibrium and gait stability. The patient is instructed to place one foot firmly and directly in front of the other, at first while looking at the floor, then while looking straight ahead, and finally while looking at the ceiling. Heel-to-toe walking should be possible under all of these conditions. Heel-to-toe walking with the eyes closed is a more difficult task that many normal persons cannot perform.

The Romberg test (Fig. 3.**1e**) is a further test of equilibrium. The patient is asked to stand with the feet together and parallel and with eyes closed, for at least 20 seconds. This should be accomplished calmly and easily, without any appreciable swaying. The test can be made more difficult by having the patient turn or incline the head to one side. It can also be performed in combination with positional testing of the arms (see below).

The functions of the vestibular system (p. 201) and cerebellum (p. 80) can be tested in a number of ways, including with the **Unterberger step test** (Fig. 3.**1f**). The patient walks in place, with the eyes closed, raising the knee to the horizontal or above with each step. After 50 steps, the patient should have rotated no more than 45° from his or her original position. Larger rotations suggest disfunction of the vestibular apparatus on the side to which the patient has turned, or of the cerebellar hemisphere on that side. In the "**star gait**" test of Babinski and Weil, the patient keeps the eyes closed and walks two steps forward and two steps back, repeatedly. Disfunction of the vestibular system manifests itself as involuntary turning to the side of the lesion. In **blind walking**, the patient first looks at the examiner, who is standing some distance away, then closes the eyes, and walks toward him or her. Vestibular lesions cause a deviation to the side of the lesion.

A number of **common gait abnormalities** are illustrated in Fig. 3.**2**.

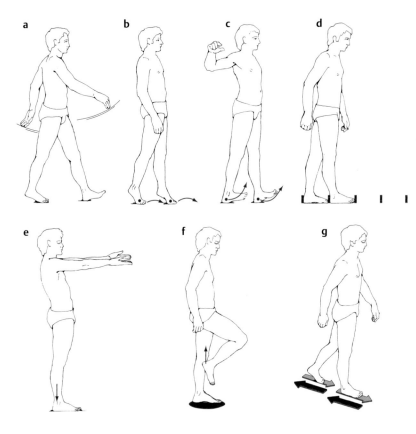

Fig. 3.**1** **Tests of stance and gait. a**
Normal gait. Note normal step length
and arm swing. **b** Walking on tiptoes.
c Walking on heels. **d** Heel-to-toe
walking. One foot is placed precisely
in front of the other. **e** Romberg test
with eyes closed, combined with postural test of the upper limbs. **f** Unterberger step test: walking in place
with eyes closed. See text for interpretation of results. **g** Babinski–Weil
test with "star gait" (*marche en
étoile*): the patient is asked to take
two steps forward and two steps
back, repeatedly, with eyes closed.
For interpretation, see text.

Table 3.**2**   **Characteristic disturbances of gait**

Designation	Abnormalities of gait	Causes, Remarks
Spastic gait (Fig. 3.**2**)	slow, stiff, with audible dragging of the soles of the feet across the ground	bilateral pyramidal tract lesion
Ataxic gait (Fig. 3.**2**)	uncoordinated, stamping, unsteady, deviating irregularly from a straight line; heel-to-toe walking impossible	cerebellar dysfunction, posterior column dysfunction, peripheral neuropathy
Spastic–ataxic gait (Fig. 3.**2**)	combination of the two above disorders; jerky, stiff, inharmonious gait	most commonly seen in multiple sclerosis
Dystonic gait	uncontrollable additional movements interfering with the normal course of gait	basal ganglionic disease causing choreoathetosis or dystonia
Hypokinetic gait (Figs. 3.**2** and 6.**33**)	slow gait, stiff, bent posture, small steps, lack of accessory arm movements; turning requires multiple small steps	most commonly seen in Parkinson disease; similar picture in the lacunar state (cerebral microangiopathy, cf. p. 102)
Small-stepped gait ("marche à petits pas")	small steps, unsteady, resembles hypokinetic gait but with more normal accessory movements	"old person's gait" most commonly seen in the lacunar state, i. e., multiple small infarcts in the basal ganglia and along the corticospinal tracts, generally caused by atherosclerosis; distinguishable from parkinsonian gait mainly by the different accompanying signs
Circumduction (Fig. 3.**2**)	increased tone in the extensors of the paretic leg, which comes forward in a gentle outward arc, with a strongly plantar-flexed foot; hardly any accompanying movement of the flexed and adducted ipsilateral arm	central (spastic) hemiparesis
Steppage gait	the advancing leg is raised high and then placed on the ground toe first, often with an audible slap	unilateral: foot drop, e. g., in peroneal nerve palsy; bilateral: e. g., polyneuropathy or Steinert myotonic dystrophy

Continued →

Table 3.**2** **Characteristic disturbances of gait** (continued)

Designation	Abnormalities of gait	Causes, Remarks
Hyperextended knee (Fig. 3.**2**)	with each step, the knee of the stationary leg is hyperextended	prevents buckling of the knee when the knee extensors are weak—unilaterally, e. g., in quadriceps weakness due to a lesion of the femoral n.; bilaterally, e. g., in muscular dystrophy
Hyperlordotic gait (Fig. 14.**3**)	exaggerated lumbar lordosis	e. g., in muscular dystrophy affecting the pelvic girdle, in boys with Duchenne muscular dystrophy
Trendelenburg gait (Fig. 3.**2**)	with each step, the pelvis tilts downward on the side of the swinging leg	severe hip abductor weakness—unilaterally, e. g., in lesions of the superior gluteal n.; bilaterally, e. g., in muscular dystrophy affecting the pelvic girdle and in bilateral hip dislocation
Duchenne gait (Figs. 3.**2** and 14.**3 b**)	with each step, the upper body tilts to the side of the stationary leg	mild or moderate weakness of the hip abductors (as in Trendelenburg gait, but less severe), or as a pain-reducing maneuver in disorders of the hip joint

Fig. 3.**2 Common gait disturbances**

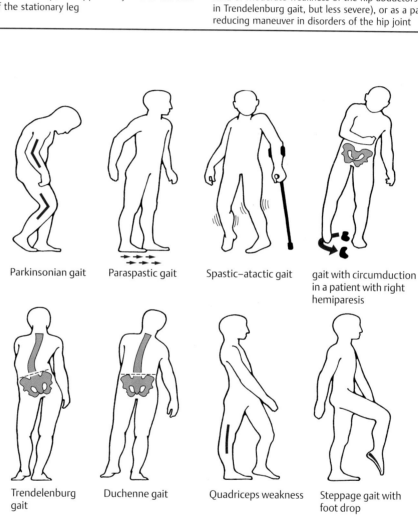

Parkinsonian gait   Paraspastic gait   Spastic–atactic gait   gait with circumduction in a patient with right hemiparesis

Trendelenburg gait   Duchenne gait   Quadriceps weakness   Steppage gait with foot drop

Examination of the Head and Cranial Nerves

Head and Cervical Spine

The examiner should first note the **general appearance** of the head and cervical spine (e. g., sunken temples in Steinert myotonic dystrophy) and the patient's facial expressions (e. g., paucity of facial expression in Parkinson disease). Young, healthy persons should be able to turn the neck and head almost 90° in either direction, so that the eye that is farther from the examiner disappears behind the root of the patient's nose. Further, the patient should be able to incline the head laterally 45° in either direction and to rotate it 60° to the right or left when the neck is maximally flexed (this rotation occurs only at the atlantoaxial and atlanto-occipital joints). Testing for **meningismus** is performed with the patient lying supine. This finding, if present, usually indicates meningeal irritation due to meningitis or subarachnoid hemorrhage, but is sometimes a reflexive response to space-occupying lesions of the posterior fossa. Meningismus consists of an isolated inhibition of neck flexion while the head can still be rotated. To test for meningismus, the examiner flexes the neck of the supine patient by bending the head forward. In genuine meningismus, the **Lasègue sign** (p. 211) is usually positive as well. If attempted passive flexion of the neck also induces flexion of the lower limbs at the knee or hip joint, this is called a positive cervical **Brudzinski sign**. This sign is often accompanied by a **positive Kernig sign**: when the patient is in the sitting position, the knee cannot be passively extended and, when the patient is supine, passive straight leg raising induces reflex knee flexion.

Auscultation of the skull may reveal a pulse-synchronous bruit over an arteriovenous fistula or an arteriovenous malformation. A carotid bruit may be due to stenosis.

The intrinsic reflexes of the facial musculature should always be examined. Tapping a finger placed over the lateral canthus of the patient's eye normally induces contraction of the ipsilateral orbicularis oculi m. This reflex normally weakens (habituates) on repeated tapping; if not, a bilateral lesion of the corticobulbar pathways is probably present. Excessively intense, bilateral contraction of the orbicularis oculi when the examiner taps on the patient's glabella (the **glabellar or nasopalpebral reflex**) also implies a bilateral corticobulbar lesion. Tapping on a tongue depressor placed on the patient's lips may induce lip protrusion (positive **snout reflex**). The **masseter reflex** (jaw jerk reflex) is elicited by gently tapping the patient's jaw from above when the patient's mouth is half open. Another way to elicit this reflex is to tap on a tongue depressor laid on the patient's mandibular teeth. The **corneomandibular reflex** ("*winking jaw phenomenon*") consists of deviation of the slightly opened jaw when the cornea is touched. Its presence on only one side, or any marked asymmetry, implies an interruption of the ascending and descending brainstem pathways terminating in the pontomesencephalic reticular formation.

Cranial Nerves

Next, the cranial nerves are examined individually. Figure 3.**3** and Table 3.**3** provide an overview of the anatomy and function of the 12 cranial nerves. The clinical syndromes associated with lesions of individual cranial nerves are presented in Chapter 11 (pp. 180 ff.). In this chapter, we will describe the main examining techniques and a selection of the important abnormal findings that can be elicited with each.

The first two cranial nerves (the olfactory and optic nn.) are, in reality, portions of the brain that have been displaced into the periphery. The remaining 10 cranial nerves structurally and functionally resemble the other peripheral nerves of the body. They have motor, somatosensory, special sensory, and autonomic functions.

CN I: Olfactory N.

Testing the sense of smell. Smell is tested individually in each nostril. The patient is asked to close his or her eyes and then to identify (or at least perceive) **aromatic substances** such as coffee, cinnamon, or vanilla that are held under the open nostril. Three-quarters of normal individuals can correctly identify coffee grounds. If there is doubt about the patient's ability to smell, asafetida (onion extract), a substance with an unpleasant stink, is used. Only a complete loss of the sense of smell (anosmia), not a mere diminution of it, is neurologically relevant. Anosmia most commonly follows severe traumatic brain injury (p. 180) but may also be due to frontal tumors, particularly olfactory groove meningioma, or postinfectious abnormalities of the nasal mucosa, e. g., after an upper respiratory "cold," or in ozena.

If it is unclear whether anosmia is of neurological origin, the patient is given a dilute ammonia solution to smell. The unpleasant **irritation** that this produces is mediated, not by the olfactory n., but by the **trigeminal n.** If the patient fails to react, then he or she is probably suffering either from an acute process affecting the nasal mucosa (e. g., acute rhinitis) or from a psychogenic disturbance. The anosmia is not neurogenic in either case.

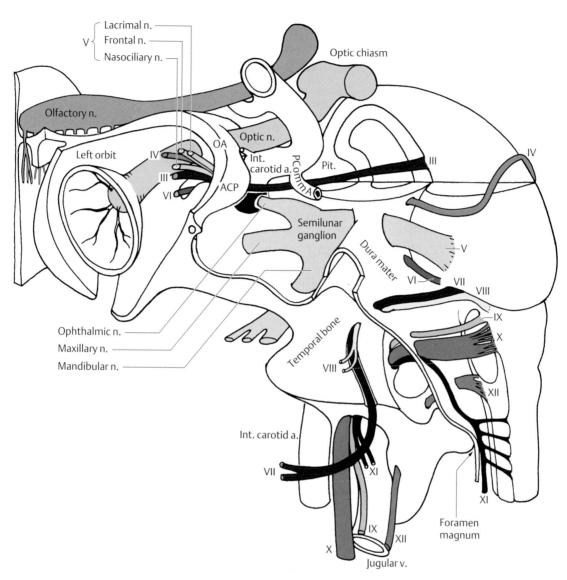

Fig. 3.3 Overview of the topographical relations of the cranial nerves and their sites of exit from the skull. ACP = anterior clinoid process, **OA** = ophthalmic a., **PCommA** = posterior communicating a., pit. = pituitary gland. **III** = oculomotor n., **IV** = trochlear n., **V** = trigeminal n., **VI** = abducens n., **VII** = facial n., **VIII** = vestibulo- cochlear n., **IX** = glossopharyngeal n., **X** = vagus n., **XI** = accessory n., **XII** = hypoglossal n. (Based on Mumenthaler, M.: Erkrankungen der Hirnnerven. In: Hornbostel H., Kaufmann W., Siegenthaler W.: *Innere Medizin in Praxis und Klinik*. Vol. II, 4th edn, Thieme, Stuttgart 1992)

Table 3.3 The 12 cranial nerves, their nuclei, and their functions

Cranial nerve	Anatomical substrates (peripheral and central); *innervated structures*	Function
I Olfactory n.	sensory neurons of the nasal mucosa (olfactory zone); olfactory fila, bulb, and tract; olfactory striae, amygdala	perception of odors (only substances dissolved in the fluid of the nasal mucosa can be perceived)
II Optic n.	retina; optic nerve, chiasm, and tract; lateral geniculate body, optic radiation, primary visual cortex on the banks of the calcarine fissure	visual perception
III Oculomotor n.	nucleus of the oculomotor n. and Edinger–Westphal nucleus (both are in the midbrain), nerve. Innervates the levator palpebrae m.; superior, inferior, and medial rectus mm.; and inferior oblique mm., as well as the constrictor pupillae m.	raising the upper lid; most of the movements of the globe (eyeball); constriction of the pupil
IV Trochlear n.	nucleus of the trochlear n. (midbrain at its junction with the pons), nerve. Innervates the superior oblique m.	depression of the adducted globe, internal rotation of the abducted globe

Continued →

Table 3.3 **The 12 cranial nerves, their nuclei, and their functions** (continued)

Cranial nerve	Anatomical substrates (peripheral and central); *innervated structures*	Function
V Trigeminal n.	pontine and spinal nuclei of the trigeminal n. (sensory root), motor nucleus of the trigeminal n. (motor root), Gasserian ganglion, three peripheral nerve branches (the ophthalmic, maxillary, and mandibular nn.). Innervates the skin and mucosa of the head and face, and the muscles of mastication (temporalis, masseter, and medial and lateral pterygoid mm.)	sensation on the face, external ear, and mucosal surfaces of the head; innervation of the muscles of mastication
VI Abducens n.	nucleus of the abducens n. (pons), nerve. Innervates the lateral rectus m.	abduction of the globe
VII Facial n.	nucleus of the facial n. (pons, motor fibers for the muscles of facial expression), superior salivatory nucleus (secretory fibers for the lacrimal, nasal, and palatal glands), nucleus of the tractus solitarius (gustatory fibers), nerve	innervation of the muscles of facial expression and the stapedius m.; lacrimation and salivation; taste on the anterior two-thirds of the tongue
VIII Vestibulo-cochlear n. (statoacoustic n., auditory n.)	sensory neurons in the cochlea (cochlear root) and in the semicircular canals, utricle, and saccule (vestibular root), peripheral afferent nerve trunk, brainstem nuclei, and projecting fibers to higher regions of the CNS	perception of sound and of bodily position, movement, and acceleration; regulation of balance
IX Glossopharyn-geal n.	nucleus ambiguus (medulla, motor fibers for the muscles of the soft palate and pharynx), nucleus of the tractus solitarius (gustatory fibers from the posterior third of the tongue, somatosensory fibers from the palatal and pharyngeal mucosa); inferior salivatory nucleus, otic ganglion (secretory fibers for the parotid gland); nerve	motor innervation of the palatal and pharyngeal muscles; somatosensory innervation of the palatal and pharyngeal mucosa; taste on the posterior third of the tongue; control of swallowing
X Vagus n.	nucleus ambiguus (medulla, motor fibers for the muscles of the soft palate and pharynx), dorsal nucleus of the vagus n., nucleus of the tractus solitarius (visceromotor and viscerosensory fibers for the thoracic and abdominal viscera), spinal nucleus of the trigeminal n. (sensory fibers from the pharynx, larynx, and external auditory canal); nerve trunk	innervation of the laryngeal musculature, speech, sensation in the external ear canal and the posterior cranial fossa, autonomic fibers to the thoracic and abdominal viscera
XI Accessory n.	nucleus ambiguus (medulla, cranial root) and spinal nucleus of the accessory n. (C1–C5, spinal root), nerve trunk, sternocleidomastoid m. and upper portion of the trapezius m.	turning the head to the opposite side, shrugging the shoulders
XII Hypoglossal n.	nucleus of the hypoglossal n. (medulla), nerve trunk, muscles of the tongue	movement of the tongue

CN II: Optic N.

Ophthalmoscopy. Inspection of the optic nerve papillae (optic discs) with the ophthalmoscope is an important technique for assessment of the optic n. *Abnormal pallor* indicates an optic nerve lesion (Fig. 3.4). In addition, **inspection of the eye grounds** can provide evidence of elevated intracranial pressure: in *papilledema*, the papillae are raised and hyperemic, and their margins are blurred. Enlarged retinal veins indicate impaired venous drainage due to intracranial hypertension (cf. Fig. 11.2, p. 183). A raised papilla with blurred margins can also be a sign of an inflammatory process affecting the optic n. (p. 182).

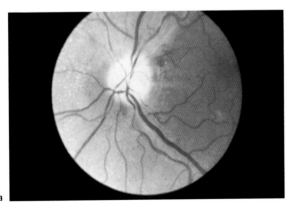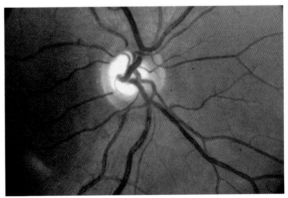

a   b

Fig. 3.4 **Optic disc (papilla) of the right eye. a** Pale, atrophic disc. **b** Normal disc (images kindly provided by the Department of Ophthalmology, University of Berne.) (For the color version of this figure, cf. Plate 1)

Testing of visual acuity for neurological purposes is usually performed with a wall chart seen from a distance. Refractive errors are corrected with eyeglasses if necessary.

Perimetry. Visual field testing is of particular importance in neurology. The visual fields can be roughly assessed in the neurologist's office or at the bedside with so-called **finger perimetry** (or digital confrontation, Fig. 3.**5**). The examiner sits directly in front of the patient and the patient fixes one eye on the examiner's nose. The examiner then moves a finger in each of the four quadrants of the visual field, testing each eye separately. The patient is asked whether he or she can see the finger. This method can reveal a major visual field defect, e. g., *bitemporal hemianopsia* or *quadrantanopsia* (p. 181). Various kinds of visual field defects, and the sites of the lesions that cause them, are depicted in Fig. 3.**6**.

If *visual neglect* is suspected, the examiner should next perform *double simultaneous stimulation* of the visual field by moving the two index fingers *at the same time* in corresponding quadrants in the two halves of the field (left and right hemifields). The patient should report seeing both fingers. If both fingers are perceived on individual testing, but only one is seen on double simultaneous stimulation, this may be due to visual neglect. *Monocular visual field defects* are revealed by separate testing of the four quadrants of the visual field in each eye with a finger starting in the periphery and moving gradually toward the center.

Smaller (monocular or binocular) visual field defects can sometimes be detected by confrontational perimetry

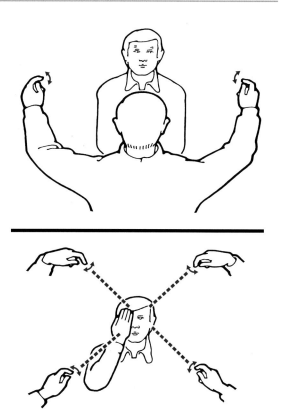

Fig. 3.**5 Testing the visual fields by digital confrontation.** Above: double simultaneous testing for the detection of visual hemineglect. Below: individual testing of all four quadrants of the visual field of each eye.

Fig. 3.**6 Visual field defects and the sites of the lesions that cause them. 1** Blindness in the left eye due to a left optic nerve lesion. **2** Bitemporal hemianopsia due to a lesion of the optic chiasm. **3** Right homonymous hemianopsia due to a lesion of the left optic tract. **4–6** Lesions at various sites in the left optic radiation: **4** Right upper quadrantanopsia due to a left temporal lobe lesion. **5** Right lower quadrantanopsia due to a left parietal lobe lesion. **6** Right homonymous hemianopsia, sparing macular vision, due to a left occipital lobe lesion.

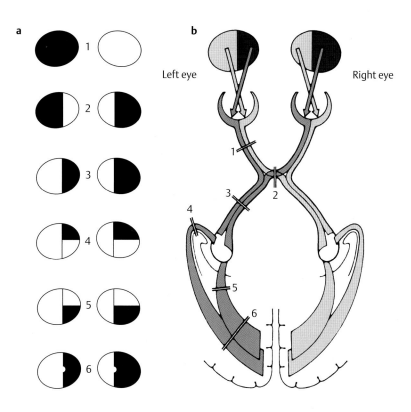

3

The Neurological Examination

with a red object, but are usually revealed only by formal testing with equipment such as the Goldmann perimeter or octopus (p. 65).

CN III, IV, and VI: Oculomotor, Trochlear, and Abducens Nn.

Inspection. The examiner should first note the position of the eyes at rest, paying particular attention to the following: *parallel position of the eyes, possible prominence of one eye*, and *symmetry of the palpebral fissures and of the pupils*. The parallel position of the eyes is best assessed by observation of the small reflected images of light sources in the examining room in the patient's eyes, which should be at an analogous position on each cornea. A prominent globe (exophthalmos) can sometimes be appreciated by viewing the eyes tangentially from above (Fig. 3.**7**).

Testing of ocular motility. The anatomy of the six extraocular muscles and the three cranial nerves innervating them is shown in Fig. 3.**8a**, while the function of the extraocular muscles is described in Fig. 3.**3** and depicted in Fig. 3.**8b**. Eye movements are tested by having the patient **keep the head stationary and follow the examiner's finger with his or her eyes**. The motility of the globes is assessed along the vertical and horizontal axes. If abnormalities of eye movement can be seen directly by the examiner, or if the patient reports double vision (diplopia), then the manner in which eye movement is

restricted (including any abnormality of the resting position of the eyes) and the type of double vision enable the examiner to determine which muscle (or muscles) is (are) paretic and, therefore, which cranial nerve is dysfunctional (**paralytic strabismus**). The eye muscles may, however, be weakened by intrinsic muscle lesions, rather than by cranial nerve palsies. A general principle for the interpretation of findings is that the positions of the eyes are farthest apart, and diplopia is therefore worst, when the patient looks in the direction of function of the paretic muscle (p. 189 ff.).

A conjugate gaze palsy (p. 188) is the inability to perform a conjugate eye movement to direct the gaze in a particular direction, either horizontally or vertically. In such patients, the lesion is not in the peripheral portion of a cranial nerve; it is located centrally, within the brain (a *supranuclear* lesion, i. e., one that lies above the nuclei of the cranial nerves that innervate the extraocular muscles). In contrast to peripheral lesions, the eyes remain parallel and there is no double vision.

When testing eye movements, the examiner should also look for *nystagmus* (see below and p. 184). Deviations from the parallel axis are best detected by observing the reflected images on the patient's cornea.

A nonparallel (skewed) position of the two eyes without diplopia implies that the patient has **concomitant strabismus**, a result of longstanding impaired vision in one eye (usually from birth or early childhood). No cranial nerve palsy is present. Concomitant strabismus can be demonstrated with the aid of a **cover test** (Fig. 3.**9**). The patient keeps both eyes open while the examiner covers one eye and asks the patient to fix his or her gaze on a particular object in the room. The cover is then rapidly switched to the other eye, so that the previously covered eye must jump into position to keep the gaze fixated on the same object. The initially uncovered eye, now covered, deviates to one side, as can be shown by switching the cover back again (*alternating concomitant strabismus*; usually *divergent*, but sometimes *convergent*).

Assessment of the pupils. The examiner should note the *shape* (round or oblong) and *size* of the pupils. Normal pupils are generally of equal size and react equally to light. Inequality of the pupils is called *anisocoria*; a small degree of anisocoria is normal in some individuals. When the examiner illuminates the pupil of one eye, there should be reflex constriction of that pupil (the **direct light response**), accompanied by an equal reflex constriction of the other pupil (the **consensual light response**). To ensure that only one pupil is illuminated, the examiner shines a flashlight on one eye while blocking the light from the other eye with his or her own hand, held in the midline over the root of the patient's nose. **Convergence** is tested by having the patient fix his or her gaze on a distant point and then look at the examiner's finger, which is held close to the face. The normal reaction is adduction of both eyes (convergence) accompanied by simultaneous reflex constriction of the pupils (the **near response**). Pathological abnormalities of the pupillary reflexes and their significance with regard to localization are presented in Figure 11.**12** on p. 194.

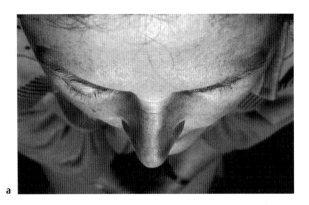

a

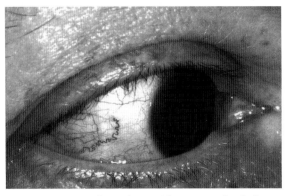

b

Fig. 3.**7 A patient with a right carotid–cavernous fistula (i. e., a fistula between the right internal carotid a. and the cavernous sinus). a** The tangential photograph reveals exophthalmos. **b** Conjunctival venous stasis is caused by elevated venous pressure.

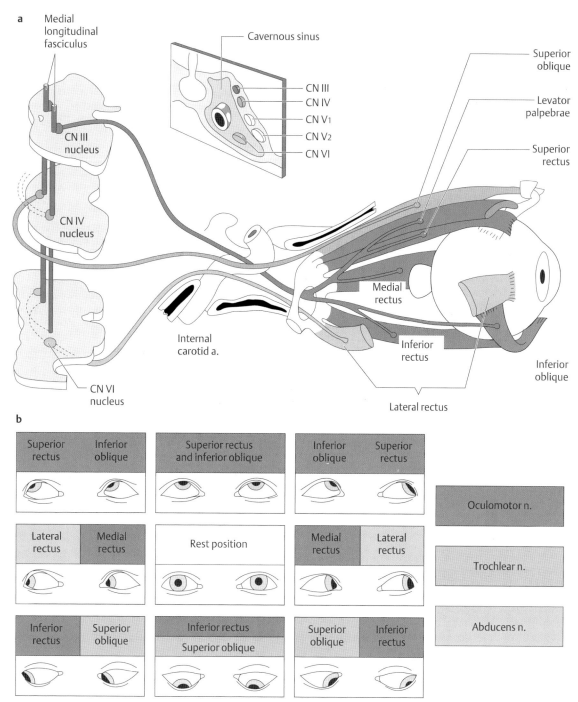

Fig. 3.**8 a The three nerves to the extraocular muscles** and the muscles innervated by each. **b** Scheme according to Hering, indicating the direction of gaze in which the main function of each eye muscle is most strongly in evidence.

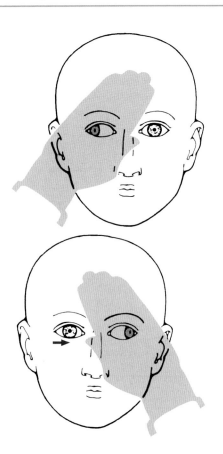

Fig. 3.**9 Cover test.** In concomitant, alternating, divergent strabismus, the covered eye (i. e., the one that is not fixating) deviates outward. When the cover is rapidly switched to the other eye, the newly uncovered eye moves to the fixating position, while the covered other eye now deviates outward with a positioning saccade (→).

CN V: Trigeminal N.

Testing sensation in the face. The somatosensory portion of this mixed cranial nerve originates in the ganglion cells of the Gasserian ganglion. The cutaneous and mucosal zones innervated by the trigeminal n. are shown in Fig. 3.**10**. Sensation should be tested with a cotton swab or a piece of tissue paper. The latter can also be used to test the **corneal reflex**: the patient is asked to look upward and the tactile stimulus is delivered to the lower edge of the cornea to avoid engendering a visually induced fright reaction. The reflex response consists of immediate closure of the eyes.

Assessment of the muscles of mastication. The motor portion of the trigeminal n. runs in its third branch (the mandibular n.) to supply the muscles of mastication, i.e., the masseter and temporalis mm. and the medial and lateral pterygoid mm. The examiner tests the function of these muscles by placing his or her fingers in front of the angle of the jaw bilaterally and asking the patient to clamp the jaw tightly (press the teeth together). In unilateral (motor) trigeminal n. paresis, the contraction of the masseter m. on the affected side is palpably weaker and the **masseter reflex** may be weaker

as well. When the patient opens the jaw, the mandible deviates to the side of the lesion because of the dominant effect of the pterygoid muscles on the healthy side.

CN VII: Facial N.

Assessment of the muscles of facial expression. The anatomy of the seventh cranial nerve is shown in Fig. 11.**15** p. 196. In assessing its function, the examiner should note any asymmetry of the face, spontaneous **facial expression** (mimesis), and contractions of the facial muscles during **movement**: the patient should be systematically asked to furrow the brow, close the eyes tightly, show his or her teeth, and whistle. In lesions of the facial n., the **corneal reflex** is weak, because the efferent arm of the reflex arc is interrupted (rather than the afferent arm, as in trigeminal lesions). The clinical findings in facial nerve palsy, and the differentiation of peripheral and central facial weakness, are presented on p. 198 and in Figs. 11.**16** and 11.**18** on pp. 197 and 198.

Assessment of taste, lacrimation, and salivation. The facial n. also contains gustatory fibers supplying taste to the anterior two-thirds of the tongue. When a facial nerve lesion is suspected, taste in this region can be tested by the application of substances with the four basic modalities of taste—sweet, salty, sour, and bitter— to the corresponding half of the tongue. Appropriate solutions to use are, for example, 20% glucose, 10% sodium chloride, 5% citric acid, and 1% quinine. (Note: "bitter" is perceived in the mucosa of the posterior third of the tongue; this sensation is thus mediated by the glossopharyngeal n., not the facial n.). Peripheral lesions of the facial n. also cause diminished lacrimation and salivation, which are usually not noticed by the patient and require special tests to demonstrate. There may also be hypersensitivity to sound (*hyperacusis*).

CN VIII: Vestibulocochlear N.

Assessment of hearing. The anatomy of the vestibulocochlear nerve is depicted in Fig. 3.**11**. The neurologist's assessment of the patient's hearing is generally limited to the determination whether (uni- or bilateral) hearing loss is present and, if so, whether it is due to **impaired conduction of sound** (middle ear process, obstruction of the external auditory canal) or to a **sensorineural deficit** (process affecting the inner ear or the cochlear portion of the eighth cranial nerve). The examiner tests hearing separately in each ear by speaking or whispering words from distances of 5 to 6 m. The patient must inactivate hearing in the ear not being tested by forcefully rubbing a finger back and forth in the external auditory canal. Total deafness, i.e., deafness even for very loud sounds, is never due to a middle ear process alone.

Differentiation of conductive and sensorineural hearing loss. These two types of hearing loss can be distinguished with the aid of the Rinne and Weber tests (Fig. 3.**12**).

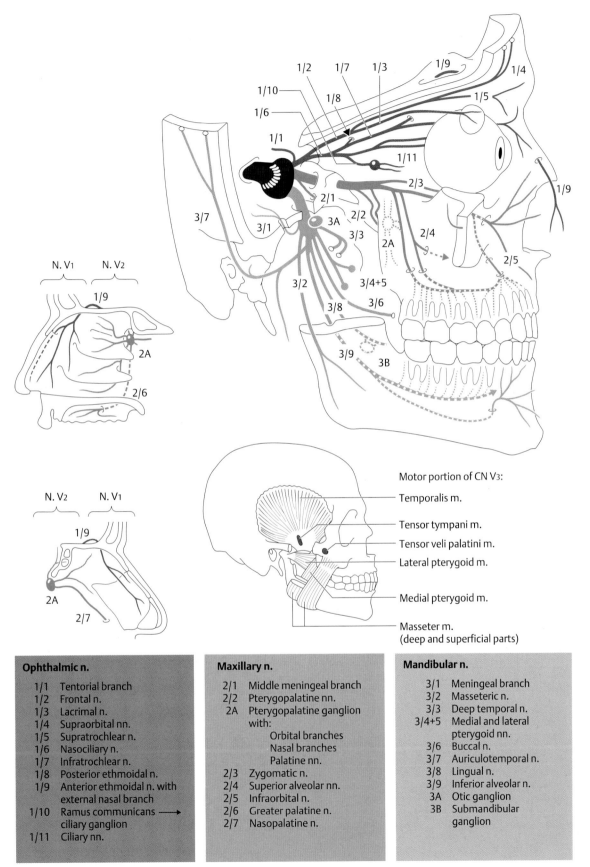

Motor portion of CN V3:

- Temporalis m.
- Tensor tympani m.
- Tensor veli palatini m.
- Lateral pterygoid m.
- Medial pterygoid m.
- Masseter m. (deep and superficial parts)

Ophthalmic n.

1/1	Tentorial branch
1/2	Frontal n.
1/3	Lacrimal n.
1/4	Supraorbital nn.
1/5	Supratrochlear n.
1/6	Nasociliary n.
1/7	Infratrochlear n.
1/8	Posterior ethmoidal n.
1/9	Anterior ethmoidal n. with external nasal branch
1/10	Ramus communicans ⟶ ciliary ganglion
1/11	Ciliary nn.

Maxillary n.

2/1	Middle meningeal branch
2/2	Pterygopalatine nn.
2A	Pterygopalatine ganglion with:
	Orbital branches
	Nasal branches
	Palatine nn.
2/3	Zygomatic n.
2/4	Superior alveolar nn.
2/5	Infraorbital n.
2/6	Greater palatine n.
2/7	Nasopalatine n.

Mandibular n.

3/1	Meningeal branch
3/2	Masseteric n.
3/3	Deep temporal n.
3/4+5	Medial and lateral pterygoid nn.
3/6	Buccal n.
3/7	Auriculotemporal n.
3/8	Lingual n.
3/9	Inferior alveolar n.
3A	Otic ganglion
3B	Submandibular ganglion

Fig. 3.**10 Anatomy of the somatosensory and motor portions of the trigeminal n.**

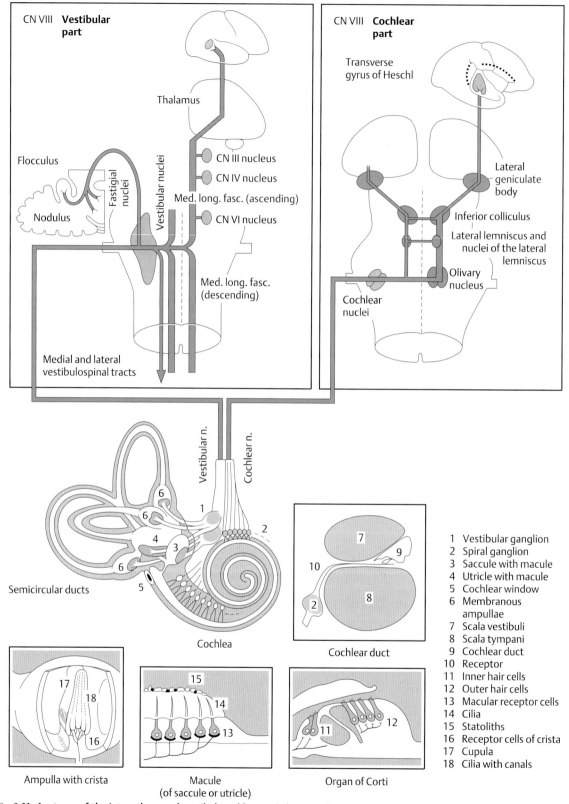

Fig. 3.**11 Anatomy of the internal ear and vestibulocochlear n.** (schematic drawing).

Fig. 3.**12 Weber and Rinne hearing tests. a Weber test:** in a patient with right-sided conductive hearing loss (picture at left), the tuning fork cannot be heard when held next to the ear (**1**). If the tuning fork is placed on the forehead (**2**), however, it is heard, and the tone is localized to the side of the hearing loss, i. e., to the right ear. In contrast, in a patient with right-sided sensorineural hearing loss (picture at right), the tone is localized to the normally hearing (left) ear. **b Rinne test:** the tuning fork is first placed on the mastoid process (**1**). As soon as the tone is no longer heard, the tuning fork is held next to the ear. If hearing is normal, the tone will now be heard again (**2**). In right-sided conductive hearing loss (middle picture), the tone will not be heard again when the tuning fork is held next to the ear (negative Rinne test). In right-sided sensorineural hearing loss, however, the tone will be heard, though for a shorter time than normal, *both* by bone conduction *and* with the tuning fork held next to the ear (positive, i. e., normal Rinne test).

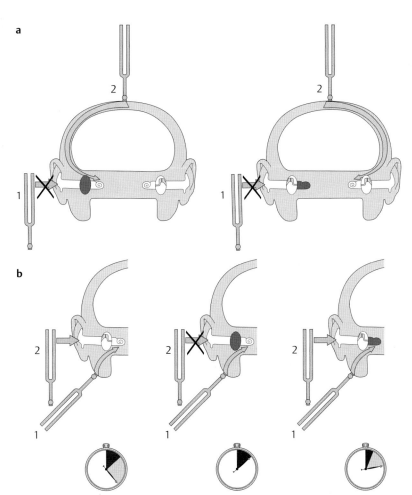

Rinne test. Air conduction of sound is better than bone conduction in normal individuals, as can be demonstrated by the following procedure: first, a vibrating tuning fork is placed on the mastoid process. As soon as the subject can no longer hear the tone, the tuning fork is removed from the mastoid process and placed next to the ear. The tone should then be heard again, and should take approximately twice as long to disappear as it did on the mastoid process. This is called a "positive," i. e., normal, Rinne test. If the time during which the tone is heard by air conduction is shorter than normal, or if the tone is not heard in this way at all, then the Rinne test is negative, indicating conductive hearing loss (that is, a middle ear process or obstruction of the external auditory canal). In patients with sensorineural hearing loss, the Rinne test is positive (normal).

Weber test. The vibrating tuning fork is placed on the middle of the forehead or on the vertex. Normally, the tone is heard equally loudly in both ears and is localized to the midline. The tone is lateralized to the worse ear in conductive hearing loss and to the better ear in sensorineural hearing loss (due to a process affecting the cochlea or the cochlear part of the eighth cranial nerve). When unilateral hearing loss has been present for many years, the Weber test no longer lateralizes.

Assessment of vestibular function. The most common symptom of a lesion affecting the labyrinth or the vestibular portion of the vestibulocochlear nerve is **vertigo**. Patients usually describe a directional or systematic type of vertigo, e. g., rotational vertigo ("like on a merry-go-round"), a feeling of turning to the side, or an "elevator" feeling. They can often state the direction of the vertigo. In contrast, dizziness of nonvestibular origin—for example, due to a brainstem lesion—is often not as well defined. Such patients may complain of giddiness, swaying, or seeing black before their eyes (see p. 201).

The objective sign of a lesion of the vestibular portion of the vestibulocochlear nerve is **nystagmus**. This is a rapid, rhythmic jerking movement of both eyes in the same direction (also called "jerk nystagmus"). A slow conjugate deviation in one direction is followed by a rapid conjugate movement that returns the eyes to the original position and then the cycle starts again. The slow deviation is the truly pathological component of nystagmus; the rapid component is a reflex correction to preserve fixation. By convention, the direction of nystagmus is given as the direction of the rapid phase. Nystagmus may be **horizontal** (toward the right or the left), **vertical** (upbeat or downbeat), or **rotatory** (clockwise or counterclockwise). Nystagmus of vestibular origin can sometimes be seen even when the patient looks straight ahead (nystagmus that beats spontaneously in this way is called *spontaneous nystagmus*); in other cases, it appears only when the examiner has the patient look to the side. In either case, nystagmus of vestibular origin always beats in the same direction (away from the side of the lesion), regardless of whether it appears when the patient looks straight ahead, to the right, and/or to the left.

Spontaneous nystagmus of vestibular origin must be distinguished from *physiological end-gaze nystagmus* and from *gaze-evoked nystagmus*. End-gaze nystagmus arises when the patient looks all the way to one side or the other (into the monocular visual field); its rapid phase beats in the direction of gaze, it is seen in both eyes to the same extent, and it disappears spontaneously after a number of beats. It is found symmetrically in normal individuals. If end-gaze nystagmus is seen on examination, the examiner should bring the test object about 10° back into the binocular visual field. The nystagmus is clinically significant only if it is still present after this maneuver (gaze-evoked nystagmus, p. 185). Some common pathological types of nystagmus are listed and described in Table 11.**1**, p. 185.

Instruments for assessing vestibular function. Frenzel goggles make nystagmus easier to observe. They contain strong magnifying lenses that render the patient unable to fixate, as well as a lamp to illuminate the globes. Nystagmus can often be suppressed by fixation and, if so, is only visible when the patient wears Frenzel goggles (head shaking is a further provocative maneuver). The magnification provided by the Frenzel lenses also makes it easier for the examiner to see fine movements.

Vestibular lesions can be assessed objectively by testing of the **rotational** and **caloric excitability** of the corresponding labyrinth. In the normal case, irrigation of the external auditory canal with warm water induces nystagmus with the rapid phase toward the irrigated ear (with cold-water irrigation, the rapid phase is toward the opposite ear). If a vestibular lesion is present, the induced nystagmus is diminished or absent.

Tests of balance and coordination. Certain abnormalities in the tests of **stance and gait** described above (Unterberger step test, Babinski–Weil test, heel-to-toe walking, p. 13) indicate dysfunction of the vestibular apparatus. In a further test, the **Bárány pointing test**, the patient is asked to stretch out his or her arm forwards and then bring it down to a target provided by the examiner, e. g., the examiner's index finger. The patient is then asked to repeat the movement with eyes closed, still trying to hit the target as accurately as possible. In unilateral vestibular lesions, the arm deviates to the side of the lesion during its downward course. The same can also be observed, however, with lesions of the ipsilateral cerebellar hemisphere.

CN IX and X: Glossopharyngeal and Vagus Nn.

The efferent fibers from the nucleus ambiguus to the muscles of the palate, larynx, and pharynx reach these structures through the glossopharyngeal and vagus nn. The larynx is innervated by two vagal branches, the su-

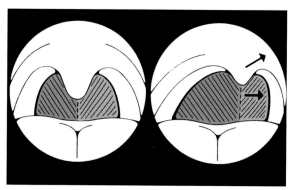

Fig. 3.**13 Palatal deviation.** In right glossopharyngeal nerve palsy, the palate and posterior pharyngeal wall deviate to the normal left side when the patient gags.

perior laryngeal n, and the recurrent laryngeal n. The glossopharyngeal n. carries somatosensory fibers from the soft palate, the posterior pharyngeal wall, the tonsillar fossa, and the middle ear, as well as gustatory fibers from the posterior third of the tongue. The vagus n. carries somatosensory fibers from the external auditory canal, part of the external ear, and the meninges of the posterior fossa. It also carries efferent parasympathetic fibers to the thoracic and abdominal viscera (cf. Table 3.**3**).

Examination of the pharynx and larynx. The motor function of the ninth and tenth cranial nerves is assessed by inspection of the palate and throat and, more importantly, by observation of the movements of these structures during **phonation** ("a–aa–ah …") and after induction of the **gag reflex** by touching the posterior pharyngeal wall with, e. g., a cotton swab. Unilateral weakness of the palatal veil and the pharyngeal muscles makes these structures deviate laterally away from the side of the lesion, as shown in Fig. 3.**13**. Hoarseness due to a unilateral recurrent laryngeal nerve palsy can sometimes be heard only when the patient sings.

CN XI: Accessory N.

Examination of the sternocleidomastoid and trapezius mm. The external (final) branch of the purely motor accessory n. supplies the sternocleidomastoid m. and the upper portion of the trapezius m. To test the sternocleidomastoid m. on one side, the examiner asks the patient to turn the head to the opposite side against resistance, then observes and palpates the muscular contraction at the anterior edge of the lateral triangle of the neck (Fig. 3.**14**).

The upper portion of the trapezius m. is examined as follows: the examiner stands in front of the patient, puts both hands on the patient's shoulders, grasps the upper edge of the trapezius m. on either side between the thumb and index finger, and asks the patient to shrug the shoulders against resistance. In unilateral accessory nerve palsy, the shrug is less powerful on the affected side and the trapezius m. is palpably thinner and weaker (Fig. 3.**15**).

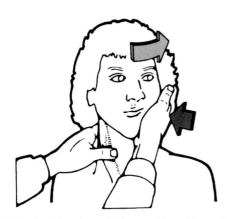

Fig. 3.**14 Testing the sternocleidomastoid m.** The patient attempts to turn the head to the left against the examiner's resistance. The right sternocleidomastoid m. contracts.

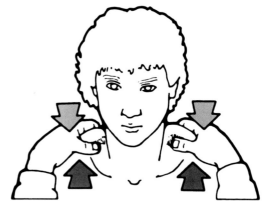

Fig. 3.**15 Testing the upper portion of the trapezius m.** The examiner places his or her hands on the patient's shoulders, grasping the upper edge of the trapezius m. on each side between his or her thumb and index finger. The patient is then asked to shrug the shoulders. Unilateral weakness, reduced contraction, or diminished volume of the trapezius m. can be palpated.

CN XII: Hypoglossal N.

The twelfth cranial nerve is a purely motor nerve to the muscles of the tongue. Lesions of this nerve produce **atrophy and weakness of the tongue**. A unilateral lesion usually produces a longitudinal furrow; when protruded, the tongue deviates to the weaker side because of the predominant force of the intact contralateral genioglossus m., which "pushes" the tongue across the midline (Fig. 3.**16**).

Phonation, Articulation, and Speech

Assessment of the patient's voice and speech is a compulsory part of the neurological examination. The examiner should pay attention to possible hoarseness, to the volume of speech (e. g., hypophonia in Parkinson disease, p. 128), and to possible disturbances of articulation (dysarthria), of the tempo of speech, and of its linguistic form and content (aphasia, p. 41).

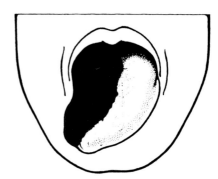

Fig. 3.**16 Atrophy and weakness of the right half of the tongue** in a lesion of the right hypoglossal n.

Examination of the Upper Limbs

General aspects. The examiner should ask the patient **which hand he or she mostly uses**, right or left. Only persons who use a pair of scissors, a knife, or a sewing needle with their left hand, or write with the left hand, are true left handers. Any abnormalities of **muscle bulk** should be noted, in particular isolated atrophy of muscle groups. **Fasciculations** must be deliberately sought: in our experience, these involuntary contractions of groups of muscle fibers, which induce no movement, can be seen under the skin only by careful observation of the unclothed patient from an adequate distance and for a sufficient length of time. The **trophic state of the skin**, the papillary pattern of the fingertips, and the configuration of the nails should also be assessed. Important positive findings include **anomalies of finger posture, tremor,** or other **involuntary movements**. The mobility of the larger joints should be tested individually and the pulses in the limbs should be felt. Vascular bruits should be listened for in the supraclavicular fossa when indicated.

Motor Function and Coordination

A number of standard tests are used to assess motor function and coordination. **Diadochokinesis** is the ability to carry out rapid alternating movements, e. g., pronation and supination of the forearm (Fig. 3.**17**). Such movements will be abnormally slow (*bradydiadochokinesia*) or irregular (*dysdiadochokinesia*) on one side or both in the presence of paresis, extrapyramidal processes, and cerebellar diseases. In the **postural test**, the patient extends both arms horizontally in front, in supination, with eyes closed (Fig. 3.**18**). An involuntary sinking, or pronation of one arm ("pronator drift"), or involuntary flexion at the elbow or wrist, indicates motor hemiparesis of central origin; conjugate deviation of both arms to one side implies an ipsilateral lesion of the labyrinth or cerebellum. In the **arm-rolling test**, the patient rapidly rotates the forearms around each other in front of the trunk (Fig. 3.**19**). Mild hemiparesis is evident as markedly diminished movement of the affected limb. In the **finger–nose test**, the patient keeps his or her eyes closed and brings the index finger slowly to the tip of the nose, in a wide arc. This can normally be done smoothly and confidently (Fig. 3.**20a**). Fluctuating deviation of the finger from the ideal arc is a manifestation of *ataxia*, indicating either a proprioceptive disturbance or a lesion in the ipsilateral cerebellar hemisphere. On the other hand, if the deviation first appears when the finger is near its target and worsens as it approaches, this is called *intention tremor* (Fig. 3.**20c**) and is caused by lesions of the dentate nucleus of the cerebellum or of its efferent projections. A positive **rebound phenomenon** consists of inadequate braking of the normal, small rebound movement that occurs when the patient isometrically contracts a muscle against the examiner's resistance and the resistance is suddenly removed (Fig. 3.**21**). If the patient is sitting, the examiner can test for rebound of the biceps brachii m. (while taking care lest the patient hit himself or herself in the face). If the patient is lying on the examining table, the patient can be asked to stretch out one arm and raise it a short distance into the air, then press strongly downward against the examiner's resistance. If the examiner suddenly lets go, a healthy subject will brake the ensuing downward movement of the arm in time, but a patient with hemiparesis or cerebellar disfunction will hit the table with it.

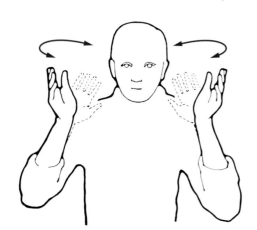

Fig. 3.**17 Testing of diadochokinesis** by rapid pronation and supination of the forearms.

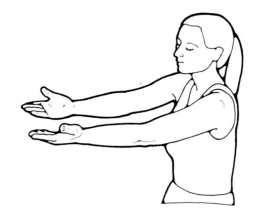

Fig. 3.**18 Positional testing of the upper limbs.**

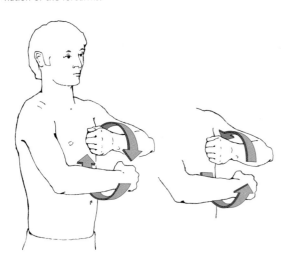

Fig. 3.**19 Arm-rolling test.** A normal subject rotates both arms to a roughly equal extent, while a patient with central hemiparesis (even if mild!) moves the nonparetic limb much more than the paretic one.

Fig. 3.**20 Finger–nose test. a** Normal, smooth, confident movement. **b** Ataxic movement **c** Intention tremor: the closer the finger comes to its target (nose), the more it deviates from the ideal line of approach.

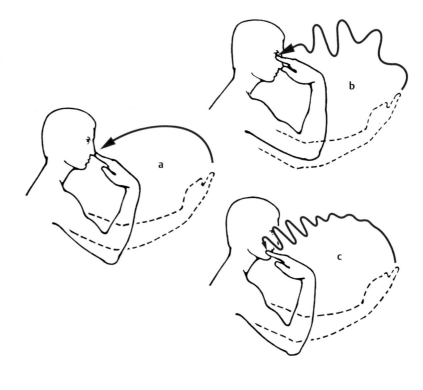

Fig. 3.**21 Rebound phenomenon** due to a cerebellar lesion. **a** Method of testing: the examiner's other hand protects the patient's face. **b** When the examiner suddenly releases the patient's actively flexed arm, the ensuing involuntary flexion should be promptly braked. **c** Braking is inadequate (the rebound phenomenon is positive) in the presence of an ipsilateral cerebellar lesion

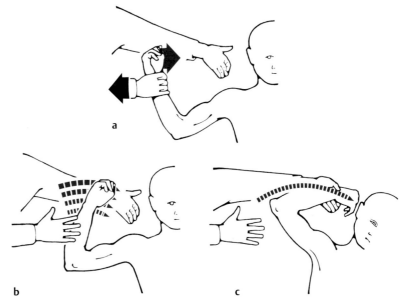

Muscle Tone and Strength

Muscle tone in the upper limbs can be tested with wide-amplitude passive movement of the radiocarpal joint or of the elbow. The movement should be rapid, but not rhythmic (so that the patient cannot predict its course). Diminished muscle tone (**hypotonia**) is a characteristic sign of intrinsic muscle lesions, peripheral nerve lesions, ipsilateral cerebellar dysfunction, and hy-

perkinetic extrapyramidal diseases. **Spasticity** is a type of elevated muscle tone produced by lesions of the pyramidal pathway (Fig. 3.**22a**). The resistance of a spastic upper limb to passive movement is usually strong at first, but may then suddenly give way ("*clasp-knife phenomenon*"); alternatively, it may increase on continued passive movement. **Rigidity** is a viscous or waxy resistance to passive movement that can be felt to an equal extent throughout the entire movement; it is

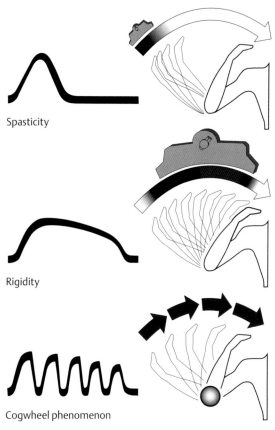

Spasticity

Rigidity

Cogwheel phenomenon

Fig. 3.**22 Abnormalities of muscle tone and the cogwheel phenomenon.**

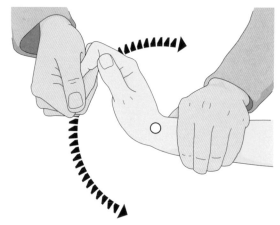

Fig. 3.**23 Testing for the cogwheel phenomenon in the radiocarpal joint.** The examiner fixes the patient's forearm with one hand, grasps the patient's fingers with the other, and moves them slowly (but not rhythmically) back and forth.

Table 3.**4 Grading of muscle strength.**
The 0–5 scale of the British Medical Research Council (MRC).

M0	=	no muscle contraction
M1	=	visible contraction not resulting in movement
M2	=	movement of the body part only when the effect of gravity is eliminated
M3	=	movement against gravity
M4	=	movement against moderate resistance
M5	=	full strength

(Grades M3 and M4 can be optionally subdivided by adding plus or minus signs)

most commonly found in Parkinson disease (Fig. 3.**22b**). The accompanying parkinsonian *cogwheel phenomenon* is best appreciated at the radiocarpal joint. The examiner should fix the patient's forearm with one hand, grasp the patient's fingertips with the other, and alternately flex and extend the radiocarpal joint, slowly and with a wide excursion, but not in perfect rhythm (Fig. 3.**23**). The examiner will then feel multiple, brief impulses of resistance at irregular intervals, giving the overall impression of a saccadic movement (Fig. 3.**22c**). Elevated muscle tone may also result from active opposition to passive movement when the patient apparently cannot relax the muscular contraction. This phenomenon, known by the German term *Gegenhalten* ("opposition"), is seen in frontal lobe lesions.

Muscle strength is tested in groups of muscles that carry out a single movement, or, if necessary, in individual muscles. The patient is asked to **contract the corresponding muscle(s) actively against the examiner's resistance**. The examiner then judges the strength of contraction at the end-point of the related movement. Thus, the examiner tests biceps strength by trying to extend the patient's flexed elbow against resistance and triceps strength by trying to flex the extended elbow against resistance. The evaluation of potential lesions of individual nerve roots or peripheral nerves requires specific testing of the particular muscles or muscle

groups innervated by these nerves (see p. 208). For the purpose of documentation, muscle strength can be graded semiquantitatively with the MRC scale shown in Table 3.**4**. Incomplete paralysis is called **paresis** and complete paralysis is called **plegia**. Further terms describe the distribution of weakness in the body: *hemiparesis* or *hemiplegia* affects one side of the body, *paraparesis* or *paraplegia* affects both lower limbs, and *quadriparesis* or *quadriplegia* affects all four limbs (less common synonyms for the last two are *tetraparesis* and *tetraplegia*). Paralysis of both arms, or *brachial diplegia*, is a rare occurrence.

Reflexes

Types of reflexes. Reflexes are processes that are induced by a specific stimulus, always take the same course, and cannot be voluntarily influenced by either the patient or the examiner. For the **intrinsic** muscle reflexes, alternatively called proprioceptive muscle reflexes, the site (muscle) of the eliciting stimulus is the same as that of the reflex contraction; for **extrinsic** (exteroceptive) reflexes, the stimulus and the response are at different sites and the afferent and efferent arms of the reflex loop, therefore, belong to different peripheral nerves or segmental nerve roots. Extrinsic reflexes become less intense (habituate) on repeated stimulation.

Pathological reflexes are usually not seen in normal individuals, or only up to a certain age; they are found in various disease processes affecting the CNS. Some pathological reflexes are of the extrinsic type. The more important reflexes, and the segmental nerve roots and peripheral nerves that mediate them, are listed in Tables **3.5–3.7**.

Table 3.**5** **The most important normal intrinsic muscle reflexes**

Reflex	Stimulus	Response	Muscle(s)	Peripheral nerve	Segment
Masseter reflex	tap on the chin or a tongue depressor laid on the lower teeth, with slightly opened mouth	brief mouth closure movement	masseter m.	trigeminal n.	V
Trapezius reflex	tap on the lateral attachment of the trapezius to the coracoid process	shoulder elevation	trapezius m.	accessory n.	XI C3–C4
Scapulohumeral reflex	tap on the medial edge of the lower half of the scapula	adduction and external rotation of the dependent arm	infraspinatus and teres minor mm.	suprascapular and axillary nn.	C4–C6
Biceps reflex	tap on the biceps tendon with bent elbow	elbow flexion	biceps brachii m.	musculocutaneous n.	C5–C6
Brachioradialis reflex ("radial periosteal reflex")	tap on the distal end of the radius with lightly bent elbow and pronated forearm	elbow flexion	brachioradialis m. (biceps brachii and brachialis mm.)	radial and musculocutaneous nn.	C5–C6
Pectoralis reflex	tap on the scapulohumeral joint from anteriorly	forward movement of the shoulder	pectoralis major and minor mm.	medial and lateral pectoral nn.	C5–T4
Triceps reflex	tap on the triceps tendon with bent elbow	elbow extension	triceps brachii m.	radial n.	C7–C8
Thumb reflex	tap on the flexor pollicis longus tendon in the distal third of the forearm	flexion of the thumb at the interphalangeal joint	flexor pollicis longus m.	median n.	C6–C8
Wrist reflex	tap on the dorsum of the wrist, proximal to the radiocarpal joint	extension of the wrist and fingers (inconstant)	wrist extensors and long extensors of the fingers	radial n.	C6–C8
Finger flexor reflex	tap on the examiner's thumb, which is laid in the palm of the patient's hand; or, tap on the flexor tendons on the volar surface of the wrist	flexion of the fingers (and of the wrist)	flexor digitorum superficialis m. (flexores carpi mm.)	median (ulnar) n.	C7–C8
Trömner reflex	patient's hand held at the middle finger; tap on the volar side of the distal phalanx of the middle finger	flexion of the distal phalanges of the fingers (including the thumb)	flexor digitorum profundus m.	median (ulnar) n.	C7–C8 (T1)
Adductor reflex	tap on the medial condyle of the femur	leg adduction	adductors	obturator n.	L2–L4
Quadriceps femoris reflex ("patellar tendon reflex," "knee-jerk reflex")	tap on the quadriceps tendon below the patella with the knee lightly flexed	knee extension	quadriceps femoris m.	femoral n.	(L2) L3–L4
Tibialis posterior reflex	tap on the tibialis posterior tendon behind the medial malleolus	supination of the foot (inconstant)	tibialis posterior m.	tibial n.	L5
Peroneus muscle reflex (foot extensor reflex)	foot lightly flexed and supinated; examiner's finger placed over the distal end of the metatarsal bones; tap on the finger, especially over the 1st and 2nd metatarsal bones	dorsiflexion and pronation of the foot	long extensors of the foot and toes, peronei	peroneal n.	L5–S1
Semimembranosus and semitendinosus reflex	tap on the tendon of the medial knee flexors (patient prone, knee lightly flexed and relaxed)	palpable muscle contraction	semimembranosus and semitendinosus mm.	sciatic n.	S1
Biceps femoris reflex	tap on the tendon of the lateral knee flexors (patient prone, knee lightly flexed and relaxed)	muscle contraction	biceps femoris m.	sciatic n.	S1–S2
Triceps surae reflex ("Achilles reflex," "ankle-jerk reflex")	tap on the Achilles tendon (knee lightly flexed, foot in right-angle posture)	plantar flexion of the foot	triceps surae m. (and other plantar flexors)	tibial n.	S1–S2
Toe flexor reflex (Rossolimo sign)	tap on the pads of the toes	flexion of the toes	flexor digitorum and flexor hallucis longus mm.	tibial n.	S1–S2

3

The Neurological Examination

Table 3.6   **The most important normal extrinsic muscle reflexes**

Reflex	Stimulus	Response	Muscle(s)	Peripheral nerve	Segment
Pupillary reflex	incident light, convergence	constriction	constrictor pupillae m.	optic and oculomotor nn.	diencephalon, midbrain, pons
Corneal reflex	gently touching the cornea from the side, e. g., with a wisp of cotton or piece of tissue paper; the eye looks medially	eye closure (and simultaneous upward movement of the globes: Bell phenomenon)	orbicularis oculi m.	trigeminal and facial nn.	midpons
Bell phenomenon (palpebrooculogyric reflex)	attempted active eye closure while the examiner holds the upper lids open	the globes normally turn upward	superior rectus and inferior oblique mm.	trigeminal and oculomotor nn.	pons
Auriculopalpebral reflex	sudden noise from a source that the patient cannot see	blink	orbicularis oculi m.	vestibulocochlear and facial nn.	caudal pons
Palatal reflex and pharyngeal (gag) reflex	touching the soft palate or the posterior pharyngeal wall with a tongue depressor	elevation of the palatal veil and symmetrical contraction of the posterior pharyngeal wall	palatal and pharyngeal musculature	glossopharyngeal and vagus nn.	medulla
Mayer reflex of the proximal interphalangeal joint	forced passive flexion of the proximal interphalangeal joints of the 3rd and 4th fingers	adduction and opposition of the first metacarpal bone	adductor pollicis m., opponens pollicis m.	ulnar and median nn.	C6–T1
Abdominal skin reflex	rapidly and lightly stroking the abdominal skin from lateral to medial	movement of the abdominal skin, including the umbilicus, toward the side of the stimulus	abdominal musculature	intercostal nn., hypogastric n., and ilioinguinal n.	T6–T12
Cremaster reflex (in males)	stroking the skin on the upper medial surface of the thigh (or pinching the proximal adductor muscles)	retraction of the testes	cremaster m.	genital branch of the genitofemoral n.	L1–L2
Gluteal reflex	stroking the skin over the gluteus maximus m.	contraction of the gluteus maximus m. (inconstant)	gluteus medius m., gluteus maximus m.	superior and inferior gluteal nn.	L4–S1
Bulbocavernosus reflex	gently pinching the glans penis; pinprick on the skin of the dorsum of the penis	contraction of the bulbocavernosus m. (visible at the root of the penis in the perineum, or palpable by rectal examination)	bulbocavernosus m.	pudendal n.	S3–S4
Anal reflex	pinprick on the skin of the perianal region or perineum, patient in lateral decubitus position with flexed hip and knee	visible contraction of the anus	external anal sphincter	pudendal n.	S3–S5

Table 3.7   **The most important pathological reflexes**

Reflex	Stimulus	Response	Significance
Orbicularis oculi reflex (glabellar reflex, nasopalpebral reflex)	tap on the glabella or on a finger applied to the lateral edge of the orbit while the orbicularis oculi m. is contracted	narrowing of the palpebral fissure by contraction of the orbicularis oculi m. (possibly bilaterally)	exaggerated in supranuclear lesions of the corticopontine pathway and in extrapyramidal diseases
Corneomandibular reflex (winking jaw)	like the corneal reflex; mouth slightly open	the jaw deviates to the side opposite the stimulus	release of an older functional synergy between the orbicularis oculi m. and the lateral pterygoid m.; due to an ipsilateral lesion of the corticobulbar pathway, lacunar state, or bulbar palsy
Marcus Gunn phenomenon (winking jaw)	opening the mouth and moving the jaw	a previously ptotic eyelid is very strongly elevated	proof that ptosis is not due to peripheral paresis or myasthenia
Bulldog reflex	placing a tongue depressor between the patient's teeth	the patient bites down so hard that the head can be lifted by the tongue depressor	release phenomenon (disinhibition) due to diffuse cortical injury, e. g., postanoxic

Continued →

Table 3.**7** **The most important pathological reflexes** (continued)

Reflex	Stimulus	Response	Significance
Orbicularis oris reflex (snout reflex, nasomental reflex)	gentle tap on a finger or tongue depressor placed on the lateral corner of the mouth or on the lips (can sometimes also be elicited from the glabella)	contraction of the orbicularis oris m. with pursing of the lips	absent or only faintly present in normal individuals; exaggerated as a result of lesions affecting the supranuclear corticopontine pathways (status lacunaris, multi-infarct dementia, extrapyramidal diseases such as Parkinson disease)
Suck reflex	slowly, gently stroking the lips	sucking and, possibly, swallowing movements; occasionally, biting; mouth opening and turning of the head toward the stimulus (termed a magnet reaction if already present when an object is brought near the mouth)	severe, diffuse brain injury, decorticate state; e. g., in apallic syndrome after anoxia or severe traumatic brain injury (normal in infants; pathological release phenomenon in later life)
Wartenberg reflex ("thumb sign")	forceful passive flexion of the 2nd through 5th fingers	flexion of the thumb	indicates a pyramidal tract lesion
Palmomental reflex (exaggerated or asymmetrical)	intensely stroking the ball of the thumb or the palm of the hand with a fingernail or wooden stick	contraction of the ipsilateral chin muscles	in diffuse cerebral injury (multi-infarct syndrome, brain atrophy, postanoxic); if unilateral, indicates contralateral brain lesion
Grasp reflex	stroking the palm	finger flexion, possibly grasping of the stimulating object	normal in infants; later a sign of diffuse brain injury (mainly in the frontal lobes); seen contralateral to a frontal lobe lesion or ipsilateral to a lesion in the basal ganglia
Grasping and groping (magnet phenomenon)	object brought near the palm of the (conscious) patient	the hand follows the presented object like a magnet, making grasping movements	
Gegenhalten	attempted passive stretching of a muscle (e. g., pushing down on the lower jaw, or forcibly extending the flexed fingers)	the patient actively and intensely contracts the muscle in question, preventing passive stretch (in the absence of generalized negativism)	in diffuse frontal lobe disease and lesions of the basal ganglia
Mass reflexes of the lower limbs in paraplegia	e. g., forceful passive flexion of the toes and forefoot (Marie–Foix handgrip)	retraction of the (otherwise plegic) lower limb by flexion at the knee and hip	reveals the intactness of the spinal reflex arc, and therefore of the peripheral nervous system (useful as a "trick" facilitating the nursing care of patients with spastic rigidity)
Babinski reflex (Fig. 3.**31**)	stroking the lateral edge of the foot from the heel to the 5th toe (or else transversely across the plantar arch)	tonic (slow) extension of the great toe, while the other toes remain in their original position or are splayed (like a fan)	indicates a lesion of the corticospinal (pyramidal) pathway on the corresponding side
Oppenheim Reflex (Fig. 3.**31**)	forcefully stroking the anterior margin of the tibia from proximal to distal (painful)		
Gordon Reflex (Fig. 3.**31**)	forcefully stroking or squeezing the calf muscles		

Intrinsic muscle reflexes of the upper limb. The intrinsic muscle reflexes are elicited by a rapid, and adequately forceful, blow on the tendon of a muscle or on the bone to which the tendon is attached. The resulting, transient stretching of the muscle excites receptors in the muscle spindles, in which afferent impulses are generated. These travel to the spinal cord and excite the α-motor neurons innervating the stimulated muscle (usually by way of interneurons at the same segmental level). The upper limb reflexes that are usually tested are the triceps, biceps, and radial periosteal reflexes (Table 3.**5**). The last-named reflex is elicited by a tap on the styloid process of the radius; this is followed by contraction, not only of the brachioradialis m., but also of the biceps and brachialis mm. The elicitation of these reflexes is illustrated in Fig. 3.**24**.

The two important *finger flexor reflexes* are essentially variations of the same reflex. The **Trömner reflex** is elicited by a rapid tap on the pads of the patient's lightly flexed fingers. The response consists of flexion of the distal interphalangeal joints of the fingers and thumb (only in the hand that was stimulated, not in the other hand). To elicit **Hoffmann sign**, the examiner gently grasps the distal phalanx of one of the patient's fingers (usually the middle finger) between his or her own thumb and index finger, then lets it snap back as the thumb slides off the patient's fingernail. The response is the same as in the Trömner reflex (Fig. 3.**25**).

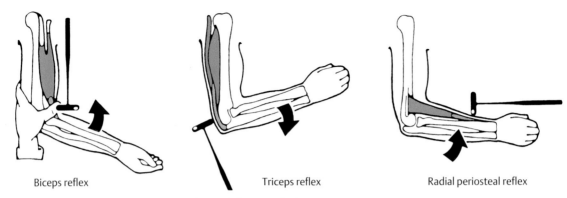

Fig. 3.**24 Elicitation of the intrinsic muscle reflexes of the upper limb.**

Biceps reflex   Triceps reflex   Radial periosteal reflex

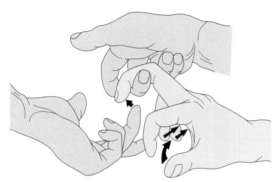

Fig. 3.**25 Elicitation of the Trömner reflex.**

Facilitating maneuvers. Initially faint or not clearly elicitable intrinsic muscle reflexes can be enhanced with various maneuvers based on the principle that preloading of the intrafusal muscle spindle fibers makes them more sensitive to stretch. Forceful contraction of practically any muscle group in the body results in a generalized sensitization of all muscle spindle fibers. Thus, all of the intrinsic muscle reflexes can be made stronger by having the patient forcefully lift his or her head from the headrest (in the supine position), clench the teeth, make fists, strongly plantar-flex the feet, or interlock the hands and pull hard (this is called the **Jendrassik handgrip**). These maneuvers are illustrated in Fig. 3.**26.**

The more common **abnormalities** of the intrinsic muscle reflexes and their significance are presented in Table 3.**8.**

Pyramidal tract signs in the upper limb. Lesions along the pyramidal pathway produce characteristic changes in the pattern of the reflexes that are normally present, as well as other, pathological reflexes that are normally absent. Evidence for a lesion of the pyramidal pathway is generally less obvious in the upper limb than in the

Table 3.8   **Significance of the more common abnormalities of the intrinsic muscle reflexes**

Abnormality	Significance	Remarks
Apparent absence of all reflexes	very weak reflexes, or inadequate examining technique	facilitation maneuvers, e. g., Jendrassik handgrip
True generalized areflexia	polyneuropathy, polyradiculopathy anterior horn cell disease myopathy Adie syndrome congenital areflexia	sensory deficit, perhaps paresis muscle atrophy without sensory deficit (same) inspect pupils often familial
Absence of an individual reflex or reflexes	nerve root lesion peripheral nerve lesion	e. g., triceps reflex (C7), Achilles reflex (S1) e. g., biceps reflex (musculocutaneous n.), Achilles reflex (femoral n.)
Very weak reflexes	usually without pathological significance	often seen in older patients
Very brisk reflexes	if generalized, often without pathological significance	particularly in younger patients
Pathologically exaggerated reflexes	"pyramidal tract signs," spasticity	compare sides (hemiparesis?) and compare upper with lower limbs (paraparesis?)
Positive Hoffmann sign and Trömner reflex	normal if symmetrical and without other, accompanying "pyramidal tract signs"	

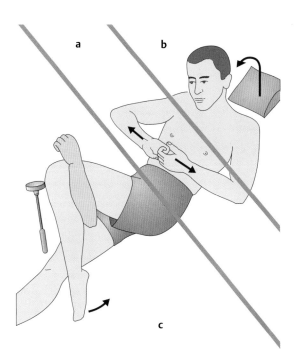

Fig. **3.26 Facilitation maneuvers** make the intrinsic muscle reflexes more intense and easier to elicit. **a** Jendrassik hand grip. **b** Same effect with active, strong raising of the head off the headrest. **c** Active plantar flexion of the foot.

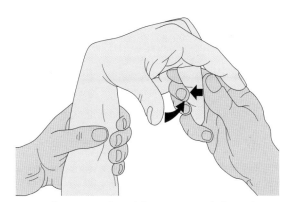

Fig. 3.**27 The Mayer reflex of the metacarpophalangeal joint** is elicited by forceful passive flexion of the middle finger. Involuntary adduction of the thumb normally follows; absence of the reflex suggests a lesion of the pyramidal pathway.

lower limb, because there are no "classic pyramidal tract signs" for the upper limb, as there are for the lower (cf. p. 38). One important clue is **exaggeration of the physiological intrinsic muscle reflexes**, especially if asymmetric. Two others are spreading of the reflex zones and unusual briskness of certain intrinsic reflexes that, under normal circumstances, are only barely elicitable, or not at all, e.g., the trapezius and pectoralis reflexes (cf. Table 3.**5**). The Trömner reflex and Hoffmann sign can also be of pathological significance if abnormally brisk or unilaterally exaggerated. **Absence of the Mayer reflex of the metacarpophalangeal joint** is also con-

sidered a pyramidal tract sign: forceful passive flexion of the middle finger at the metacarpophalangeal joint is normally followed by reflex adduction of the metacarpal bone of the thumb (Fig. 3.**27**), but not if there is a lesion in the pyramidal pathway. Another pyramidal tract sign is flexion and opposition of the thumb when the examiner forcefully pulls on an actively flexed finger.

Sensation

Sensory testing takes time, patience, and good cooperation from the patient. Its general purpose is to identify any sensory deficit that may be present, delimit its site and extent precisely, and determine which sensory modalities are affected. The pattern of findings obtained in this way usually permits classification of the causative lesion as central, radicular, or peripheral. During the examination, the clinician must keep in mind what he or she is looking for with each examining technique in each part of the body where it is being applied.

The sense of touch (*esthesia*) is tested with the patient's eyes closed. The examiner lightly touches various sites on the patient's body with a finger, a feather, a piece of tissue paper, or the like. Precise quantitative testing can be performed with graded instruments, such as von Frey hairs or an adjustable Wartenberg pinwheel, but is not necessary in routine practice. (Sharp pinwheels can also transmit infectious diseases such as hepatitis and AIDS; sterilization before each use is mandatory!) It generally suffices to describe a deficit as either a deficient sense of touch (*hypesthesia*) or an absent sense of touch (*anesthesia*). Depending on the clinical situation, the examiner may want to measure sensation quantitatively in a particular dermatome or in the distribution of a particular peripheral nerve, or to compare sensation on mirror-image sites on the body.

Two-point discrimination, stereognosis. The *epicritic* component of the sense of touch (ultimately derived from Greek *krites*, "judge") is tested on the pads of the fingers, e. g., by determining the patient's ability to discriminate two simultaneous stimuli located close together. This can be done with a pair of calipers or simply with the two points of an unfolded paper clip. The two pointed ends are placed on the skin simultaneously, initially very close together, and then at increasing distances until the patient reports feeling two separate stimuli. The threshold distance is usually larger when the stimuli are simultaneous than when they are successively applied; on the fingertips, it should be no more than 5 mm. Epicritic sensation can also be tested by having the patient identify a coin by touch, or "read" a number written on the patient's fingertip. Normal performance on these tests also requires intact **stereognosis.**

Vibration and position sense. Vibration sense (*pallesthesia*) is tested with a vibrating 64- or 124-Hz tuning fork solidly placed on various bony prominences of the body, i. e., sites where the bone is covered only by skin. The intensity of vibration can be graduated, if desired, with the aid of special adjustable tuning forks, such as the Rydel–Seiffer model, which allows grading in eighths. This is mostly unnecessary, as there is an easier method: as soon as the patient reports that the vibration is no longer felt, the examiner tests his or her own vibration sense with the same tuning fork at an analogous position. If the examiner still clearly feels the vibration, then the patient unquestionably has a deficit of vibration sense (the rarely used scholarly terms are *pallhypesthesia* for a partial deficit, *pallanesthesia* for a total deficit). Milder deficits can usually be detected only in the periphery (e. g., at the ankles), while more severe ones are evident further up the trunk. Vibration sense usually declines by one- or two-eighths over the course of normal aging.

The examiner tests **position sense** by passively moving some part of the patient's body (in the hands, usually the middle finger) and asking the patient in which direction it is being moved. The patient should not, of course, be able to observe the movement visually.

Temperature sense (*thermesthesia*) should be tested particularly when a central lesion is suspected, because the pain and temperature pathways run separately from those of the other sensory modalities in the spinal cord and brainstem, and do not join them until the level of the thalamus (p. 74).

A lesion that affects the spinothalamic tract in the spinal cord or brainstem, but spares the other sensory pathways, produces a *dissociated sensory deficit*: pain and temperature sensation are impaired in the corresponding part of the body, but the sense of touch is preserved. A partial deficit of temperature sense is called *thermhypesthesia*, a total one *thermanesthesia*.

To test the sense of temperature, the examiner fills two test tubes or special-purpose metal containers with cold and warm water and applies them to different parts of the patient's body. Thermal stimuli can be delivered in graded fashion, if desired, by varying their temperature, area, and duration.

The ability to feel pain (*algesia*) should be tested by pinching a fold of skin, never by pinprick. A partial deficit is called *hypalgesia*, a total one *analgesia*.

Allesthesia or *allocheiria* is the perception of a tactile stimulus somewhere other than the site at which it was delivered. This phenomenon can occur in normal individuals and is of uncertain significance. (*Alloesthesia* and *allochiria* are variant spellings.)

Examination of the Trunk

The back and spine are examined with the patient standing. **Inspection** may reveal scoliosis or an alteration of the normal lordosis or kyphosis of particular segments of the vertebral column. Protruding ribs on one side (often visible only when the patient bends forward) are a sign of torsional scoliosis. As one looks at the patient from behind, there is a triangular gap to either side of the patient's waist, formed by the dependent arm, the rib cage, and the upper border of the pelvis; asymmetry of this gap is a further sign of scoliosis. A plumb line from the spinous process of C7 should overlie the natal cleft; deviations should be measured and documented (preferably in centimeters, rather than finger breadths). One should also look for stepping of the lumbosacral vertebrae (e. g., in spondylolisthesis, p. 260) or tenderness of the spinous processes to pressure or percussion. Techniques for testing the **mobility of the cervical spine** were described above in **Examination of the Head and Cranial Nerves** (p. 16). The mobility of the thoracolumbar spine is tested by having the patient bend the trunk forward, backward, and to either side, and then rotate it to either side. On **forward bending** with extended knees, young patients should be able to touch the ground (finger-to-ground distance 0 cm). Spinal mobility can be quantified with the two **Schober tests**: the small Schober index pertains to the lumbosacral spine, the large Schober index to the thoracic spine. To measure the small Schober index, place a mark on the patient's skin 10 cm above the spinous process of L5, have the patient bend forward as far as possible, and measure the distance again; it should now be at least 15 cm. The large Schober index is measured similarly, starting from a point 30 cm below

the spinous process of C7, which on maximal forward bending should move to at least 32 cm below it. Any diminution of the normal cervical lordosis is best seen when the patient stands with shoulders and heels to the wall and bends the head as far back as possible. The back of the patient's head normally touches the wall; if not, the distance from the occipital protuberance to the wall should be measured in centimeters. An abnormality of this type is found, e. g., in ankylosing spondylitis.

Reflexes. The **abdominal skin reflexes** are extrinsic muscle reflexes. They are tested by rapid stroking of the abdominal skin (e. g., with a wooden stick) from lateral to medial, at three different segmental levels, on either side. They can be enhanced, if necessary, by having the patient lift his or her head off the headrest. Diminution of the abdominal skin reflexes indicates a lesion of the pyramidal pathway. A diminished or absent reflex at only one level on one side suggests a segmental peripheral lesion. Total bilateral absence is usually an artifact of deficient examining technique, but may also be caused by an obese or flaccid abdominal wall (e. g., after pregnancy). "True" bilateral absence of all abdominal skin reflexes is seen in bilateral lesions of the pyramidal pathway; an accompanying sign in such patients is unusual briskness of the **intrinsic reflexes of the abdominal musculature**. These are tested by tapping at the sites of muscle attachment, e. g., at the costal margin or the symphysis pubis. Alternatively, the examiner can place his or her own hand on the abdomen and tap on it. The **cremaster reflex** is tested (in males) by stroking the medial surface of the thigh or by forceful pressure with a finger near the origin of the adductor muscles. The **anal reflex** is tested by stimulating the perianal skin, e. g., with a pointed wooden stick. This induces reflex contraction of the anal sphincter. The anal reflex is sometimes easier to appreciate on rectal examination with a gloved finger (with which the examiner can also assess sphincter tone); it is abolished by lesions of the cauda equina and conus medullaris (p. 143 ff.).

Sensation. Sensation on the trunk is tested to localize a possible *sensory level* due to a spinal cord lesion. A sensory level is a segmentally delimited sensory deficit. If caused by a bilateral lesion of one or more spinal nerve roots, it is limited to one or a few dermatomes; if caused by spinal cord transection, it covers the entire body from the toes up to the rostral border of the injured spinal segment. The segmental height of a sensory level should be located as precisely as possible by testing both from above and from below.

Examination of the Lower Limbs

The procedure here is essentially the same as in the upper limbs (cf. **Examination of the Upper Limbs**, pp. 27 ff.). Particular attention should be paid to the **examination of the peripheral pulses**, because pathological processes frequently affect the circulation of the lower limbs. The pedal and popliteal pulses should be palpated; the pulses in the abdominal vessels should be examined by auscultation, as should those of the femoral a., both in the groin and in the proximal adductor canal. The **Ratschow test** is a provocative test of the blood supply to the leg: the examiner holds up both legs of the supine patient and the patient rotates the feet back and forth. A normal individual can do this for several minutes without difficulty, but, if arterial insufficiency is present, pain soon develops in the feet. In addition, when the legs are brought back to the horizontal position, the skin takes a longer time than normal to regain its usual pink color (in patients of light complexion) and venous refilling is likewise delayed.

Coordination and Strength

The following motor tests should be performed: in the **heel–knee–shin** (HKS) test, the patient closes the eyes, brings the heel of one leg through the air in a wide arc to place it on the opposite knee, then slides the heel down the shin to the front of the ankle, and finally back up to the knee (Fig. 3.**28**). Unsteadiness indicates ataxia. In the **postural test**, the patient lies supine, raises the lower limbs so that the hips and knees are at right angles, and holds them in this position (Fig. 3.**29**). The examiner looks for possible sinking of a leg, indicating (mild) paresis. **Strength**, too, should be tested in the supine patient. Additional special tests are used for individual muscle groups. For example, a patient with quadriceps weakness has trouble stepping up onto a stool or chair, or standing up from a sitting position (if the weakness is bilateral). The dorsiflexors of the feet and toes should always be tested, because these distal muscles are frequently weakened early in the course of many different neurological disorders. Great toe dorsiflexion, for example, is weak in L5 radiculopathy. In suspected polyneuropathy, it may be useful to palpate the con-

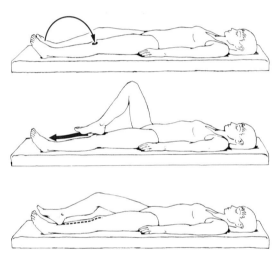

Fig. 3.**28 The heel–knee–shin test.** With eyes closed, the patient brings one heel to the opposite knee, then slides it down the shin.

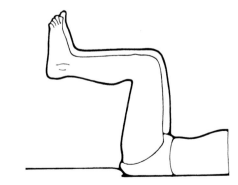

Fig. 3.**29 Postural test of the legs in the supine position.**

tractions of the muscles of the dorsum of the foot and to compare the patient's ability to spread the toes on the two sides.

Reflexes

Intrinsic muscle reflexes. The **quadriceps reflex** (patellar tendon reflex) and **Achilles' reflex** are the most important intrinsic muscle reflexes of the lower limb. They should be tested in every patient (Fig. 3.**30**). In some situations, it may also be advisable to test the *adductor re-*

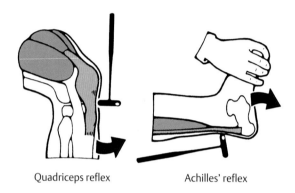

Quadriceps reflex   Achilles' reflex

Fig. 3.**30 Testing of the quadriceps and Achilles' reflexes.**

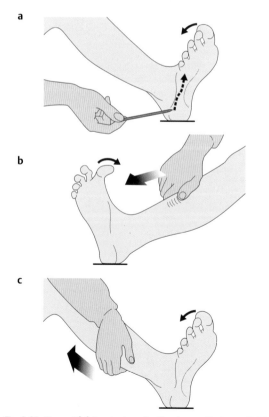

a

b

c

Fig. 3.**31 Pyramidal tract signs in the lower limbs. a** Babinski sign. **b** Oppenheim reflex. **c** Gordon reflex.

flex or the *knee flexor reflexes*. The latter are elicited by tapping the biceps femoris tendon (lateral border of the popliteal fossa) and the semimembranosus and semitendinosus tendons (medial border of the popliteal fossa). The inconstantly present *tibialis posterior reflex* is elicited by a tap on the tendon of this muscle behind the medial malleolus, while the foot is held in mild pronation. The response consists of supination.

Pathological reflexes. There are a number of important pathological reflexes in the lower limb whose presence implies a lesion of the pyramidal pathway. Chief among these is the **Babinski reflex** or "Babinski sign" (Fig. 3.**31a**). To elicit it, the examiner forcefully strokes the lateral plantar surface of the patient's foot, proceeding from the heel toward the toes. The pathological response is a slow, tonic dorsiflexion of the great toe, usually accompanied by fanning of the other toes. (Babinski himself called these phenomena "*signe de l'orteil*"—the great toe sign— and "*signe de l'éventail*"—the fan sign.) The same response can sometimes be elicited by stroking other parts of the foot, particularly the anterior ball of the foot from lateral to medial. The *Oppenheim sign* is the Babinski phenomenon evoked by a painfully intense stroke along the edge of the tibia, from the knee downward (Fig. 3.**31b**); the *Gordon sign* is the same phenomenon evoked by pressing or forcefully squeezing the calf muscles (Fig. 3.**31c**). The *Rossolimo sign* (toe flexor reflex) consists of flexion of the second through fifth toes in response to a tap, from the plantar side, on their distal phalanges; it is a somewhat unreliable indicator of a pyramidal tract lesion. These additional pathological reflexes need not be sought if the "classic" Babinski reflex is present, but only when it is absent or equivocal despite other clinical evidence of a pyramidal tract lesion. "*Mute soles,*" i. e., the lack of any toe movement at all when the Babinski reflex is tested, is a preliminary stage of the Babinski reflex in some patients and clinically meaningless in others. Mute soles in deeply comatose patients are associated with a poorer prognosis.

All of the important reflexes of the lower limbs are summarized in Tables 3.**5**–3.**7**, including the normal intrinsic and extrinsic muscle reflexes and the pathological reflexes.

Sensation

The earliest and most sensitive evidence of a mainly distal sensory deficit in the lower limbs, e. g., in polyneuropathy, is an impairment of **vibration sense**. Normal persons can feel vibration in all joints down to the distal interphalangeal joints of the toes. They can also recognize numbers drawn on the skin of the lower leg and usually on the pad of the great toe as well (**stereognosis**). **Position sense** in the great toe is tested by holding it on both sides and alternately dorsiflexing and plantar-flexing it; the patient should be able to state in which direction the toe was moved. Position sense is impaired, for example, by posterior column lesions.

Examination of the Autonomic Nervous System

Many clinical tests of the autonomic nervous system have been devised; not a few are rather cumbersome. We will merely mention some of them here: *testing of pupillary reactivity* after the local application of various substances, *measurement of the rise in blood pressure* after the administration of ephedrine, *observation of changes in blood pressure* with orthostasis or on a tilt table, *observation and measurement of sweating* after warming of the body or observation of local sweating with the aid of pilocarpine iontophoresis, *measurement*

of the pulse on inspiration and expiration or after the administration of 1 mg of atropine, assessment of voiding and erectile function (in males), etc. Such tests are generally used only in selected patients to answer specific questions. All patients, however, should be asked about possible disturbances of autonomic function when the history is taken (urination, defecation, sexual function, sweating).

Neurologically Relevant Aspects of the General Physical Examination

Many internal illnesses have neurological symptoms, sometimes as the main or sole manifestation of disease. The clinician performing a neurological examination should pay special attention to any potential symptoms or signs of a general, not exclusively neurological condition.

The patient's **general appearance** may suggest a wasting illness, such as a malignant neoplasm, or an endocrinopathy. Abnormal pallor of the **skin** may be a sign of anemia and a straw-yellow coloration may indicate pernicious anemia due to vitamin B12 deficiency. The

skin should also be carefully inspected for evidence of neurocutaneous diseases, vasculitic processes, or collagen vascular disease, which, taken together, are not at all uncommon. Findings to look for include the café-au-lait spots of neurofibromatosis (von Recklinghausen disease), abnormal shape and quality of the nails, herpetic vesicles, etc. The **cardiovascular examination** is very important: the *blood pressure* must be measured, *pulses* felt in the upper and lower limbs, and *vascular bruits* listened for, particularly in the neck, the supraclavicular fossae, the abdomen, and the groin bilaterally. The patient should also be examined for possible organomegaly or lymphadenopathy.

Neuropsychological and Psychiatric Examination

Psychopathological Findings

Many neurological illnesses are associated with psychiatric disturbances of greater or lesser severity. The organic neurological clinical picture is only complete once any psychopathological abnormalities that may be present have been thoroughly assessed and documented.

The examiner should first determine whether the patient is awake and alert. If not, he or she will be unable to receive and process incoming stimuli in the normal way. The patient may have a *disturbance of consciousness* of varying degrees of severity, ranging from drowsiness to coma, as described in Table 3.**9**.

In addition to the patient's level of consciousness and attention, the examiner should assess his or her *orientation, concentration, memory, drive, affective state,* and *cognitive ability*. The overall psychopathological picture is composed of these elements. If mental functioning is disturbed by an underlying neurological illness (so-called *psycho-organic syndrome* or *organic brain syn-*

drome), the manifestations often progress in a characteristic sequence, regardless of the etiology. At first, short-term and long-term memory, concentration, and attention are impaired; the patient is easily fatigued and has difficulty processing new information or performing complex tasks. Later, the patient becomes progressively disoriented, first to time, then to place, and then to person. Reactive depression is common at this stage. Ultimately, all spontaneous activity ceases; the patient loses interest, lacks drive, and in the end becomes permanently confused. Disturbances of this type can often be discerned in the patient's behavior, growing increasingly evident to the examiner over the course of the clinical interview and physical examination. Further historical data from the patient's family are often helpful. The **MiniMental Status Test** (Table 3.**10**) is widely used to assess cognitive function. For congenital psycho-organic abnormalities (mental retardation) and acquired forms (dementia), see p. 137.

Table 3.**9** **Degrees of impairment of consciousness, and other abnormal states of consciousness**

Designation	Features
Normal consciousness	oriented to place, time, and person (self), answers questions promptly and appropriately, follows commands correctly
Drowsiness	mostly awake, responds to questions and commands slowly but usually correctly (after repetition if necessary), moves in response to a sufficiently intense stimulus, usually oriented and coherent
Somnolence	mostly asleep, arousable with a moderately intense stimulus, generally requires repetition of questions or commands but then responds correctly, reacts slowly and after a delay but usually correctly
Stupor	asleep unless awakened, can only be awakened with a strong (auditory) stimulus or perhaps only with a mechanical stimulus, cannot answer questions or follow commands or does so only after intense repetition, and then only incompletely
Coma	unconscious, cannot be awakened, does not respond to a verbal or auditory stimulus, may respond to painful stimuli of graded intensities with specific (localizing) self-defense, nonlocalizing withdrawal of a limb, or abnormal flexion or extension responses, depending on the grade of coma (see also Table 2.**54**)
Confusion	inappropriate spontaneous behavior and responses to questions and commands, deficient orientation to place, time, and/or person (self); the confused patient may be fully conscious, less than fully conscious, or agitated (see below)
Agitation	motor unrest, inappropriate spontaneous behavior, cannot be quieted by verbal persuasion, more or less disoriented, does not follow commands appropriately

Table 3.**10** **MiniMental Status Test** (after Folstein et al.)

Name of patient: ....

Date of birth: ....

Date of examination: ....

    1 point for each correct answer

Orientation in time

  1. "What day of the week is it?" ....

  2. "What is today's date?" ....

  3. "What is the current month?" ....

  4. "What is the current season?" ....

  5. "What year is it?" ....

Orientation to place

  6. "Where are we (hospital, old age home, etc.)?" ....

  7. "On what floor?" ....

  8. "In what city?" ....

  9. "In what state (province, canton, etc.)?" ....

10. "In what country?" ....

Retentiveness
"Please repeat the following words."
(To be spoken at one word per second; to be performed only once)

11. "Lemon, ...

12. Key, ...

13. Ball." ....

Attention and calculations

14. "Please count from 100 backward by sevens" (serial-7 test) ....

15. one point for each correct subtraction, ...

16. maximum five points ....

17. ....

18. ....

Recent memory

19. "Which three words ....

20. did you repeat earlier?" ....

21. one point for each word correctly recalled ....

Continued →

Table 3.**10**   **MiniMental Status Test** (after Folstein et al.) (continued)

Language, naming

22. "What is this?" (show a pencil)   . . . .

23. "What is this?" (show a watch)   . . . .

24. "Please say after me: 'No ifs, ands, or buts.' "   . . . .

Language comprehension, motor execution

25. "Take this piece of paper in your hand, ...

26. fold it down the middle, ...

27. and put it on the ground." (each command to be given only once)   . . . .

Reading

28. "Please do what it says on this card." (Show card—"Close your eyes")   . . . .

Writing

29. "Write any sentence." (the patient is given a piece of paper and something to write with)   . . . .

Drawing

30. "Please copy this drawing."
(all 10 edges of the two pentagons must be drawn,
and the pentagons must overlap, for the patient
to receive one point for this task)   . . . .

Level of wakefulness: . . . .

Total points achieved: . . . .

Neuropsychological Examination

> The neuropsychological examination is designed to detect **cognitive deficits** (particularly in the areas of language, recognition, and the performance of motor tasks) and **disorders of perceptual processing** that may be due to a focal cortical lesion.

The localizing significance of various neuropsychological deficits is illustrated in the diagram of Fig. 3.**32**.

Aphasia. Language disorders due to cortical disfunction are called aphasia and are generally caused by left-sided lesions. A basic distinction is drawn between abnormalities of language production (**motor aphasia** or Broca aphasia) and of language comprehension (**sensory aphasia** or Wernicke aphasia). In Broca aphasia, there is a paucity of spontaneous speech, even though the "organic apparatus" for speech production (phonation, respiration, vocal muscles) remains intact. In Wernicke aphasia, speech comprehension is impaired despite intact hearing and processing of nonlinguistic auditory signals.

Fig. 3.**32 Cognitive deficits** that typically result from focal brain lesions (diagram adapted from A. Schnider).

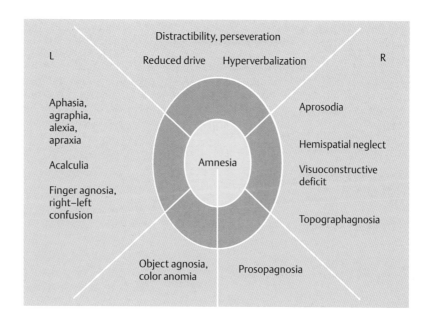

The examiner begins to assess the patient's spontaneous speech while taking the history; if necessary, the patient can be given specific language tasks, e. g., "Describe this picture." Various kinds of abnormality may be noted. The patient's utterances may be found to be unusually poor in meaning-bearing words and overloaded with connectives and "function words." Sentences may be faultily constructed (*paragrammatism*). The flow of speech may be either considerably greater than normal or slow and hesitant (*telegraphic speech*). Individual words may be deformed in certain characteristic ways (e. g., sound substitutions or *phonematic paraphasias*, such as "cog" for "dog"), or words may be used in place of other words from the same semantic category (*semantic paraphasias*, e. g., "table" for "chair"). Some words may be replaced by invented pseudowords (*neologisms*). Impaired language comprehension may be manifested by the patient's inability to point out various objects in the room, including parts of his or her own body, when these are named by the examiner. Complex commands are an even more sensitive functional test. The patient can be asked, for example, to place a certain named object in between two other named objects, or to interpret a complicated sentence, such as the following: "Not in the closet, but on top of it, was where he had placed his hat. Where was the hat?" Aphasic patients often make errors in the repetition of spoken sentences and in the naming of objects or parts of the body that are shown to them. Reading and writing may also be impaired.

Disturbances of spatial processing are usually caused by right-hemispheric lesions. Evidence for such a disturbance is present if the patient has unusual difficulty in spontaneously drawing or copying three-dimensional figures (cube, house, etc.). Deficits of this kind are often accompanied by neglect of the left side of space and the left half of the patient's own body (hemispatial neglect).

Apraxia. Disturbances in the goal-directed execution of complex actions or sequences of actions are known as **apraxia**. If the individual components of a *single* action cannot be put together correctly, the patient is suffering from **ideomotor apraxia**. Different parts of the body can be affected individually. In facial apraxia, for example, the patient may be unable to follow a command to execute certain motor tasks with the face, e. g., drinking through a straw or clicking the tongue. A patient with ideomotor apraxia of the upper limbs may be unable to salute or to mime the action of slapping someone in the face; a patient with ideomotor apraxia of the lower limbs may be unable to kick an imaginary football. In **ideational apraxia**, individual actions can be performed, but cannot be combined into more complex sequences. A patient might thus be unable to ready a letter for mailing, as this requires several steps: folding the letter, putting it in the envelope, sealing the envelope, and putting a stamp on it. Cortical lesions causing apraxia are usually on the left side.

Agnosia is an inability to recognize and correctly interpret incoming stimuli in a particular sensory modality even though sensation as such is intact. A patient with **visual agnosia**, for example, has no visual impairment but cannot recognize objects on sight; the patient can name an object only after feeling or hearing it (e. g., the jangling of a bunch of keys).

Special types of agnosia include an inability to recognize colors (*color agnosia*) or faces (*prosopagnosia*). The responsible lesion is in the visual association cortex, i. e., in the occipital or occipitotemporal region, in one or both hemispheres. Stereognosis is tested by putting a familiar object (key, pair of scissors) in the patient's hand and asking him or her to palpate it and name it (with eyes closed). An inability to do this despite intact sensation is called **tactile agnosia**. Further special types of agnosia are *finger agnosia* and *autotopagnosia* (difficulty recognizing parts of one's own body). *Anosognosia* is the denial or trivialization of one's own neurological deficits, e. g., hemiplegia or even blindness.

Higher cognitive functions. More than just the basic neuropsychological functions described above must be intact so that the individual can thrive in his or her social environment and cope adequately with the demands of everyday life. A person's fund of knowledge, memory, intelligence (by which we mean a capacity for abstract thought and problem solving), personality, and social behavior are all of vital importance, as are his or her mood and motivation. The assessment of these higher cognitive functions requires a careful weighing of historical information (particularly from persons in the patient's social environment: family, friends, colleagues), in addition to certain standardized neuropsychological tests. There are specific tests for the patient's fund of knowledge, logical thinking, and cognitive skills such as the recognition of differences, the formation of categories, and the interpretation of symbolic information, e. g., proverbs. These so-called higher "integrative" functions depend not only on an intact cerebral cortex, but also on other, deeper regions of the brain.

Special Considerations in the Neurological Examination of Infants and Young Children

Most of the techniques presented above for the neurological examination of adults cannot be used in infants or small children. In this age group, the important clinical indicators of nervous system function are **body posture**, **spontaneous motor behavior**, and the **reflex motor responses** induced by certain specific stimuli.

In taking the clinical history, the examiner must inquire about any problems that may have occurred during the child's gestation and delivery. In the physical examination, attention should be paid to any constant, fixed postures of the limbs or asymmetry of the skull (plagiocephaly). The tension of the fontanelles should also be assessed by inspection and palpation.

Reflexes

General aspects. The primitive motor functioning of healthy infants and toddlers is mainly controlled by a number of reflex mechanisms. These reflexes can be affected by neurological disease so that they are absent, or exaggerated, or persist beyond the age at which they normally disappear.

Postural reflexes control the posture of the body and its relation to the ground. **Positioning reflexes** return the body to a "normal" position after a perturbation; the vestibular system plays an important role in these reflexes. Finally, **statokinetic reactions** and **equilibrium reactions** provide the body in motion with important protective movements and righting responses.

The manner of eliciting the reflexes described in this section is illustrated in Fig. 3.**33**.

Reflexes reflecting the state of maturation of the infantile CNS. A wide variety of reflexes can be pathologically altered in developmental disorders of the CNS. We will only present the more important ones here.

The **doll's-eyes phenomenon** is induced by turning the head from side to side or up and down, in an awake, supine infant. The eyes make a compensatory movement in the opposite direction and thus stay in their original position with respect to outside space. This vestibular reflex is demonstrable at birth and persists for the first six weeks of life.

The **foot placement reflex** is elicited by holding the infant upright under the axillae (while supporting the head) and allowing the dorsum of a foot to touch the edge of the table. A normal newborn infant will flex the hip and knee and put the foot on the table. This reflex disappears in the first few weeks of life.

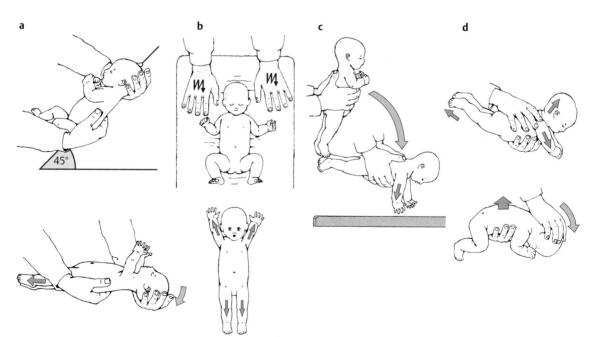

Fig. 3.**33 Reflexes in the infant. a** Moro reflex: the infant is held by the examiner in a diagonal, half-supine position, with one hand under the trunk and one hand supporting the head. When the examiner suddenly tips the infant toward the horizontal, momentarily reducing the supportive pressure on the occiput, the infant extends its upper and lower limbs. **b** The same response can be induced in a supine infant if the examiner suddenly strikes and depresses the mattress. **c** Parachute reflex: the examiner suddenly tips the infant forward, from a vertical position toward the horizontal. Normally, the arms are extended, as if to break the infant's fall. **d** Landau reflex: an infant held around the trunk in a prone position tends to keep the limbs extended and the head tilted upward. When the head is passively tilted downward, the normal response is flexion of the limbs (positive Landau reflex). (Modified from Lietz, R.: *Klinische-neurologische Untersuchung im Kindesalter*, 2nd edn, Deutscher Ärzteverlag, Cologne, 1993).

The **stepping reflex** is seen when the examiner holds the infant under the axillae so that the soles of the feet just touch the surface of the examining table and then slowly moves the infant forward. The infant will then make stepping movements with the feet. This reflex, too, is elicitable only in the first few weeks of life.

In the **tonic hand-grasp reflex**, the infant forcefully grasps the examiner's index finger when it is placed in the palm of the hand. The grasp is so tight that the infant can even be held up by the examiner's finger. In the analogous foot-grasp reflex, there is tonic flexion of the toes on stimulation of the sole of the foot. The tonic hand-grasp reflex is present in the first two months of life, then gradually diminishes till it totally disappears, usually in the third month of life, and no later than the fourth.

To elicit the **Moro reflex**, the examiner holds the infant in a diagonal, half-supine position, with one hand under the trunk and one hand supporting the head. The infant is then suddenly tipped toward the horizontal, while the support under the occiput is momentarily released. The body flexes as if in fright and the arms are first extended and then brought forward as if in a hug (Fig. 3.**33a**). A similar response can be elicited in a supine infant by suddenly striking and depressing the mattress (Fig. 3.**33b**). The Moro reflex is no longer seen after the third or fourth month of life. Its absence in the first few months of life is usually associated with severe brain damage.

Support reactions are tested by pressing on the infant's palms or soles. The infant extends the corresponding limb as if to support its weight with it. Support reactions are present at birth in the legs and develop in the arms over the first four or five months of life. Cerebral lesions make these reactions abnormally intense.

The positioning reflexes are evoked by a combination of afferent input from the vestibular system and from receptors in the skin, joints, and muscles. In the **parachute reflex**, the vestibular system plays the most important role: the examiner holds the infant around the trunk with both hands, lifts it off the examining table, holds it at about a 60° angle, and then suddenly tips the infant forward into a horizontal position, near the surface of the table (or crib). Infants aged about four months or older will extend their arms, downward and in mild abduction, and open their hands, as if to break the fall (Fig. 3.**33c**).

In the **Landau reflex**, the examiner first lifts the infant into the air in a prone position; the infant will respond by extending the limbs and head. The examiner then flexes the infant's head, and the infant flexes the limbs as well (Fig. 3.**33d**). This reflex should be demonstrable from the fourth to the 18th month. In infants with cerebral damage, the Landau reflex appears late or not at all, or else it persists longer than normal.

To elicit the **asymmetric tonic neck reflex (nuchal reflex)**, the examiner slowly turns the supine infant's head to one side, while preventing any movement of the shoulders. The arm and leg are then extended on the side to which the head is turned and flexed on the other side (fencing posture). This reflex is present in newborns and disappears at the age of four months. Persistence after the sixth month is pathological.

The **Babinski sign** (p. 38) is normally present in infants and usually disappears when the child learns to walk. It is absent in all healthy children from the age of two years onward.

The diagram in Fig. 3.34 represents the **stages of normal motor development in infancy and early childhood**. Some abnormal findings that may suggest a cerebral motor disorder at different times in the first year of life are listed in Table 3.**11**.

Table 3.**11** **Findings suggesting a cerebral motor disorder in the first year of life**

- High-risk birth (prematurity, cyanosis at birth, abnormal Apgar scores)
- Abnormal flaccidity or fixed lumbar lordosis
- Tendency to opisthotonus
- Feeding difficulties
- Spasticity with resulting difficulty in changing diapers
- Squint
- No head lifting in the prone position at age three months or older
- No head control in the sitting position at age four months or older
- Persistence of certain reflexes
- No free sitting or flattening of the lumbar kyphosis at age nine months or older

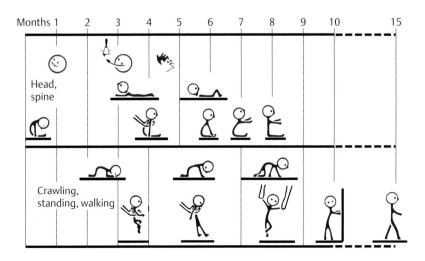

Fig. 3.**34 Stages of normal motor development in infancy and early childhood.**

4 Ancillary Tests in Neurology

Fundamentals

> Neurological conditions can often be correctly diagnosed from the history and physical examination alone, but ancillary tests of various kinds are nonetheless vitally important, in many patients, to confirm the diagnosis and identify the etiology precisely. In this section, we will discuss **imaging studies** including conventional radiographs, CT and MRI, **electrophysiological tests** (including EEG, EMG, electroneurography, and evoked potentials), and ultrasonography, as well as the laboratory testing of bodily fluids (blood, CSF) and the histopathological or cytological study of biopsy specimens.

Whenever an ancillary diagnostic test is proposed, the **specific indication for the test** should be considered carefully and critically:
- Only after thorough and meticulous clinical history taking and neurological examination.
- Only after the formulation of a clinical differential diagnosis, in which all of the competing diagnoses are ranked by probability.
- The study that should be performed is the one whose result is most likely to be important for further diagnostic and therapeutic management,

- but only if this will be of clear benefit to the patient,
- and only if the risks of performing the study do not outweigh any potential benefit that its findings might bring.
- Multiple studies providing the same diagnostic information should not be performed merely for repeated confirmation of the findings.
- A study should not be performed if, regardless of its result, another study will have to be performed that is likely to yield at least as much information.
- Only very rarely should studies be performed to confirm a diagnosis that is already practically certain.
- If a genetic study is contemplated, the potential consequences should be discussed thoroughly with the patient and his or her family before the study is performed.
- The costs must not be forgotten.

Because of the high expense of some diagnostic tests—in particular, certain types of imaging study and some of the newer molecular biological studies—the physician is obliged to be cost conscious and order them only when necessary. It is understood, however, that an essential test should not be left out just because of the expense.

Imaging Studies

Conventional Skeletal Radiographs

Even though newer techniques are available, conventional radiograph images can still be of diagnostic use, with or without tomographic (sectional) views. Plain radiograph views of the skull and spine are occasionally indicated for neurological diagnosis.

Skull radiographs are performed for very few purposes nowadays and are hardly ever indicated. (They cannot be used as a substitute for CT in head trauma; if a CT is indicated, but unavailable for some reason, then the patient should probably be transported to a center where a CT can be performed.) Plain films of the skull enable visualization of:
- fractures (though much less well than on CT, see Fig. 4.1),
- congenital malformations of the bony skull, and
- various developmental disorders.

Skull radiographs are useless in the diagnostic evaluation of headache or intracranial processes.

Plain radiographs of the spine are sometimes useful for the demonstration of:
- fractures,
- bony tumors (which, however, are more easily seen by CT or MRI—cf. Fig. 4.2),
- degenerative diseases and slippage (olisthesis) of the spine,
- infections involving bone,
- axial skeletal deformities,
- dynamic abnormalities (abnormal mobility or instability of individual spinal segments; their demonstration requires special radiological techniques, so-called "functional studies").

Most findings of these types, with the notable exception of dynamic spinal abnormalities, can be more readily seen in a CT or MRI scan.

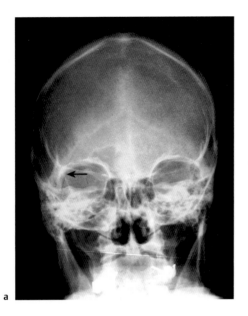

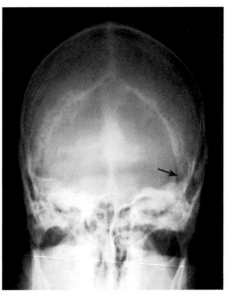

Fig. 4.**1 Skull fracture** seen in a plain skull radiograph. The a–p (**a**) and p–a (**b**) images both reveal a fracture line medial to the lamb-doid suture on the right (arrow).

a

b

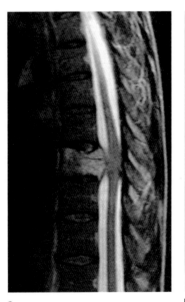

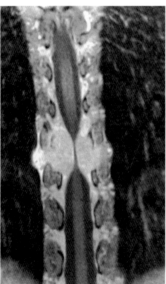

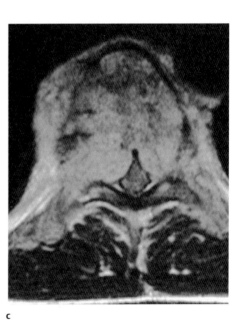

a   b   c

Fig. 4.**2 Chordoma of the T7 vertebral body** in a 48-year-old woman. **a** The spinal cord is posteriorly displaced and compressed. **b** An image in the frontal plane after the administration of contrast medium shows the tumor compressing the spinal cord from both sides. **c** At the level of the tumor, the subarachnoid space is completely obliterated by tumor.

Computed Tomography (CT)

Technique. CT yields horizontal (axial) sectional images in which the bone and soft tissues are well seen. The images can also be digitally reconstructed in other planes if desired. The technique of CT involves a rotating roentgen ray beam that penetrates the tissue from many different directions. In older CT machines, each plane of section was scanned individually by the rotating beam; in the current generation of scanners, multiple beams travel in a continuous spiral. The beam is attenuated to different degrees by tissues of different radiodensities and its amplitude after attenuation is measured by a circular array of detectors and amplifiers. From the resulting pattern of attenuation, the radiodensity at each location in the interior of the brain can be calculated (for example, at each of 512 × 512 pixels; this requires highly specialized computer software). Finally, a visual image is created in which the radiodensity at each location in the tissue is depicted on an analogue gray scale. Different types of tissue have different radiodensities and therefore appear distinct in the CT image (Fig. 4.**3**). Blood vessels, too, can be visualized.

Fig. 4.**3 Normal CT scan of the head. a** Note the symmetrical, normal-sized frontal and occipital horns of the lateral ventricles. The cerebral cortex and deep white matter can be distinguished from each other, and the falx cerebri can be seen in both the frontal and occipital regions. A number of blood vessels can be seen. Also note the bilateral calcifications of the choroid plexus of the lateral ventricles. **b** Some of the blood vessels around the base of the brain (arrows) are well seen after the administration of contrast medium.

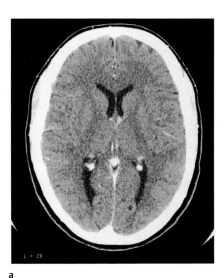

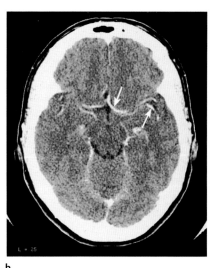

a   b

Spiral CT. As mentioned above, the latest generation of scanners uses one or more roentgen ray beams rotating in a spiral, i. e., the roentgen ray tube(s) swivels around the patient's head while the table is slowly advanced, at constant velocity. The resulting spiral data set is numerically converted into axial sections. This technique shortens the time required for each scan and thereby reduces the **radiation load** to the patient. It also enables three-dimensional reconstruction of bony structures, as shown in Fig. 4.**4**. The administration of intravenous contrast medium increases the sensitivity and specificity of CT scanning: penetration of contrast medium into brain tissue (*contrast enhancement*) indicates disruption of the blood–tissue barrier or the blood–CSF barrier. Blood vessels can also be selectively imaged (*CT angiography*).

Each CT examination is associated with a radiation load to the patient roughly equaling that of a conventional chest radiograph. CT is less expensive than MRI. The comparative indications and advantages of these two techniques are presented in Table 4.**1**.

Table 4.**1   Comparative indications of CT and MRI of the head**

Location and type of pathology	CT	MRI
Brain atrophy	+++	+++
Acute infarct	++	+++
Older infarct	++	+++
Lacunar state	+++	+++
Intraparenchymal hemorrhage	++	+++
Subarachnoid hemorrhage	+++	+
Aneurysm	+	++
Venous thrombosis	+	+++
Brain tumor (cerebral hemispheres)	++	+++
Pituitary tumor	+	+++
Brain metastases	+++	+++
Carcinomatous meningitis	–	++
Hydrocephalus	+++	+++
Traumatic brain injury	+++	++
Acute subdural or epidural hematoma	+++	+
Meningoencephalitis	++	+++
Abscess	++	+++
Parasitic cyst(s)	+	+++
Arachnoid cyst	++	+++
Posterior fossa	+	+++
Pathology of the white matter	+	+++
Multiple sclerosis	–	+++
Atlanto-occipital joint	+	+++
Skull lesions	+++	+

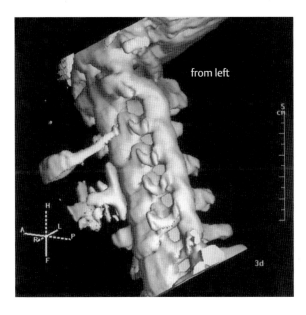

from left

Fig. 4.**4 Three-dimensional reconstruction of the cervical spine by spiral CT** (gyroscan; courtesy of PD Dr. H. Spiess, Neuroradiological Institute, Talstrasse, Zurich, Switzerland).

Magnetic Resonance Imaging (MRI)

MRI is a cross-sectional imaging technique that does not rely on the use of ionizing radiation.

Technique. The underlying physical principles of MRI are as follows: the most common atomic nuclei in all tissues of the body are hydrogen nuclei (protons). They are positively charged and possess an intrinsic magnetic property known as "spin," which can be imagined as a rotation of the proton around its own axis. Each proton thus has its own, small magnetic field. A proton to which an external magnetic field is applied orients itself in the field like a compass needle (Fig. 4.5). When the protons in a particularly bodily tissue are oriented in this way, and then excited with a radiofrequency pulse at a particular frequency (the resonance or Larmor frequency), they will take on energy and reorient themselves opposite the field. Once the exciting pulse is switched off, the protons release the energy that they previously absorbed as they return to their original orientation. The released energy can be detected with a radio antenna or coil and is the **magnetic resonance signal**. The signals from different points in a slab of tissue are distinguished from one another by means of gradient fields, i.e., smaller magnetic fields overlying the main field. The MR

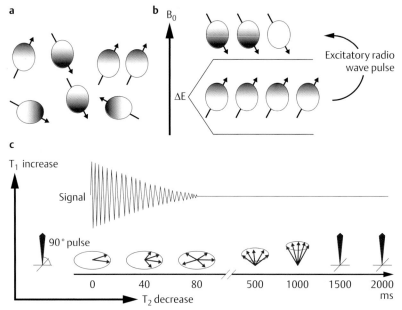

Fig. 4.**5 Physical principles of magnetic resonance imaging** (after Edelmann and Warach). **a** The magnetic axes of the protons are randomly distributed over space. **b** If a magnetic field B_0 is applied to the protons, they align themselves either parallel or antiparallel to the field. A proton aligned parallel to B_0 has a lower energy than one aligned antiparallel to it; therefore, most protons have a parallel alignment at first. If radio waves of a specific frequency (the Larmor frequency) are now applied, protons can absorb the energy they need to "flip" from the lower-energy to the higher-energy state, thereby becoming antiparallel to the field B_0. The flipped protons then gradually return to the parallel, lower-energy state (relaxation). The speed of relaxation is determined by two tissue-specific constants called T_1 and T_2. **c** After the 90° excitatory pulse is delivered, the protons precess in the transverse plane. They are in phase at first, and therefore give off a maximally intense signal. Very small inhomogeneities of the magnetic field make the protons precess at slightly different speeds, resulting in "dephasing" and loss of signal intensity. This process, which takes only a few milliseconds, is called T_2 relaxation. The MR signal is usually measured during T_2 relaxation. The restoration of magnetization parallel to B_0 is a somewhat slower process, called T_1 relaxation. A number of techniques (e. g., gradient echo, spin echo) are used to generate the largest possible MR signal.

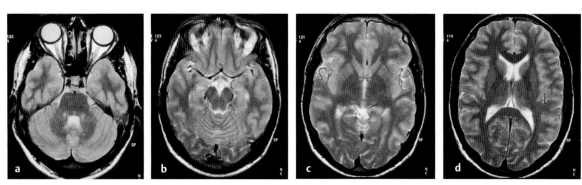

Fig. 4.**6 a–h Normal MRI of the brain** in 5 mm sections from the base of the brain to the vertex.

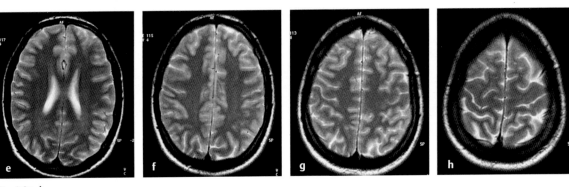

Fig. 4.**6 e–h**

image is a gray-scale map of the different intensities of MR signal coming from the tissue (Fig. 4.6) and can be computed in any desired plane of section. Gadolinium–DTPA can be given intravenously as a contrast medium for MRI.

The MR signal intensity of tissue is a function of its local physical and chemical properties, which determine, for example, the length of time that the hydrogen nuclei need to return to their initial orientation (T_1 and T_2 relaxation times). The signal intensity is further influenced by the technical parameters of the scanner (e. g., the strength of the applied magnetic field and the frequency of the emitted impulses). The MRI signal characteristics of various normal and pathological tissues in the brain are listed in Table 4.2.

MR angiography. When the spin-echo technique is used in MRI scanning, flowing blood gives rise to a signal

Tabelle 4.**2 MRI signal intensities of normal and abnormal structures** (after Edelmann)[1]

Tissue	T_1-weighted image	T_2-weighted image
Cerebrospinal fluid	Dark	Very bright
Brain		
White matter	Bright	Slightly dark
Gray matter	Slightly dark	Slightly bright
MS plaque	Intermediate to dark	Bright
Bland infarct	Dark	Bright
Tumor/metastasis	Dark	Bright
Meningioma	Intermediate	Intermediate
Abscess	Dark	bright
Edema	Dark	Bright
Calcification	Intermediate or bright	Intermediate or dark
Fat	Very bright	Intermediate to dark
Cyst		
Containing mostly water	Dark	Very bright
Containing proteinaceous fluid	Intermediate to bright	Very bright
Containing lipids	Very bright	Intermediate to dark
Bone		
Cortical bone	Very dark	Very dark
Yellow bone marrow	Very bright	Intermediate to dark
Red bone marrow	Intermediate	Slightly dark
Bone metastasis		
Lytic	Dark	Intermediate to bright
Sclerotic	Dark	Dark
Cartilage		
Fibrous	Very dark	Very dark
Hyaline	Intermediate	Intermediate
Intervertebral disk		
Normal	Intermediate	Bright
Degenerated	Intermediate to dark	Dark
Muscle	Dark	Dark
Tendons and ligaments		
Normal	Very dark	Very dark
Inflamed	Intermediate	Intermediate
Torn	Intermediate	Bright

Continued →

Tabelle 4.**2** **MRI signal intensities of normal and abnormal structures** (after Edelmann)[1]

Tissue	T_1-weighted image	T_2-weighted image
Contrast enhancement with gadolinium–DTPA		
Low concentration	Very bright	Bright
High concentration	Intermediate to dark	Very dark
Hematoma		
Hyperacute	Intermediate	Intermediate to bright
Acute	Intermediate to dark	Dark to very dark
Subacute	Bright rim, intermediate	Bright rim, dark center, later all bright
Chronic	Dark rim, bright center, later all dark	Dark rim, bright center, later all dark

[1] Bright = hyperintense, dark = hypointense, intermediate = isointense in comparison to brain tissue

only if it is excited by two radio wave pulses arriving one after the other at the same location. If the blood rapidly passes through the imaging plane, the bit of blood that received the first excitatory pulse has already flowed away by the time the second pulse arrives and no signal is generated—the vessel appears dark (there is a "flow void"). However, if the blood flows slowly enough to receive both pulses in the imaging plane, the vessel appears bright. When gradient-echo sequences are used, flowing blood always appears bright, while stationary tissue appears dark. Computer algorithms can combine the individual sectional images, processing them to generate a projectional image resembling a conventional angiogram; this is a **magnetic resonance angiogram** (Fig. 4.**7**). With MR angiography, an occluded carotid artery, for example, can be diagnosed noninvasively. Contrast-enhanced MR angiography is currently being performed increasingly often. In this technique, the signal is produced not by the flowing of the blood per se, but by the contrast medium in the bloodstream.

The indications for MRI and CT scanning of the brain and spinal cord are listed and compared with each other in Table 4.**1**.

Angiography with Radiological Contrast Media

Diagnostic imaging of the cerebral blood vessels is indicated when a vascular stenosis, occlusion, or malformation is suspected as the cause of a neurological illness.

Methods. Conventional arteriography, also known as **angiography with radiological contrast media**, is indicated for certain special purposes, e. g., the preoperative visualization of intracranial aneurysms or arteriovenous malformations. This type of study involves the introduction of an intra-arterial catheter by way of the femoral a. along a guide wire all the way up to the great vessels supplying the brain. Contrast medium is injected into these vessels while fluoroscopic images are simultaneously obtained. The image changes from one second to the next, as the contrast medium distributes itself in the vascular system of the brain. All of the images are digitized and an image obtained before any contrast medium was injected is subtracted from each to generate a **digital subtraction angiogram**, which shows nothing but the blood vessels supplying the head and brain (both extra- and intracranial). Contrast medium can be injected into the carotid a. to display the anterior circulation (Fig. 4.**8**), or into the vertebral a. to display the posterior circulation (Fig. 4.**9**).

The **blood vessels of the spinal cord** can also be studied angiographically, e. g., for the diagnosis and treatment of spinal arteriovenous malformations or fistulae.

Intravenous angiography has largely been abandoned.

The potential complications of angiography include hemorrhage or dissection at the femoral puncture site, the detachment of atherosclerotic plaques from arterial walls by the tip of the catheter, and the induction of vasospasm with consequent cerebral ischemia, possibly leading to stroke. The contrast media that are used can also have side effects.

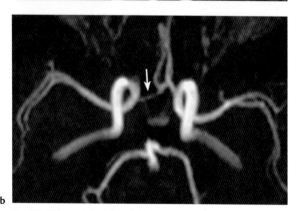

Fig. 4.7 **MR angiography of the intracranial vessels. a** Coronal and **b** axial projections. The arteries in this study are normal except for hypoplasia of the main stem of the right anterior cerebral a. (arrow).

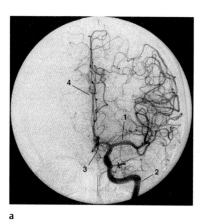
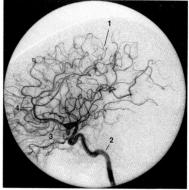
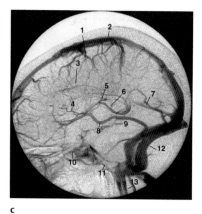

a   b   c

Fig. 4.**8 Normal digital subtraction angiogram of the in-tracranial anterior circulation** (carotid distribution). **a** Anteroposterior projection. **b** Lateral projection. **c** Venous phase, lateral projection. **a and b:** 1 MCA = middle cerebral a., 2 ICA = internal carotid a., 3 ACA = anterior cerebral a., 4 pericallosal a. **c:** 1 Superior cerebral vv. (rolandic and Trolard), 2 superior sagittal sinus, 3 inferior sagittal sinus, 4 septal v., 5 thalamostriate v., 6 internal cerebral v., 7 straight sinus, 8 v. of Labbé = inferior anastomotic v., 9 basal v. of Rosenthal, 10 cavernous sinus, 11 inferior petrosal sinus, 12 lateral sinus, 13 jugular v.

Fig. 4.**9 Selective angiography of the left vertebral a. a** Arterial phase, anteroposterior projection. **b** Arterial phase, lateral projection.

1 posterior cerebral a.
2 superior cerebellar a.
3 anterior inferior cerebellar a. (AICA)
4 left vertebral a.
5 basilar a.
6 posterior inferior cerebellar a. (PICA)

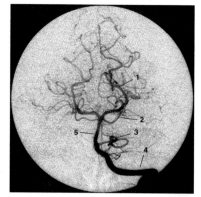
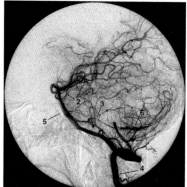

The general rule, when a diagnostic study of the blood vessels is desired, is to choose the type of study that is expected to yield sufficient information for effective diagnosis and treatment while putting the patient at the lowest risk. MR angiography (Fig. 4.**10**) and Doppler ultrasonography (Fig. 5.**61**) now suffice for most purposes.

The indications of cerebral angiography are listed in Table 4.**3**.

Table 4.**3   Indications for angiography of the intracranial vessels**

Visualization of saccular aneurysms

Visualization of arteriovenous malformations and fistulae

Detailed representation of saccular aneurysms (after diagnosis by MRI, as an aid to treatment by neurosurgical or interventional neuroradiological methods)

Detailed representation of arteriovenous malformations (after diagnosis by MRI, as an aid to treatment by neurosurgical or interventional neuroradiological methods)

Visualization of other vascular anomalies:
- moya–moya
- agenesis of vessels and other developmental anomalies
- vascular stenosis or occlusion
- arterial dissection

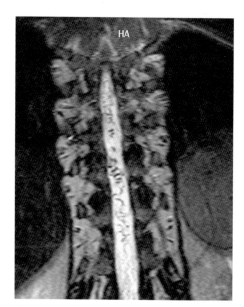

Fig. 4.**10 Arteriovenous malformation on the surface of the cervical spinal cord.** The malformation is visible in this T_2-weighted MR image as a void in the midst of the bright CSF signal of the subarachnoid space.

Myelography and Radiculography

Technique. Radiculomyelography (the visualization of intraspinal structures with contrast medium) is generally performed after the injection of 10–15 ml of water-soluble contrast medium into the subarachnoid space via lumbar puncture—or, rarely, via suboccipital puncture. The passage of contrast medium through the subarachnoid space, including the nerve root sleeves, can then be followed on the radiologic image and any obstructions to the flow of contrast medium can be identified (e. g., spinal tumors). The nerve roots appear as filling voids within the nerve root sleeves. The bony spine is seen on the myelographic images as well and can be evaluated at the same time.

The indications for myelography and radiculography are listed in Table 4.4 together with those of other, competing types of study. CT and MRI have now replaced radiculomyelography for many of its earlier indications.

Findings. Some of the more common myelographic findings are depicted schematically in Fig. 4.11. Further myelographic images can be found elsewhere in this book: lumbar intervertebral disk herniation, Fig. 12.7, p. 212; cervical myelopathy, Fig. 7.8, p. 148; spinal cord tumors, Figs. 7.4–7.7, p. 147.

Diagnostic Techniques of Nuclear Medicine

CSF Scintigraphy/Isotope Cisternography

Technique. The subarachnoid space is entered with a fine needle in the suboccipital or lumbar region and a radiolabeled substance, e. g., human albumin labeled with ^{131}I, is injected into the cerebrospinal fluid. The radioactive contrast medium should be detectable one to two hours later in the basal cisterns, four to six hours later over the cerebral convexity, and 24 hours later in the superior sagittal sinus. In normal individuals, it is never detected in the lateral ventricles.

The indications for this type of study are, for example, the localization of a fistula through which CSF is leaking from the subarachnoid space into the nasal cavity (where it can be detected on a nasal tampon), or the demonstration of malresorptive hydrocephalus, in which contrast medium can be seen to enter the lateral ventricles (Fig. 4.12).

Table 4.4   **Indications for contrast myelography as compared with other imaging techniques**

Condition/suspected pathology	Plain radio-graphs	CT	MRI	Contrast my-elography, radiculogra-phy, myelo-CT	Remarks
Pain without neurologic deficit	++				
Clinically localizable radiculopathy		+++	++		Plain films may be useful, e. g., in vertebral body tumors
Clinically evident lumbar radiculopathy with unclear CT findings				++	
Suspected radiculopathy, but no clear segmental localization		+	+++		
Suspected spinal cord compression		++	+++		
Suspected spinal stenosis	++	++	+++		
Clinically evident spinal stenosis			++	+++	
Suspected myelopathy due to cervical spondylosis		+	+++	+	
Suspected myelitis or demyelination			+++		

+++ =   most suitable study, usually adequate for diagnosis;
++   =   study generally useful;
+   =   study occasionally necessary or indicated in addition to other tests

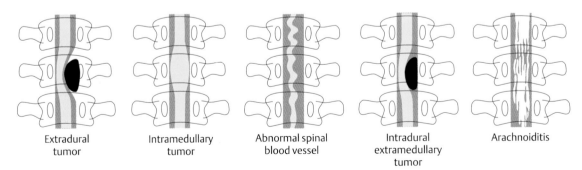

| Extradural tumor | Intramedullary tumor | Abnormal spinal blood vessel | Intradural extramedullary tumor | Arachnoiditis |

Fig. 4.11 **Typical findings in contrast myelography** (schematic diagram).

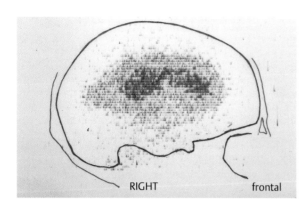

Fig. 4.**12 CSF scintigram in a patient with malresorptive hydrocephalus.** After injection of iodine-131-labeled human albumin into the cisterna magna, the radioactive contrast medium refluxes into the lateral ventricles, because of slow CSF flow.

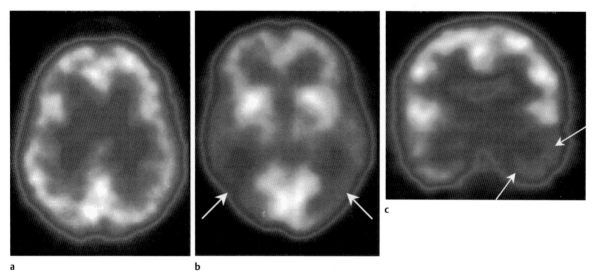

Fig. 4.**13 SPECT studies. a** Normal study. **b** SPECT in a patient with Alzheimer disease. Hypoperfusion is seen bilaterally in the parietal and temporal lobes, particularly on the right. Cf. normal finding in a. **c** This SPECT study in a patient with medically intractable complex partial seizures, performed after the intravenous administration of 180 MBq of ^{131}I-iomazenil, reveals diminished binding to benzodiazepine receptors in the left temporal region.

SPECT

Technique. Single photon emission computed tomography uses either a 99m-technetium compound or [133]I-amphetamine as a tracer. The purpose of this type of study is to measure regional cerebral blood flow.

Indications. SPECT can be performed to demonstrate reduced perfusion of the brain, e. g., in stroke or in Alzheimer disease, which is associated with reduced activity in the temporoparietal region (Fig. 4.**13a**, **b**). It can also be used to detect focal pathological processes of other kinds, e. g., epileptogenic foci (Fig. 4.**13c**).

PET

Technique. Positron emission tomography uses the short-lived positron-emitting radionuclides ^{11}C, [14]O, or [18]F. This type of study can therefore only be performed near a cyclotron in which these isotopes are produced. PET can be used to produce quantitative tomographic images of regional cerebral blood flow (rCBF), cerebral blood volume (CBV), oxygen consumption (the cerebral metabolic rate for oxygen = CMR_{O_2}), and glucose consumption (CMR–Glu).

Indications. With PET, physicians can perform biochemical studies in vivo. The radioactive labeling of substances metabolized in the human brain makes it possible to measure their concentration and kinetics in specific brain areas. Thus, for example, the localization and concentration of injected DOPA can be studied in patients with suspected Parkinson disease.

Electrophysiological Studies

Fundamentals

Electrophysiological processes are an intrinsic part of all cellular activity (p. 4). Differences in electrical potential and changes in these differences over time can be amplified, displayed on an oscilloscope, and recorded on paper or in digitized form. **Electroencephalography** records the activity of cortical neurons and neuronal populations and **electromyography** that of muscle cells. The conduction of spontaneous or induced impulses in peripheral nerves is assessed by **electroneurography**. Repeated stimulation of the receptors of a particular sensory system (e. g., the retina, by visual stimuli) and simultaneous measurement of the resulting cortical activity enables determination of the conduction velocity within the sensory system in question (**evoked potential studies**). The complex electrophysiological phenomena that occur during sleep are registered by **somnography** (sleep studies). These electrophysiological diagnostic techniques offer a practically riskfree means of assessing the functional state of the nervous system, though some of them are rather unpleasant for the patient. Despite the absence of risk, they should only be performed for strict indications, in accordance with the general principles outlined above on p. 45.

The techniques discussed in this chapter are in widespread use and belong to the diagnostic armamentarium of any clinical neurophysiologist.

Electroencephalography (EEG)

Principle. The surface EEG registers fluctuations in electrical potential that are generated by the cerebral cortex. These represent the sum of the excitatory and inhibitory synaptic potentials.

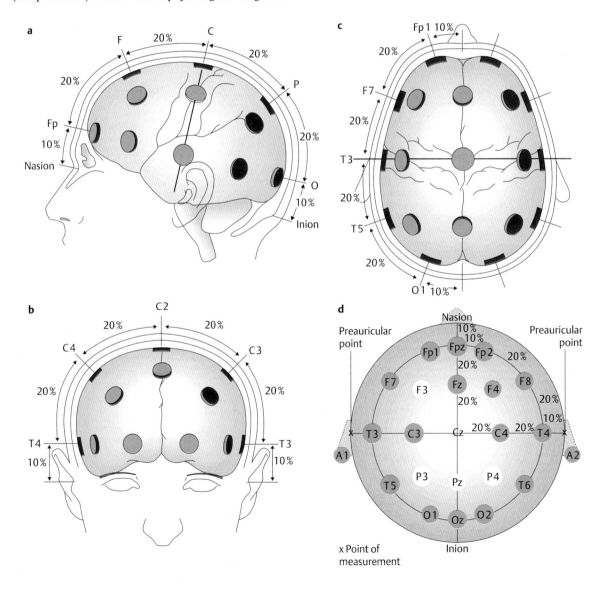

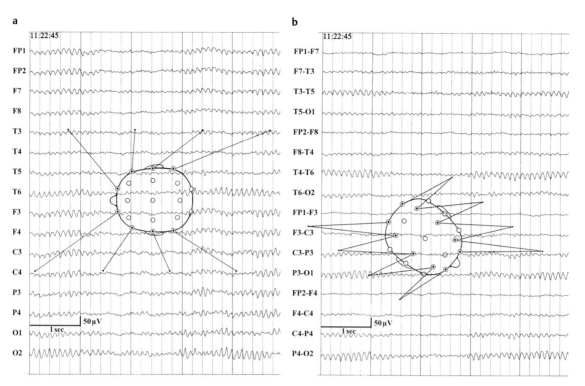

Fig. 4.**15 Normal EEG. a** Monopolar recording, **b** bipolar recording.

Technique. Electrodes are placed on the scalp according to the internationally standardized 10–20 system (Fig. 4.**14**). The potential fluctuations at each electrode are recorded, either in bipolar mode (i. e., differences in potential between adjacent electrodes) or in unipolar mode (i. e., differences in potential between each electrode and a reference electrode). Their magnitude at the scalp is 10–100 μV. They are amplified and recorded on paper in 12 parallel channels. Fluctuations in electrical potential are classified by frequency. Certain maneuvers, e. g., opening and closing the eyes, hyperventilation, and rhythmic photic stimulation, affect the EEG tracing in characteristic ways and may induce pathological waves in patients with epilepsy.

Evaluation. A mainly occipital alpha rhythm is the major component of the EEG tracing in a normal, awake individual. There is a progressive slowing of frequencies during sleep, depending on the sleep stage (depth of sleep). The following EEG changes indicate a pathological process in the brain:

◁ Fig. 4.**14 Placement of EEG electrodes according to the 10–20 system** (a–c from Masuhr K.F., Neumann M.: Neurologie, Hippokrates, Stuttgart 1992; d from Künkel H.: Das EEG in der neurologischen Diagnostik, in Schliack H., Hopf H.C.: *Diagnostik in der Neurologie*, Thieme, Stuttgart 1988). **a** Lateral view. The electrodes are placed at fixed percentage intervals between the nasion and the inion. **b** Frontal view. The preauricular points serve as reference points for the placement of the central transverse row of electrodes. C2 is the intersection of the central transverse and longitudinal rows. **c** Superior view. **d** Names of the electrodes in the 10–20 system.

General changes. Slowing of the background rhythm in the awake patient is abnormal, as is acceleration of background activity (e. g., in the form of a beta rhythm). The latter is often due to medication use.

Focal findings. Slowing of background activity (e. g., in the form of theta or delta waves) limited to a circumscribed area of the brain reflects focal cortical disfunction. Findings of this type are often due to structural lesions of the brain (e. g., tumors).

Sharp waves and spikes. These characteristically shaped abnormal potentials are seen in persons with epilepsy. During a seizure, characteristic seizure-related potentials appear (spikes with a prolonged following wave—the "spike and wave" pattern). Pathological EEG changes are not necessarily demonstrable between seizures; thus, a normal interictal EEG does not rule out epilepsy.

An example of a normal EEG is shown in Fig. 4.**15** and the most important graphoelements of the EEG are shown schematically in Fig. 4.**16**.

Indications. The main indications for EEG are summarized in Table 4.**5**. EEG changes are also seen in many other processes affecting the brain. The most important pathological EEG rhythms are shown in Fig. 4.**16**.

Polysomnography

Technique. Polysomnography is a special application of EEG in which the EEG is recorded simultaneously with a number of other electrophysiological parameters. It is used to assess sleep and sleep disturbances. The EEG

Table 4.5 **The main indications for electroencephalography**

Confirmation of the diagnosis of epilepsy

Determination of the type of epilepsy that is present

Brief, episodic impairment of consciousness of unknown etiology

Longer-lasting disturbances of consciousness, delirium

Metabolic disturbances

Creutzfeldt–Jakob disease

Sleep studies (e. g., in suspected narcolepsy)

Designation	Morphology	Definition
1 β rhythm	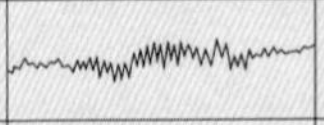	Regular sequence of waves at 14–30 Hz
2 Spindles	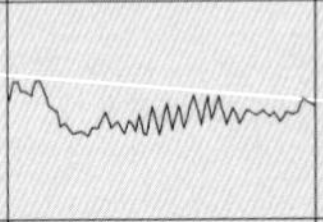	Regularly waxing and waning waves at 14–30 Hz
3 α rhythm	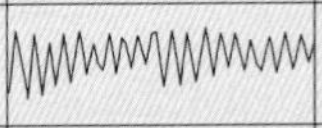	Regular sequence of waves at 8–13.3 Hz
4 ϑ rhythm	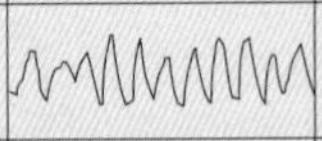	Regular sequence of waves at 4–7 Hz
5 δ rhythm	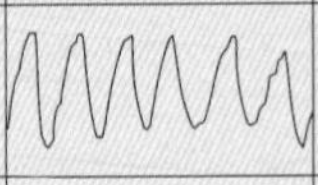	Regular sequence of waves at 1–3.5 Hz
6 δ activity	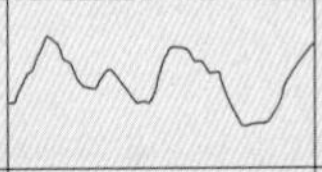	Irregular sequence of polymorphic waves at 1–3.5 Hz
7 Subdelta wave	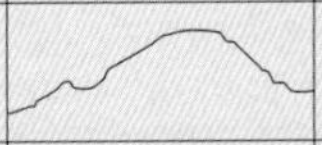	Wave with duration > 1 s
8 Steep waves (steep potential)	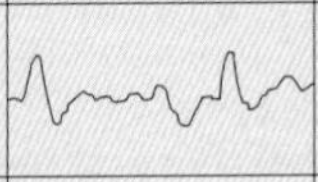	Conspicuous, blunt, steep individual waves
9 Sharp waves (sharp potential)	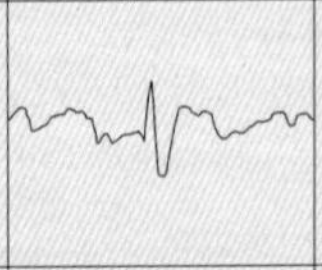	Sharp and steep waves of 80–250 ms duration, ascending phase usually steeper than descending phase
10 Spike	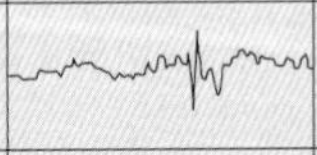	Sharp and steep wave of duration < 80 ms
11 Polyspikes	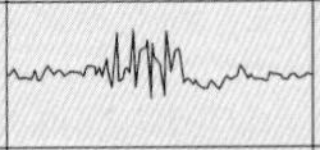	Compact series of spikes
12 Spike–wave complex	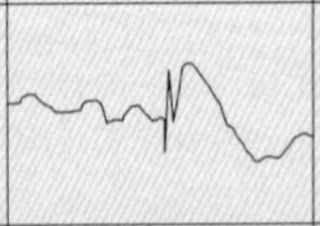	Complex consisting of a spike and slow wave
13 Rhythmic spikes and waves	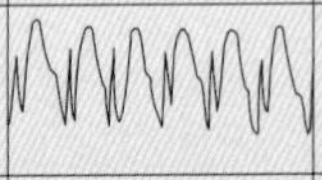	Sequence of regular spike–wave complexes at about 3 Hz
14 Sharp and slow waves	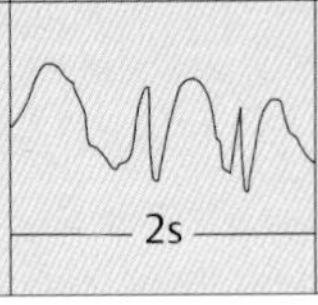	Sequence of complexes of sharp waves and slow waves of 500–1000 ms duration, often rhythmic
	2s	

Fig. 4.16 **The most important graphoelements in EEG:** designations, morphology, and definitions (from Schliack H., Hopf H.C.: *Diagnostik in der Neurologie*, Thieme, Stuttgart 1988).

changes that normally occur during sleep are related to the progression of the individual through various sleep stages, including deep or REM sleep (REM = "rapid eye movement"). The recorded parameters include eye movements (by electro-oculography), respiratory excursion, airflow in the nostrils, muscle activity (by surface EMG), cardiac activity (by ECG), and the partial pressure of oxygen (by transcutaneous pulse oximetry) (Fig. 4.17). These are displayed together with the EEG in a polygraph recording (**polysomnogram**).

Indications. The most important indication for a sleep study is a clinical suspicion of sleep apnea syndrome (p. 171) on the basis of a characteristic history obtained from the patient or bed partner, together with related physical findings and a low partial pressure of oxygen measured during sleep by pulse oximetry. The typical polysomnographic finding in such patients is shown in Fig. 4.18. Polysomnography is also indicated for the diagnosis of narcolepsy, as well as for the assessment of excessive fatigue and daytime somnolence.

Evoked potentials

General principles. Evoked potentials are used to assess the integrity of individual functional systems (visual, auditory, somatosensory, or motor). The system under study is activated with a repeatedly delivered stimulus. The resulting fluctuations of electrical potential in the brain can be detected by summation of the potentials that are recorded when the excitatory stimulus has been delivered a large number of times. Evoked potentials provide evidence of whether impulse conduction in the system in question is intact from the site of stimulation all the way to the cerebral cortex. Sometimes a partial or total conduction block can be localized precisely between two relay stations for neural transmission within a particular system. In addition, evoked potentials may reveal subclinical lesions. The most important types of evoked potential for clinical practice are outlined in the following paragraphs.

Visual evoked potentials (VEP). The patient fixates on a video screen displaying a checkerboard pattern in which the white and black fields are regularly and periodically inverted, while electrical potentials are recorded through a needle electrode in the scalp at the occiput. Evoked potentials are obtained by summation; the largest fluctuation is a positive wave that appears 100 milliseconds after the stimulus. Delay of this wave is found early in the course of optic neuritis and persists thereafter (Fig. 4.19).

Auditory evoked potentials (AEP). A click stimulus delivered periodically to one ear induces the generation of neural impulses that travel along the auditory nerve to the brainstem, the thalamus, and finally the cerebral cortex. The electrophysiological response is measured from the vertex of the head in relation to a reference electrode on the earlobe. The normal AEP contains five different waves, each of which is generated by a different structure along the chain of impulse transmission.

Fig. 4.**17 Recording scheme for polysomnography.**

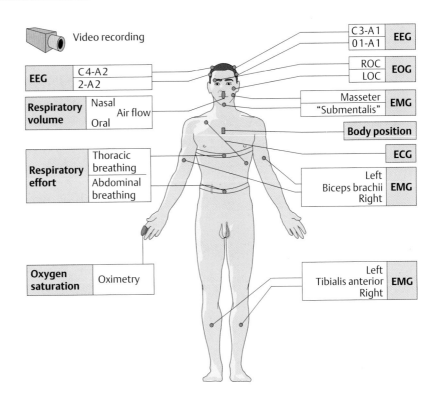

Fig. 4.**18 Hypnogram.** Polysomnography in a patient with REM-sleep-associated obstructive sleep apnea syndrome. **1** EEG frequency analysis. **2** Rapid eye movement (REM) sleep. **3** Submental muscle activity measured through a surface electrode. **4** Sleep stages. AWK = awake, REM = REM sleep, 1–4 = sleep stages 1–4. **5** Time axis. **6** Nasal/oral air flow and count (cnt) of apneic and hypopneic episodes per minute. **7** Transcutaneously measured oxygen saturation (upper curve) and frequency of desaturations by 4% or more (lower curve). **8** ECG (bpm = beats per minute) and number of tachycardias, bradycardias, or extrasystoles. **9** Surface EMG from the masseter m. **10** Surface EMG from the right tibialis m. **11** Surface EMG from the left tibialis m. **12** Body position.

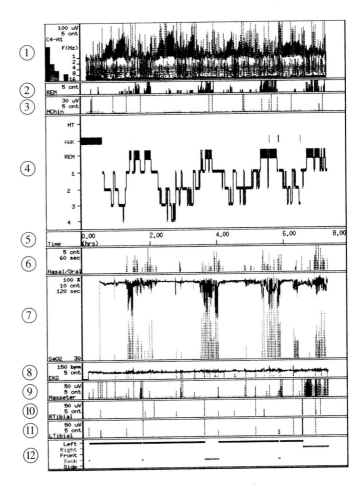

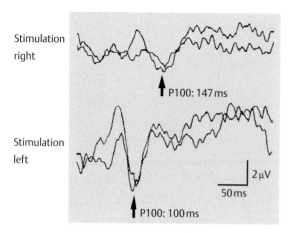

Stimulation right

↑ P100: 147 ms

Stimulation left

2 µV

50 ms

↑ P100: 100 ms

Fig. 4.**19 Visual evoked potentials (VEP).** A 38-year-old woman with multiple sclerosis and right optic neuritis. The cortical response on the right side is significantly delayed compared to the normal left side.

Somatosensory evoked potentials (SSEP). When a repetitive electrical stimulus is applied to the skin, impulses are generated at the terminal sensory branch of a peripheral nerve and conducted centrally via the peripheral nerve, nerve root, posterior columns/spinothalamic tract, medial lemniscus, and thalamocortical connections. A lesion at any point along this pathway can alter the evoked potentials, which are recorded first over Erb point (for the median n.) or the lumbar spine (for the tibial n.), and then through a scalp electrode in the parietal region on the side opposite the stimulation. An example of delayed conduction in the central somatosensory pathway is shown in Fig. 4.**20**.

Motor evoked potentials (MEP). In this technique, a rapidly alternating magnetic field produced by a ring-shaped magnetic impulse generator induces a stimulating electrical current in the motor cortex. Action potentials are then generated in the cortex and travel down the pyramidal pathway to the muscles. Surface electrodes placed on an arm or leg muscle are used to record the summed motor potentials. These potentials are larger and easier to record when the subject lightly contracts the corresponding muscle beforehand. An abnormality of the MEP implies a lesion in the peripheral or central portion of the motor pathway (see Fig. 4.**21**). Epilepsy, cardiac pacemakers, and ferromagnetic intracranial implants are contraindications for transcranial magnetic stimulation for any purpose, including MEP.

Electromyography

Principle. Electrical activity is recorded from a muscle through bipolar needle electrodes, first at rest, and then with light and maximal voluntary muscle contraction. The recorded potentials are displayed visually on an oscilloscope and also converted into audible signals from a loudspeaker. When the muscle is lightly contracted, the potentials arising from individual motor units can be observed. (A motor unit is the set of muscle fibers innervated by a single motor anterior horn cell by way of its multiple axon collaterals.) When the muscle is strongly or maximally contracted, a large number of motor unit potentials come together to form an interference pattern.

Insertional activity and spontaneous activity. The resting muscle is normally electrically silent; when the needle is inserted, there are normally only a few positive sharp waves or fibrillations. **Pathological spontaneous activity** of a muscle is manifested as *prolonged insertional activity* as well as *pathological fibrillation potentials* and *positive sharp waves* (Fig. 4.**22**). This spontaneous activity reflects denervation of the muscle. *Fasciculations* and *complex repetitive discharges* are further forms of pathological spontaneous activity, as are *myotonic repetitive discharges.*

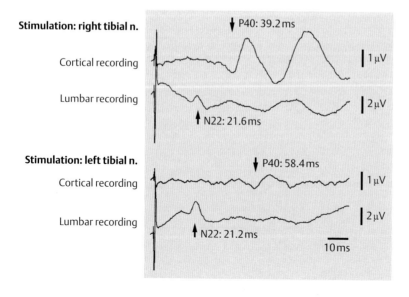

Stimulation: right tibial n.

Cortical recording

↓ P40: 39.2 ms

1 µV

Lumbar recording

2 µV

↑ N22: 21.6 ms

Stimulation: left tibial n.

Cortical recording

↓ P40: 58.4 ms

1 µV

Lumbar recording

2 µV

↑ N22: 21.2 ms

10 ms

Fig. 4.**20 Somatosensory evoked potentials of the tibial n.** A 44-year-old woman with multiple sclerosis. Normal lumbar N22 potential on both sides. The cortical P40 potential appears at a normal latency of 29.2 ms on the right, but is significantly delayed on the left, with a latency of 58.4 ms, and also abnormally small. These findings indicate impaired conduction in the spinothalamic pathways.

Fig. 4.**21 Motor evoked potentials** in a 61-year-old man with cervical syringomyelia. Recording of motor potentials from the abductor digiti minimi m. after electrical stimulation of the ulnar n. at the wrist, the forearm, and the C8 root (tracings **a–c**). After cortical stimulation (**d**), the recorded motor evoked potential is reduced in amplitude and somewhat delayed. The calculated central motor conduction time (CMCT) of 9.2 ms is prolonged in comparison to the normal value of 8.7 ms. These findings suggest impaired conduction in the pyramidal tract in the cervical spinal cord.

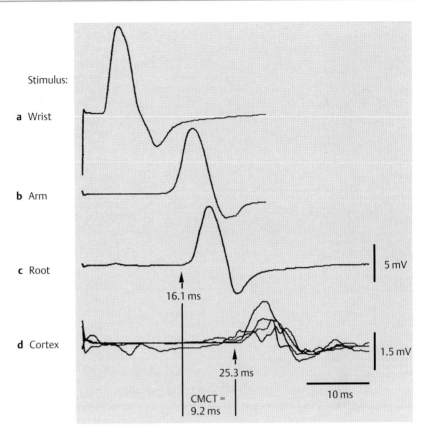

Stimulus:

a Wrist

b Arm

c Root

d Cortex

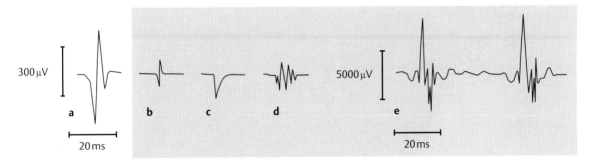

Fig. 4.**22 Different types of potentials in an electromyogram.** **a** Normal motor unit potential. **b** Fibrillation potential in denervation. **c** Positive sharp waves in denervation. **d** Fragmented polyphasic low-amplitude potential, as seen in reinnervation. **e** Abnormally prolonged and high-amplitude motor unit potential ("giant potential") in chronic anterior horn cell disease.

Electrical activity with voluntary contraction. Muscle action potentials are observed when the muscle is voluntarily contracted. The amplitude and duration of individual motor unit potentials are proportional to the size of the motor unit, i. e., the number of muscle fibers it contains. The more strongly a muscle is contracted, the more motor units will be recruited. When a large number of motor units are active, their potentials can no longer be seen individually. Instead, they summate to form a (complete) interference pattern (Fig. 4.**23a**).

The size and shape of electromyographic potentials are altered by many different types of neuromuscular disease. **Myopathy** is characterized by a diffuse loss of individual muscle fibers throughout the affected muscle(s). Each motor unit potential is therefore of lower amplitude and shorter duration (Fig. 4.**23d**). In principle, all of the motor units are still present, but they contain fewer muscle fibers than before; thus, on maximal voluntary contraction of the muscle, the interference pattern is full, but of lower than normal amplitude. In contrast, in a **neuropathic process** (*chronic denervation* of a muscle), the motor units are larger than normal because of repeated denervation and reinnervation. When the nerve fiber to a particular motor unit degenerates, axon collaterals sprouting from the nerves of adjacent motor units take over the muscle fibers of the denervated unit, so that the surviving motor units actually contain more muscle fibers than before. Their

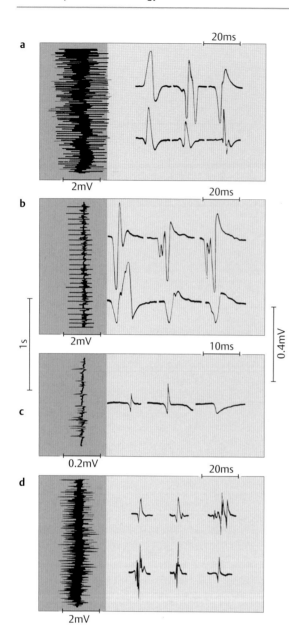

Fig. 4.23 **Various EMG findings. a** Normal electromyogram with full interference pattern. **b** Individual oscillations in the reinnervation stage after a peripheral nerve injury. **c** Total denervation. Fibrillation potentials and positive sharp waves are seen. **d** Myopathy. Despite muscle weakness, there is a complete interference pattern. The individual potentials making up the interference pattern are of low amplitude; some of them are polyphasic and fragmented.

motor unit potentials are usually polyphasic and of increased amplitude and duration (Fig. 4.**23b**). Because of the reduced number of motor units, maximal voluntary contraction of a denervated muscle yields a markedly attenuated interference pattern, in which the individual action potentials of the remaining motor units appear as large oscillations.

Electrical activity at the motor end plate. Abnormalities of the motor end plate affecting neuromuscular transmission are also revealed by EMG. On repetitive electrical stimulation of a peripheral motor nerve, the recorded muscle action potential becomes smaller with each stimulus (decrement phenomenon, Fig. 4.**12**, p. 53).

Indications. In disorders affecting muscle, EMG can be used to determine whether the underlying pathological process is located in the muscle itself (myopathic process), in the nerve innervating it (neuropathic process), or at the neuromuscular junction. It can also be used to grade the severity of muscle denervation and the extent of reinnervation. In combination with electroneurography (see below), EMG is a very important type of ancillary study for the diagnosis of neuromuscular diseases. The indications for these two methods are listed side by side in Table 4.**6**.

Electroneurography

Principle. Electroneurography is a method of measuring the **motor and sensory conduction velocities** of peripheral nerves. The result of measurement is always the

Tabelle 4.6   **Indications for EMG and ENG**

Condition/suspected pathology	EMG (needle myography)	ENG	Remarks
Suspected anterior horn cell disease	++	Negative	
Suspected nerve root lesion	+	++ (F wave)	Imaging studies may be more important
Suspected plexus lesion (differentiation from peripheral nerve lesion)	+	++ (F wave)	
Focal peripheral nerve lesion	++	++	Severity of injury, signs of regeneration, localization of injury
Polyneuropathy	+	++	
Myopathy	++	Normal	
Ischemic muscle damage	++		
Myasthenia gravis	++		Repetitive stimulation, jitter phenomenon

++ = indicated test
+ = may be additionally useful

conduction velocity of the most rapidly conducting fibers in the nerve being studied. The technique involves stimulating and recording electrodes placed at some distance from each other along the course of a peripheral nerve. The measured conduction velocity is then the temporal interval between the delivery of the stimulus and the beginning of the recorded response, divided by the distance between the electrodes. Normal values in the arms are 50–70 m/s, in the legs 40–60 m/s. The amplitude and duration of the recorded response are a function of the number of functioning axons and the degree of dispersion of their conduction velocities. A case illustrating the usefulness of ENG is presented in Fig. 4.24 (localized compression of the common peroneal n. at the head of the fibula).

F wave. When a peripheral motor nerve is stimulated, the resulting impulses travel not only orthodromically (in the normal direction of transmission, i. e., distally, toward the muscle), but also antidromically (toward the spinal cord). The antidromic impulse reaches the ganglion cells of the anterior horn and is then sent back to the periphery in the manner of an echo. This echo is the so-called "F wave." Thus, *two* orthodromic impulse waves go down the peripheral nerve, the original wave due to the stimulus and the F wave; compared with the original wave, the F wave is later and smaller in amplitude. Sometimes it is not seen at all. If the F wave is delayed by a longer interval than usual, this may indicate slowed conduction in the plexus or nerve roots.

Other Electrophysiological Studies

Other types of electrophysiological study are used less commonly in neurological diagnosis. We will only briefly mention a few of them here.

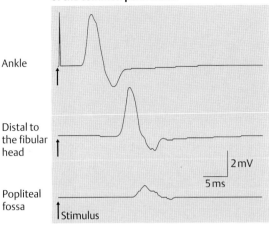

Motor neurography of the common peroneal n.

Fig. 4.**24 Electroneurography of the right common peroneal n.** in pressure palsy at the fibular head. The farther the stimulating electrode is from the recording electrode (in the peroneal muscles), the longer the latency until the summed muscle potential appears. When the stimulus is delivered in the popliteal fossa, the amplitude of the summed potential collapses. This implies that conduction is blocked in all axons between the popliteal fossa and the stimulation site distal to the fibular head. The finding is typical in pressure palsy.

Oculography is a study of the electrical potentials accompanying eye movements. It can be used for objective documentation of gaze saccades and pathological eye movements. When oculography is used to study vestibular disturbances, it is called **electronystagmography**. **Retinography** is mainly used to determine whether the lesion causing a visual disturbance is in the retina or in the optic nerve.

Ultrasonography

There are two main types of ultrasound study: **Doppler sonography** and **duplex sonography**.

Principle. The 19th-century Austrian physicist Christian Doppler discovered that the frequency of a wave changes when its source and receiver are in relative motion. Thus, when ultrasound pulses are directed at erythrocytes in flowing blood, the ultrasonic waves reflected back from the erythrocytes are altered in frequency to a degree that depends on the flow velocity. In fact, the Doppler shift is directly proportional to the flow velocity.

Technique. The ultrasound probe contains both a transmitter and a receiver of ultrasonic waves. The angle of insonation should be as steep as possible to minimize angle-dependent variations in the measured values and thus keep the results as consistent as possible from study to study. There are two types of Doppler system: *continuous-wave (CW)* systems detect all moving wave

reflectors within the cone of insonation, while *pulsed-wave (PW)* systems detect only those at a particular depth, which can be chosen by the examiner. In CW Doppler studies, the signals of different vessels may overlie one another.

The Doppler signal can be represented graphically as a frequency spectrum that changes over time (Fig. 4.25). It can also be transduced into an audible signal. Ultrasound waves are reflected to varying extents by different types of tissue with different acoustic resistance; thus, the profile of reflected echo intensities can be used to construct a two-dimensional sectional image of the insonated tissue. The so-called B image ("*brightness mode*") or **echotomogram** is a gray-scale representation of the tissue (Fig. 4.25a). The combination of Doppler flow measurement with B imaging is called **duplex ultrasonography**. The velocity of blood flow can be color-coded and displayed as an overlay on the B image; this is called **color duplex ultrasonography** (Fig. 4.26).

4

Ancillary Tests

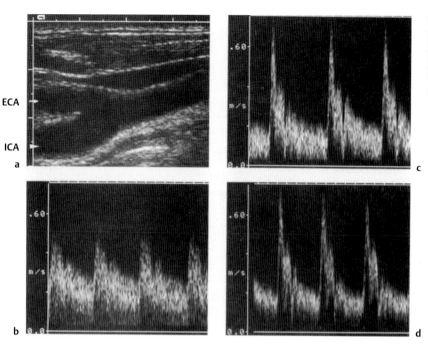

ECA

ICA

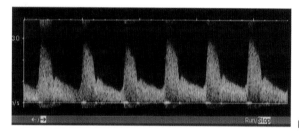

Fig. 4.**25 Doppler study of a normal carotid bifurcation. a** Two-dimensional sectional image (B image) of the carotid bifurcation. **b–c** Doppler frequency-time spectra in the common carotid (**b**), internal carotid (**c**), and external carotid arteries (**d**).

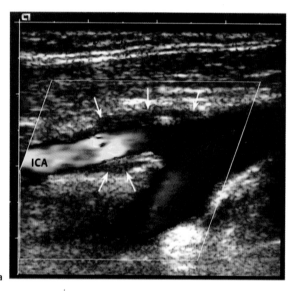

ICA

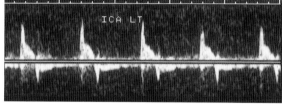

Fig. 4.**26 Color-coded duplex ultrasonography of carotid stenosis. a** Duplex ultrasonography of the carotid bifurcation. Rapid flow is coded as bright, slow flow as dark. Flow is abnormally rapid in the internal carotid a. (ICA) because the lumen is narrowed. Atherosclerosis can be seen in the thickened vessel wall (arrow). **b** Flow spectrum of the internal carotid a. showing elevated maximal systolic and end-diastolic velocities (from the laboratory of the Neurological and Neurosurgical Clinics, University of Berne, Switzerland). ECA = external carotid a., CCA = common carotid a.

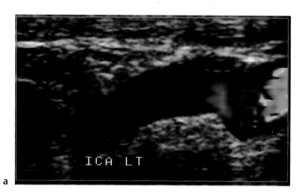

ICA LT

Fig. 4.**27 Color-coded duplex ultrasonography of an occlusion of the left internal carotid a.** 3 cm above the carotid bifurcation. **a** Blood flow can be seen up to the bifurcation. In the internal carotid a. (ICA LT), there is only minimal movement of the blood column. **b** Doppler ultrasonography reveals no more than a brief forward flow in early systole at greatly reduced maximal speed; backward flow is already seen in early diastole.

Fig. 4.**27 c** ▷

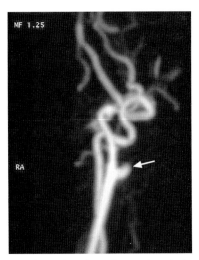

Fig. 4.**27 c** MR angiography reveals occlusion of the internal carotid artery.

Indications. The velocity and flow profile (laminar or turbulent) of the blood flowing within a particular vessel depend, among other things, on the vessel's caliber and on the nature of its wall. Ultrasound studies aid in the detection of vascular stenosis and occlusion, vessel wall irregularities, abnormalities of the speed and direction of blood flow, and turbulent flow. Insonation of the extra- and intracranial vessels (e. g., of the middle cerebral a. through the thin bone of the "temporal window," or of the basilar a. through the foramen magnum) yields an informative picture of the current state of blood flow in the brain (Fig. 4.**27**). This diagnostic technique is inexpensive, non-invasive, and free of risk.

4

Ancillary Tests

Other Ancillary Studies

Cerebrospinal Fluid Studies

Technique. Cerebrospinal fluid is usually obtained by lumbar puncture (LP) below the level of the conus medullaris, i. e., at L4–5 (occasionally at L3–4 or L5–S1). Suboccipital puncture is fraught with a much higher rate of complications and is performed only when meningitis is suspected and no fluid can be obtained by lumbar puncture ("dry tap"), or when LP is contraindicated because of a known purulent process in the lumbar region. LP is performed with sterile technique on a patient in the lateral decubitus position (or, occasionally, sitting up). The recommended positioning is shown in Fig. 4.**28**. The physician performing the puncture measures the CSF pressure with a manometer and visually assesses the color of the fluid. The laboratory tests to be performed include cell count, glucose and protein content, and others (esp. cultures), depending on the clinical situation. The most important CSF tests are listed in Table 4.**7**.

Normal CSF values are listed in Table 4.**8** together with the corresponding serum values.

Indications. Lumbar puncture is useful in the diagnosis of diseases affecting the meninges, the brain and spinal cord, and the nerve roots, which can manifest themselves with changes in the biochemical or cellular properties of the cerebrospinal fluid. The most important abnormal CSF findings are listed in Table 4.**9**.

Table 4.**7**   **Clinically relevant CSF studies**

Routinely performed tests

pressure

color (turbidity? xanthochromia? bloody tinge?)

cell count and differential

protein

glucose

Tests to be performed under special circumstances

immunoglobulins

IgG–albumin index

oligoclonal bands

measurement of specific IgG, IgA, and IgM against Borrelia, parasites, and viruses

cultures: bacterial, fungal, viral, mycobacterial

gram and Ziehl–Neelsen staining, touch prep

VDRL and FTA tests for syphilis

cytological examination for malignant cells

DNA amplification (polymerase chain reaction) in suspected tuberculosis or viral diseases

cystatin C in amyloid angiopathy

antineuronal antibodies in suspected paraneoplastic syndromes

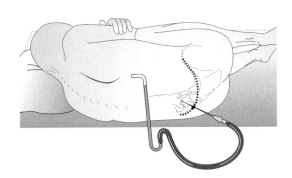

Fig. 4.**28 Patient position for lumbar puncture.**   ▷

Contraindications. Intracranial hypertension is the most important contraindication to lumbar puncture. Before any LP is performed, the patient's optic discs should be inspected with an ophthalmoscope to rule out papilledema. Nor should an LP ever be performed if the platelet count is below 5000/μl. It should only rarely be performed, for strict indications and with extreme caution, in anticoagulated patients or when the platelet count is below 20 000/μl.

Complications of lumbar puncture are rare overall. If the patient harbors an intracranial mass causing elevated intracranial pressure, CSF removal may be followed by herniation of parts of the brain into the ten- torial notch or the foramen magnum, potentially resulting in death. If an intraspinal mass is present, preexisting paraparesis may worsen after LP. After the procedure is performed, persistent leakage of CSF out of the subarachnoid space through the puncture hole(s) in the dura mater may result in symptomatic intracranial hypotension with orthostatic headache. Other possible complications include iatrogenic infection and epidural hematoma, potentially causing cauda equina syndrome.

Tissue Biopsies

Muscle biopsy is justified in patients with neuromuscular disease when the clinical history, physical examination, and electromyographic, chemical, and/or genetic studies fail to yield a sufficiently precise diagnosis. The biopsy should be performed under local anesthesia in a muscle that is known to be affected by the disease process, but is not so atrophic as to reduce the chance of a diagnosis. In many cases, a needle biopsy alone suffices. Depending on the clinical situation, histochemical and/or electron-microscopic study of the tissue specimen may be indicated in addition to conventional histological staining.

Nerve biopsy is performed under local anesthesia. A relatively unimportant sensory nerve is chosen for biopsy, usually the sural n. The ensuing sensory deficit on the lateral edge of the foot is generally an acceptable price to pay for a firm diagnosis, but the patient must be informed of it before granting his or her consent to the procedure. Part of the specimen is used to make a teased preparation in which nerve fibers and their myelin sheaths can be seen over a certain length of nerve. More importantly, very thin cross-sections of the nerve are prepared, which can be microscopically examined for various abnormalities, including disordered myelination or inflammatory changes of the vasa nervorum.

Brain biopsy is performed by a neurosurgeon, usually with stereotactic technique, for very strict indications.

Table 4.8 **Normal CSF values and corresponding serum values in adults[1]**

	CSF	Serum
Pressure	5–18 cm H_2O	
Volume	100–160 ml	
Osmolarity	292–297 mosm/l	285–295 mosm/l
Electrolytes		
Na	137–145 mmol/l	136–145 mmol/l
K	2.7–3.9 mmol/l	3.5–5.0 mmol/l
Ca	1.0–1.5 mmol/l	2.2–2.6 mmol/l
Cl	116–122 mmol/l	98–106 mmol/l
pH	7.31–7.34	7.38–7.44
Glucose	2.2–3.9 mmol/l	4.2–6.4 mmol/l
CSF/serum glucose ratio[1]	>0.5–0.6	
Lactate	1–2 mmol/l	0.6–1.7 mmol/l
Total protein	0.2–0.5 g/l	55–80 g/l
Albumin	56–75%	50–60%
IgG	0.010–0.014 g/l	8–15 g/l
IgG index[2]	< 0.65	
Leukocytes	< 4/μl	
Lymphocytes	60–70%	

[1] Because there is normally an equilibrium between CSF and serum, it is advisable to measure CSF and serum values at the same time.
[2] IgG index = [CSF IgG (mg/l) × serum albumin (g/l)]/[serum IgG (mg/l) × CSF albumin (mg/l)]

Table 4.9 **CSF analysis: main indications and findings**

Condition/suspected pathology	Appearance	Cell count and type	Protein	Pressure	Special remarks
Purulent meningitis	turbid	↑↑ mostly granulocytes	↑	possibly ↑↑	LP is urgent—the most important diagnostic study
Chronic meningitis	clear	↑ mostly lymphocytes	↑	possibly ↑	
Encephalitis	clear	↑ mostly lymphocytes	possibly ↑	possibly ↑	
Subarachnoid hemorrhage	bloody—xanthochromic	↑ erythrocytes	possibly ↑	possibly ↑	xanthochromia in 6 hours to 6 days
Intracerebral hemorrhage	xanthochromic	possibly ↑ erythrocytes	normal	↑	LP not indicated
Subdural hematoma	xanthochromic	usually normal	↑	normal, ↑, ↓	LP not indicated
Low CSF pressure syndrome	clear	normal	↑ to ↑↑	↓↓↓	aspirate if no spontaneous CSF flow

Its purpose is the histological diagnosis of (potentially treatable) structural alterations of the brain whose presence has been revealed by imaging studies, but whose precise nature is nonetheless unclear. Examples are brain tumors and inflammatory processes.

Perimetry

Perimetry is used to detect visual field defects (p. 181).

Goldmann perimetry is a dynamic method in which moving spots of light of variable size and intensity are presented in the patient's visual field, starting in the periphery and moving toward the center. The findings associated with different types of visual field defect are illustrated in Fig. 3.**6**, p. 19.

Static computed perimetry is performed with the so-called Octopus apparatus. The brightness of a stationary light source is increased until the patient can see it. The measured brightness thresholds at all tested points in the visual field can be displayed visually as raw numbers, on a gray scale, or as a pseudo-three-dimensional visual field "landscape." Illustrative findings in a case of homonymous quadrantanopsia are shown in Fig. 4.**29**.

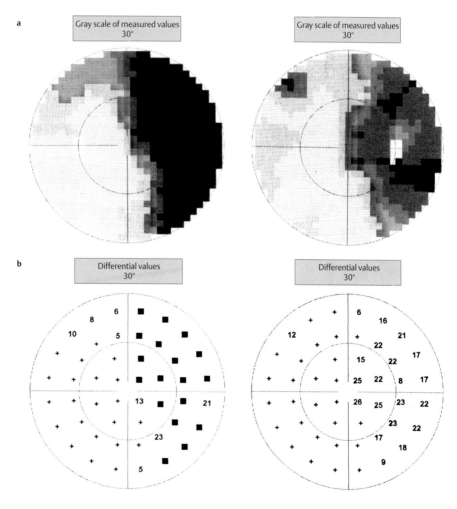

Fig. 4.**29 Automatic (Octopus) perimetry in right homonymous hemianopsia. a** Gray-scale representation of the visual field defect. **b** Differential value chart representing the loss of light sensitivity at each point in the visual field, measured in decibels (dB), as compared to the average local sensitivity in a normal control population. There is no measurable loss at the points marked with solid black squares. See also Fig. 3.**6**.

Topical Diagnosis and Differential Diagnosis of Neurological Syndromes

Fundamentals

The neurological deficits produced by a lesion in any given area of the nervous system are characteristic of the area involved and relatively independent of the type of lesion. Thus, the **clinical manifestations** of neurological disease are determined above all by **the site of the lesion**. A thorough knowledge of these relationships is essential in clinical practice. The first step in diagnostic assessment is always the *localization* of the disease process in the nervous system. This can usually be done with great precision based on the information obtained in the clinical interview and neurological examination. The *etiology* is then sought in a second step with the aid of further information (course of the disease over time, any accompanying nonneurological manifestations, results of ancillary tests).

In this chapter, we will show how the clinical manifestations of neurological disease can be used to make inferences about the site of the lesion and its possible etiologies. We will first describe the typical findings of lesions affecting individual functional systems (the motor and somatosensory systems) and then those of lesions in particular areas of the brain. The manifestations of diseases affecting the spinal cord and peripheral nerves will be discussed in the relevant, later chapters.

Muscle Weakness and Other Motor Disturbances

Anatomical Substrate of Motor Function

It is a useful simplification to consider the motor system as consisting of the following components (Fig. 5.1):

First (central) motor neuron (neurons in the precentral gyrus). The axons travel in the corticobulbar and corticospinal tracts through the internal capsule and cerebral peduncle and terminate either in the cranial nerve nuclei of the pons and medulla (corticobulbar pathway) or on the anterior horn cells of the spinal cord (pyramidal pathway). **Lesions of the first motor neuron** in the precentral gyrus, or at any other site, produce the following deficits:

- *spastic weakness* (elevated muscle tone, diminished raw strength, and impaired fine motor control);
- *increased intrinsic muscle reflexes, spreading of reflex zones, and pathological reflexes* (Babinski, Oppenheim, and Gordon, pathologically brisk Hoffmann sign and Trömner reflex, inextinguishable or asymmetrically persistent clonus); *diminished or absent extrinsic muscle reflexes* (e. g., abdominal skin reflex);
- *no muscle atrophy* (though there may be mild atrophy of disuse in the later course of disease);
- *asymmetry of the reflexes* if the lesion is unilateral.

The second (peripheral) motor neuron originates in one of the motor relay stations mentioned above (the motor cranial nerve nuclei or the anterior horn cells of the spinal cord). It consists of a cell body (ganglion cell) and an axon that travels by way of a spinal nerve root, plexus, and peripheral nerve to the skeletal muscle. Each ganglion cell, together with its axon and the muscle fibers that it innervates (there may be many, or only a few), comprises a single motor unit. The following deficits are associated with a **lesion of the peripheral motor neuron**:

- *flaccid weakness* (diminished muscle tone and raw strength);
- *diminished* or *absent intrinsic muscle reflexes*;
- *muscle atrophy* becoming evident about three weeks after injury and progressing thereafter.

Motor end plate and muscle. In addition to the first and second motor neurons, normal motor function requires effective impulse transmission from the peripheral nerve to the muscle fiber, followed by fiber contraction. A lesion or **functional disturbance** of either or both of these elements causes *flaccid weakness* usually accompanied by *atrophy and diminished reflexes* (p. 275).

Because every movement, as we have seen, is the product of a complex interaction of many different ana-

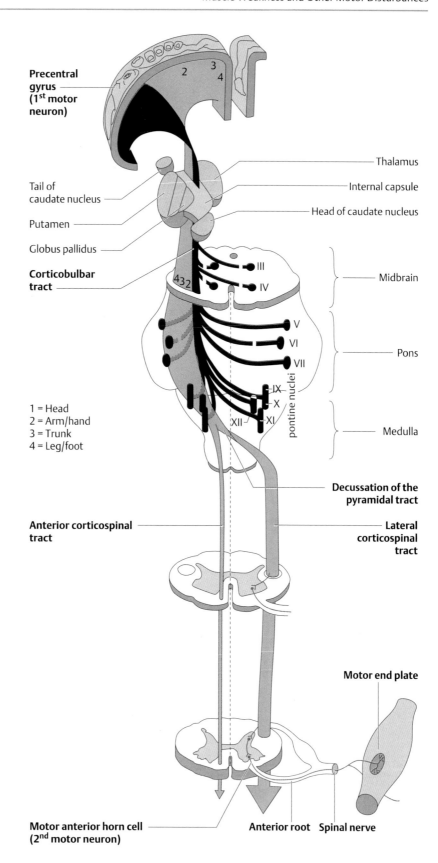

Fig. 5.**1 Anatomical substrate of movement** (modified from Liebsch, R.: *Intensivkurs Neurologie.* Urban & Schwarzenberg, Munich, 1996, and Mumenthaler, M.: *Neurologische Differenzialdiagnose*, 4th edn, Thieme, Stuttgart, 1992).

Precentral gyrus (1st motor neuron)

Thalamus

Tail of caudate nucleus

Internal capsule

Putamen

Head of caudate nucleus

Globus pallidus

Corticobulbar tract

III
IV

Midbrain

V
VI
VII

Pons

IX
X
XII XI

pontine nuclei

Medulla

1 = Head
2 = Arm/hand
3 = Trunk
4 = Leg/foot

Decussation of the pyramidal tract

Anterior corticospinal tract

Lateral corticospinal tract

Motor end plate

Motor anterior horn cell (2nd motor neuron)

Anterior root   **Spinal nerve**

5

Topical Diagnosis and Differential Diagnosis

tomical structures, motor processes are subject to a wide range of pathological disturbances. Typical findings of lesions of individual components of the motor system are listed in Table 5.1. The following table, in contrast, begins with certain typical constellations of motor deficits, then lists the likely site(s) of the lesion producing each, and finally some of the possible etiologies. Table 5.2 thus reflects the "classic" threefold paradigm of clinical thinking, from the physical findings to the site of the lesion to the diagnosis.

Table 5.**1**   Aspects of motor function and their localizing significance

Criterion	Motor neuron in anterior horn	Spinal nerve root or peripheral nerve	Central motor pathway (corticobulbar and corticospinal)	Extrapyramidal system	Cerebellum
Raw strength	↓	↓	↓	normal	normal
Tone	↓	↓	↑	possibly rigid, possibly ↑	↓
Muscle atrophy	++	++	∅ (except for possible atrophy of disuse)	∅	∅
Intrinsic muscle reflexes	↓ or absent	↓ or absent	↑	normal	normal
Extrinsic muscle reflexes	↓ or absent	↓ or absent	↓	normal	↓
Pyramidal tract signs	∅	∅	+	∅	∅
Coordination	↓	↓	↓	normal or ↓	↓ ↓
Distribution of weakness	no rule	corresponding to the affected root or nerve	global	no weakness	no weakness
Fasciculations	++	rare	∅	∅	∅

Table 5.**2**   Patterns of distribution of weakness and their localizing significance

Pattern of distribution of weakness	Type of paralysis	Anatomical substrate	Causative illnesses; remarks
Focal, isolated, usually asymmetrical weakness of individual muscles or muscle groups	● flaccid	● peripheral nerve lesion	● when a purely motor nerve is involved, usually high-grade paresis of the muscle(s) that it innervates; when a mixed nerve is involved, there are additional sensory and/or autonomic deficits
	● flaccid	● nerve root lesion	● paresis and reflex deficits (if any) in the segmentally innervated muscle(s), usually accompanied by a sensory deficit in the dermatome of the affected nerve root
	● flaccid	● loss of anterior horn ganglion cells	● initial stage of spinal muscular atrophy; fasciculations are usually seen in the muscles innervated by the lost anterior horn cells
	● flaccid	● muscle ischemia	● compartment syndromes, e. g., tibialis anterior syndrome; sensation intact, muscle contracted
Symmetrical, mainly proximal weakness	● flaccid	● myopathy	● initial stage of limb girdle muscular dystrophies
	● flaccid	● loss of anterior horn ganglion cells	● initial stage of certain types of spinal muscular atrophy
Symmetrical, mainly distal weakness	● flaccid	● myopathy	● initial stage of certain types of muscular dystrophy or myotonia, e. g., Steinert myotonic dystrophy (in such cases usually beginning distally, and involving mainly extensor muscles)
	● flaccid	● lesion of distal portion of multiple peripheral nerves	● polyneuropathy; often accompanied by paresthesiae and sensory deficits

Continued →

Table 5.**2** **Patterns of distribution of weakness and their localizing significance** (continued)

Pattern of distribution of weakness	Type of paralysis	Anatomical substrate	Causative illnesses; remarks
Hemiparesis: ● **hemiparesis including the face**	● spastic	● lesion of the contralateral motor cortex or cortico-bulbar and cortico-spinal pathways as they pass through the corona radiata and internal capsule, down to the level of the cerebral peduncle	● ischemic stroke, intracerebral hemorrhage, tumor, trauma, infection, or inflammation; the weakness is usually mainly distal (the ends of the limbs, esp. the hands, have a larger cortical representation) and accompanied by impairment of fine motor control and sensation
● **hemiparesis sparing the face (no weakness of the muscles of facial expression)**	● spastic	● lesion of the contralateral caudal portion of the brain-stem	● focal lesion, usually microinfarct (contralateral hemiparesis usually accompanied by sensory deficits and caudal cranial nerve deficits, see below)
	● spastic	● hemisection of the spinal cord at a high cervical level, on the side of the paretic limbs	● e. g., trauma or compression by a tumor; may be accompanied by ipsilateral hypesthesia and contralateral (dissociated) deficit of pain and temperature sensation below the level of the lesion, as well as segmentally delimited flaccid paresis at the level of the lesion (because of anterior horn cell involvement)
Special form: crossed unilateral weakness (face on one side, body on other side)	● spastic	● brainstem lesion (medulla, pons, or midbrain)	● combination of ipsilateral cranial nerve deficit and contralateral hemiparesis; if the affected cranial nerve is a motor nerve, there may be flaccid weakness in the muscles it innervates
Quadriparesis/global weakness:	● spastic	● lesion of the cerebral cortex of both hemi-spheres	● e. g., hypoxic brain injury after cardiorespiratory arrest
	● spastic	● lesion of the deep cerebral white matter of both hemispheres	● e. g., multiple sclerosis
	● spastic	● (partial) transverse lesion of the brain-stem interrupting all corticospinal projections	● e. g., locked-in syndrome
	● spastic	● high cervical spinal cord transection	● e. g., trauma or compression by tumor; accompanied by sensory deficit in all modalities below the level of the lesion (sensory level) and segmentally delimited flaccid weakness at the level of the lesion
	● mixed spastic/flaccid	● loss of central motor neurons and anterior horn ganglion cells	● amyotrophic lateral sclerosis
	● flaccid	● loss of anterior horn ganglion cells at many different spinal cord levels	● acute anterior poliomyelitis, advanced stage of spinal muscular atrophy
	● flaccid	● lesion of multiple nerve roots at multiple segmental levels	● e. g., advanced stage of Guillain–Barré syndrome (acute or chronic recurrent)
	● flaccid	● myopathy	● advanced stage of various types of muscular dystrophy, generalized form of myasthenia; myositis
	usually no objective evidence of weakness	● disease of an internal organ ● psychogenic ● depression	● e. g., thyroid dysfunction

Continued →

5

Topical Diagnosis and Differential Diagnosis

Table 5.**2**   **Patterns of distribution of weakness and their localizing significance** (continued)

Pattern of distribution of weakness	Type of paralysis	Anatomical substrate	Causative illnesses; remarks
Paraparesis	• spastic	• bilateral parasagittal lesion (cortical representation of the lower limbs in the precentral gyri)	• often in falx meningioma; sometimes accompanied by sensory deficits in the lower limbs due to simultaneous involvement of the postcentral gyri; there may also be neuropsychological abnormalities and urinary dysfunction
	• spastic	• thoracic spinal cord transection	• e. g., trauma or compression by tumor; sensory level, possible segmentally delimited weakness at the level of the lesion
	• spastic	• disease process affecting the corticospinal tracts bilaterally	• spastic spinal paralysis; purely motor deficit (no sensory deficit)
	• flaccid	• acute lesion of multiple lumbar nerve roots	• initial stage of Guillain–Barré syndrome (often with ascending weakness); cauda equina syndrome due to massive lumbar intervertebral disk herniation
	• flaccid	• lesion of multiple peripheral nerves of the lower limbs	• polyneuropathy; usually in combination with sensory deficits and reflex deficits (e. g., Achilles' reflex)
	• flaccid	• myopathy	• e. g., initial stage of myotonic dystrophy

Motor Regulatory Systems

The smooth, precise, and economical execution of a movement requires a properly functioning "regulatory system" in addition to the effector components discussed above. The regulatory system must do the following:

- *integrate proprioceptive input* from the peripheral nerves, posterior columns (fasciculus gracilis and fasciculus cuneatus), thalamus, and thalamocortical pathways, along with further input from the vestibular apparatus and the visual system, and use this "feedback" data to optimize each phase of the movement at every moment;
- *plan the force and amplitude of the movement* (extrapyramidal system and cerebellum);
- coordinate the activity of all of the muscles taking part in a movement and, in particular, ensure the *effective complementary functioning of agonist and antagonist muscles* (extrapyramidal system, cerebellum, and spinal cord).

A loss of function of one or more components of this regulatory system impairs the execution and coordination of movement. Disturbances of this type are typically manifest as:

- ataxia,
- hypokinesia,
- involuntary movements.

Ataxia is an impairment of the smooth performance of goal-directed movement (*repeated deviation from the ideal line of a movement*). The different types of ataxia have specific clinical features, depending on the nature and location of the underlying lesion:

Cerebellar ataxia is characterized by irregularity of the entire course of a movement. A lesion in a *cerebellar hemisphere* produces ataxia in the ipsilateral limbs, while a *vermian* lesion mainly produces truncal ataxia

(ataxia of stance and/or gait). On the other hand, involvement of the *dentate nucleus* or its *efferent fibers* causes intention tremor: in targeted movements, the deviation from the ideal line of approach increases as the limb approaches the target (Fig. 3.**20**, p. 29).

Central sensory ataxia results from impaired position sense due to lesions of the *somatosensory cortex,* the *thalamus,* or the *thalamocortical pathways.*

Posterior column ataxia is produced by lesions of the afferent somatosensory pathways in the dorsal portion of the spinal cord (*fasciculus gracilis* and *fasciculus cuneatus*—also known as the columns of Goll and Burdach). It is most apparent when the patient walks; it is regularly accompanied by impaired proprioception and position sense. Patients can compensate for posterior column ataxia to some extent with visual cues; this form of ataxia is thus appreciably worse in the dark, or when the patient's eyes are closed, than in a well-lit room with the patient's eyes open.

> **!** *The distinguishing characteristic of spinal, as opposed to cerebellar, ataxia is that it is mainly evident when visual input is removed.*

Peripheral sensory ataxia is caused by disease processes affecting the peripheral sensory nerves, e. g., *polyneuropathy*, and is associated with loss of reflexes and impaired epicritic sensation.

Other types of ataxia. *Frontal lobe lesions* sometimes cause contralateral ataxia; *motor weakness* can also impair motor coordination, causing ataxia. *Psychogenic ataxia* is typified by its irregularity and by the lack of constant, objectifiable neurological deficits. Patients with psychogenic ataxia do not fall.

Hypokinesia is generalized slowing of all types of movement.

It is typically found in (hypokinetic) Parkinson disease (p. 128). Spontaneous movements are sparse or absent, automatic accessory movements cease (e. g., arm movements during walking), and all voluntary movements are slowed. The muscles are rigid and the cogwheel phenomenon is usually demonstrable (p. 30).

It is also found in *depression* as a sign of generally diminished drive; in such cases, it is not accompanied by any other neurological deficit.

Involuntary movements come in many varieties, the more important of which are listed in Table 5.3. The phenomenology and localizing significance of each type of involuntary movement are described.

Table 5.**3** **Involuntary movements and movement disorders**

Designation	Manifestations	Localization; Remarks
Spontaneous muscle activity not producing movement		
• Fibrillations	phasic contractions of individual muscle fibers, not visible to the naked eye, only demonstrable by EMG	due to contractions of individual muscle fibers; pathological at rest or as prolonged insertional activity in the EMG (p. 58)
• Fasciculations	brief, irregular contractions of individual groups of muscle fibers, visible to the naked eye	due to contractions of individual motor units; always pathological; especially typical of chronic lesions affecting the anterior horn ganglion cells
• Myokymia	visible waves of contraction passing across many different fiber bundles in a muscle or group of muscles	unknown
Hyperkinetic phenomena		
• Myorrhythmia	rhythmic twitching in a muscle group (always the same one) producing movement; frequency usually 1–3 Hz	central nervous system
• Myoclonus	nonrhythmic, rapid, large-amplitude, sometimes very intense twitching of one or more muscles, producing visible movement	cerebral cortex, cerebellum; seen physiologically in persons who are falling asleep (hypnagogic myoclonus)
• Tremor	rhythmic oscillation (usually fine, sometimes coarse), at a frequency that remains roughly constant for the affected individual, of more or less constant localization; may be observed at rest (rest tremor) or with action (action tremor; e. g., postural tremor, kinetic tremor, intention tremor)	central nervous system (mainly cerebellum, extrapyramidal system)
• Chorea	brief and relatively rapid, shooting muscle contractions, mainly distal, nonrhythmic, irregular, of varying localization, sometimes putting the joints into extreme positions for a brief period of time	basal ganglia/striatum
• Athetosis	like chorea, but slower, writhing movements with longer-lasting hyperflexion or hyperextension of the joints	basal ganglia
• Ballism	brief, shooting muscle contractions, mainly proximal and therefore causing pronounced movement (flinging movements of the limbs, jactation)	subthalamic nucleus
• Dystonia	involuntary, longer-lasting muscle contraction that slowly overcomes the resistance of the antagonist muscles, usually leading to turning movements and bizarre postures of individual parts of the body (trunk, limbs, head)	basal ganglia
• Tics and ticlike movements	irregular muscle contraction limited to certain parts of the body, rapid, but not lightninglike	psychogenic

Continued →

Table 5.**3**   **Involuntary movements and movement disorders** (continued)

Designation	Manifestations	Localization; Remarks
Other		
● Spasms	muscle contractions of variable frequency and intensity, occurring at irregular intervals, occasionally painful; two examples are ● hemifacial spasm (Fig. 11.19) and ● blepharospasm	facial nerve lesion, extrapyramidal disorder (a type of dystonic movement disorder); very rarely psychogenic
● Cramps	long-lasting, tonic contractions of individual muscles or muscle groups, fixed position of the joints, usually painful, often in the calf	of muscular origin

Sensory Disturbances

Anatomical Substrate of Sensation

It is another useful simplification to consider the somatosensory system as consisting of the following components (Fig. 5.**2**, Table 5.**4**):

The peripheral part of the somatosensory system contains sensory (afferent) nerves and receptors that are specialized for the perception of the individual modalities of somatic sensation.

Sensory receptors in the periphery are classified into three principal types. **Exteroceptive receptors** (exteroceptors) transduce physical stimuli from the external environment (e. g., *mechanoreceptors, thermoreceptors*). **Proprioceptive receptors** (proprioceptors) inform the nervous system about head and body posture, the positions of the joints, and tension in muscles and tendons (*muscle spindles* and *Golgi tendon organs*). Finally, the **nociceptors**, which subserve pain, occupy an intermediate position between the extero- and proprioceptors. The density of somatosensory receptors is greatest in the skin, but they are also found in most other tissues of the body, including the viscera (but not in the brain or spinal cord!).

Afferent sensory nerve fibers run in the **peripheral nerves**, **plexuses**, and **posterior spinal nerve roots**. These are the axons of the first somatosensory neurons, whose cell bodies lie in the spinal ganglia (dorsal root ganglia). All other sensory neurons have their cell bodies within the central nervous system.

The central part of the somatosensory system comprises all of the somatosensory pathways and nuclei of the **spinal cord, brainstem,** and **cerebral hemispheres**. These can be classified, according to their function, as follows:

Posterior column system. The centripetal processes of the pseudounipolar spinal ganglion cells (first sensory neuron) that subserve **epicritic sensation** carry information from both exteroceptors (tactile sense, stereognosis and vibration) and proprioceptors (position sense). They travel by way of the posterior columns to the nucleus gracilis and nucleus cuneatus of the medulla, without any intervening relay in the spinal cord. These medullary nuclei contain the second sensory neurons, whose axons, in turn, form the medial lemniscus, which travels onward to the thalamus.

Lesions affecting the posterior column system impair all of the "high-resolution" somatosensory modalities:
● diminished ability to recognize objects by touch (*astereognosia*) and *impaired two-point discrimination*;
● impaired vibration sense (*pallhypesthesia* or *pallanesthesia*) and *impaired position sense and kinesthesia*;

Table 5.**4**   **The somatosensory system**

peripheral portion	● receptors	exteroceptors (mechano- and thermoreceptors) proprioceptors (body posture, joint position, tension in muscles and tendons) nociceptors
	● nerve fibers	peripheral nerves, plexuses, posterior roots
central portion	● spinal cord	posterior columns anterolateral columns spinocerebellar tracts
	● brainstem	posterior column fibers terminate in synaptic relay stations in the medulla (nucleus gracilis, nucleus cuneatus); the efferent fibers of these nuclei ascend in the brainstem as the medial lemniscus and terminate in the thalamus the spinothalamic tracts ascend the spinal cord in the anterolateral columns (fasciculi) and terminate in the thalamus the spinocerebellar tracts terminate in the cerebellum.
	● cerebral hemispheres	thalamus thalamocortical tracts somatosensory cortex

Fig. 5.**2 Anatomical substrate
of somatic sensation.**

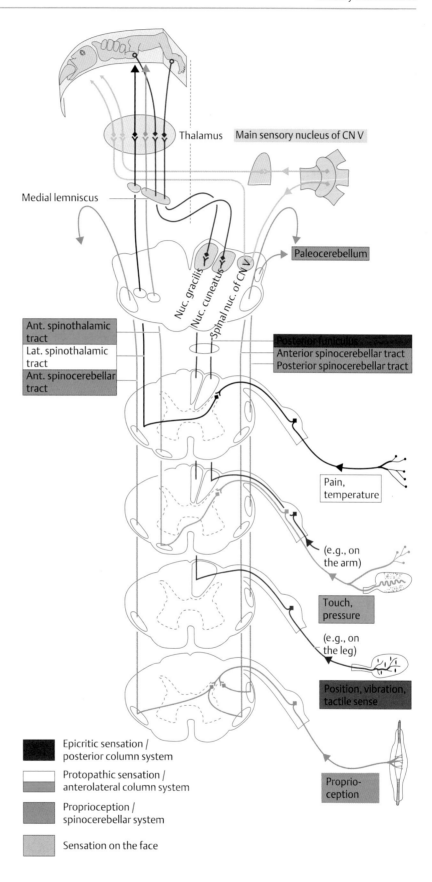

Thalamus

Main sensory nucleus of CN V

Medial lemniscus

Paleocerebellum

Nuc. gracilis

Nuc. cuneatus

Spinal nuc. of CN V

Ant. spinothalamic tract

Lat. spinothalamic tract

Ant. spinocerebellar tract

Posterior funiculus

Anterior spinocerebellar tract

Posterior spinocerebellar tract

Pain, temperature

(e.g., on the arm)

Touch, pressure

(e.g., on the leg)

Position, vibration, tactile sense

Proprio-ception

Epicritic sensation /
posterior column system

Protopathic sensation /
anterolateral column system

Proprioception /
spinocerebellar system

Sensation on the face

- unsteady stance and gait (*spinal ataxia,* see below) due to the lack of proprioceptive feedback regarding the posture and movements of the head, trunk, and limbs.

Anterolateral column system. The centripetal processes of the pseudounipolar spinal ganglion cells (first sensory neuron) that subserve **protopathic sensation** (pain, temperature sensation, coarse touch and pressure) form synapses onto second sensory neurons in the posterior horn of the spinal cord. The axons of these cells cross the midline in the anterior spinal commissure and then ascend in the spinal cord and through the brainstem to terminate in the thalamus. Fibers related to pain and temperature sensation travel in the lateral spinothalamic tract, fibers related to coarse touch and pressure in the anterior spinothalamic tract.

Lesions affecting the lateral spinothalamic tract in the spinal cord or brainstem, or the corresponding thalamic nuclei, produce a *dissociated sensory deficit*: pain and temperature sensation are impaired below the level of the lesion, while touch remains intact. The deficit is contralateral to the lesion because the lateral spinothalamic tract is crossed.

Thalamocortical system. The axons of the second neurons of both the posterior column system and the anterolateral column system terminate in the thalamic nuclei that contain the third neurons of the somatosensory system. These neurons, in turn, send their axons by way of the posterior limb of the internal capsule to the primary somatosensory cortex (postcentral gyrus) and the neighboring association areas. The third neurons thus belong to the so-called thalamocortical system. **Lesions** of this system produce a contralateral hemisensory deficit, which usually affects all of the somatosensory modalities, though sometimes to different extents.

The spinocerebellar system conveys information regarding **tension and stretch of muscles and tendons** from the muscle spindles and Golgi tendon organs to the paleocerebellum. The main spinal pathways used by this system are the posterior spinocerebellar tract (which exclusively carries information from the ipsilateral half of the body) and the anterior spinocerebellar tract (which carries information from both sides of the body). The paleocerebellum, in turn, gives off multiple efferent pathways, which influence muscle tone to ensure the *smooth cooperative functioning of agonist and antagonist muscle groups in standing and walking.* The paleocerebellum thus plays an important role in the regulation of balance, though its activity is wholly unconscious. **Lesions of the spinocerebellar pathways** and paleocerebellum cause *ataxia of stance and gait* (see above).

Table 5.**5** is analogous to Table 5.**2**; it provides an overview of the typical constellations of somatosensory deficits and their pathoanatomical basis. We have not mentioned any specific diagnoses in this table in order to keep it perspicuous. Some of the typical clinical findings are illustrated in Fig. 5.**3**.

Tabelle 5.5 **Patterns of distribution of somatosensory deficits**

Pattern of distribution of deficit	Sensory qualities affected	Anatomical substrate; remarks
sharply delimited, unilateral, focal, asymmetrical	- all	- **lesion of the peripheral (sensory) nerve trunks;** maximal sensory deficit in the autonomous zone of the affected nerve; hypesthesia generally more pronounced than hypalgesia; concomitant impairment of sweating in the area of the deficit
less sharply delimited, unilateral, segmental, asymmetrical	- all	- **lesion of the spinal nerve roots;** hypalgesia more pronounced than hypesthesia in monoradicular lesions
gradually increasing from proximal to distal, bilaterally symmetrical (stocking-and-glove distribution)	- diminished vibration and position sense at first; the remaining sensory qualities may be lost as the deficit progresses	- **polyneuropathy;** sometimes also seen in polyradiculopathy
segmental, bilaterally symmetrical	- pain and temperature sense	- **lesion of the anterior commissure of the spinal cord, which contains the decussating fibers of the lateral spinothalamic tract;** exclusively at a particular segmental level, without damage to ascending pathways
unilateral below a given spinal cord level	- pain and temperature sense	- **lesion of the contralateral lateral spinothalamic tract**
	- vibration and position sense	- **lesion of the ipsilateral posterior columns**
	- all qualities other than pain and temperature on the side of the lesion; pain and temperature contralaterally	- **lesion of one-half of the spinal cord,** regularly producing ipsilateral spastic hemiparesis below the level of the lesion, as well as unilateral segmental flaccid paresis at the level of the lesion and on the same side as the lesion

Continued →

Tabelle 5.**5** **Patterns of distribution of somatosensory deficits** (continued)

Pattern of distribution of deficit	Sensory qualities affected	Anatomical substrate; remarks
bilateral below a given spinal cord level	• all	• **lesion of the entire cross-section of the spinal cord;** regularly accompanied by spastic paraparesis below the level of the lesion and by bilateral segmental flaccid weakness at the level of the lesion The sensory deficits of both uni- and bilateral spinal cord damage are found below the level of the most severe anatomical lesion.
unilateral, including the face	• all	• **lesion of the contralateral thalamus, or of the ascending thalamocortical projection passing through the internal capsule;** contralateral parietal cortex (rare)
	• pain and temperature sense	• **thalamic lesion** on the side opposite the sensory deficit; may be accompanied by spontaneous pain on the affected side of the body, as well as abnormally prolonged pain in response to a stimulus that usually produces only brief pain (= hyperpathia); very rarely due to a cortical lesion
unilateral, sparing the face	• all	• circumscribed lesion of the contralateral dorsal internal capsule, or unilateral high cervical cord lesion (see above)

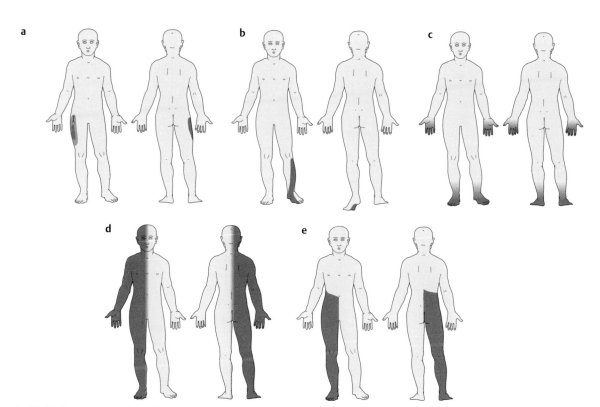

Fig. 5.**3 Typical patterns of distribution of somatosensory deficits. a Peripheral nerve lesion:** meralgia paraesthetica due to a lesion of the lateral femoral cutaneous n. **b Radicular lesion:** typical sensory deficit in L5 radiculopathy. **c Polyneuropathy:** distal, stocking-and-glove sensory deficit. **d Central lesion:** contralateral hemisensory deficit. **e Spinal cord lesion** at the T6 level: hemihypesthesia below the level of the lesion.

5

Topical Diagnosis and Differential Diagnosis

Disturbances of Consciousness

Anatomical substrate. Intact consciousness requires normal functioning of the *cortex of both cerebral hemispheres.* The "driving force" of cortical activity, however, is located in a lower center, i. e., in a collective of neurons in the brainstem called the *reticular formation,* which sends impulses toward the cerebral cortex by way of the intralaminar thalamic nuclei. The reticular

formation and its ascending projections are known collectively as the *ascending reticular activating system.*

Impairments of consciousness may thus be caused either by the simultaneous impairment of function of *both* cerebral hemispheres, or by damage to the reticular formation in the brainstem, and/or to its ascending projections (uncoupling of the cortex from the activating input of the reticular formation). Depending on their severity, impairments of consciousness are termed **somnolence, stupor,** or **coma** (Table 3.9, p. 40). Coma, the most severe impairment of consciousness, can also be more finely graded, according to any of several semi-quantitative schemes that have been proposed. The best known of these is the Glasgow Coma Scale (GCS, Table 6.6, p. 88).

Causes. Consciousness may be impaired either by a structural lesion of brain tissue, or else indirectly by a systemic disturbance of some kind (metabolic, toxic, or anoxic coma; see below). If a **structural lesion** is the cause, there are often accompanying focal neurological deficits whose presence enables the clinician to infer the probable site of the lesion. The direct cause of the impairment of consciousness is often not the lesion itself, but rather the cerebral edema surrounding it (cf. Table 5.6). Focal neurological signs are usually absent in purely **metabolic, toxic,** or **anoxic coma.**

Bilateral cortical dysfunction can also be the result of an **epileptic seizure** or an **infectious/inflammatory process** such as meningitis or encephalitis (in which case meningism is usually present). Finally, there are also purely psychogenic states (**psychogenic stupor**) that may superficially resemble an organic impairment of consciousness. The more important causes of impaired consciousness are listed in Table 5.6. Here we have classified all impairments of consciousness into four basic clinical situations and listed the common etiologies for each.

Differential diagnosis. We will now briefly describe three other types of disturbance of consciousness that must be distinguished from coma.

Apallic syndrome/coma vigil ("persistent vegetative state"). This condition is usually due to severe and extensive brain damage. It is characterized by a *complete uncoupling of midbrain and diencephalic activity from cortical activity* and thus by a *complete dissociation of wakefulness and consciousness.* (The term "apallic" signifies "without cerebral cortex.") The vegetative functions (breathing, cardiovascular regulation, sleep–wake cycle) are preserved, though possibly abnormal to some extent. Cognitive or goal-directed motor activity is entirely lacking. Unlike the comatose patient, the apallic patient lies in bed with eyes open, staring blankly into the distance, not fixating the gaze on anything, and not responding to verbal or noxious stimuli. At other times, the patient is in a sleeplike state, with eyes closed. Muscle tone is elevated, and automatisms and primitive reflexes are sometimes observed in the perioral area. Common types of autonomic dysfunction seen in apallic

Table 5.6 Causes of impaired consciousness

Clinical situation	Possible causes
Impaired consciousness or coma without focal signs or meningism (purely toxic/metabolic or anoxic coma)	**various metabolic disorders** ● hypo- or hyperglycemia ● uremia ● liver failure ● endocrine dysfunction ● electrolyte disturbances ● metabolic acidosis or alkalosis **intoxications** (e. g., alcohol, medications, carbon monoxide) **acute heart failure or diminution of the circulating blood volume (anoxic encephalopathy)** ● myocardial infarction ● atrial fibrillation ● cardiac tamponade ● hypovolemic shock ● cardiorespiratory arrest etc. Focal neurological signs are absent only if cerebral ischemia and hypoxia have not yet caused irreversible structural damage in the CNS
Impaired consciousness or coma without focal signs, with meningism	**meningitis** **subarachnoid hemorrhage**
Impaired consciousness or coma with focal signs (structural lesion)	**supratentorial lesions** (*acute:* infarct, trauma, intracranial hemorrhage, subdural/ epidural hematoma; *subacute/ chronically progressive:* infections, tumors); impairment of consciousness is often due to edema in the brain tissue around the lesion and the resulting intracranial hypertension and capillary hypoxia, sometimes accompanied by midline shift and herniation, with secondary brainstem damage **infratentorial lesions** (*acute:* infarct, trauma, hemorrhage; *subacute/chronically progressive:* infections, tumors)
Transient impairment of consciousness, possibly accompanied by involuntary motor phenomena	**generalized epileptic seizure**

patients include tachycardia, excessive sweating, and rapid breathing.

Akinetic mutism is often due to *extensive, bilateral frontal lobe damage* or to a lesion affecting the projections of the ascending reticular activating system to the frontal lobes, e. g., a *bilateral thalamic or midbrain lesion.* Swallowing and extrinsic muscle reflexes are intact and the patient's eye movements are usually normal, yet spontaneous verbal or motor expressions are lacking. The patient still appears to be awake and can sometimes be induced to speak or move with intensive prompting.

Locked-in syndrome is not a disturbance of consciousness, though it can be mistaken for one. The patient is awake and alert, but can express him- or herself only through vertical eye movements and eyelid movements, because all four limbs are paralyzed, as well as all of the muscles innervated by the lower cranial nerves. The unwary clinician may have the false impression of a comatose patient who does not respond to external stimuli. A detailed description of the locked-in syndrome and its causes is found in the next section.

Dysfunction of Specific Areas of the Brain

Up to this point, we have described the characteristic neurological deficits produced by lesions of individual functional components of the nervous system. "Normally," however, more than one functional component is affected. There is often simultaneous impairment of motor function, cooordination, sensation, and possibly consciousness. The individual clinical signs and symptoms described above often appear together in particular constellations (= syndromes) that are characteristically associated with the region of the nervous system in which the lesion is located and largely independent of the nature of the lesion itself.

We will now describe the major syndromes of individual regions of the brain.

Syndromes of the Individual Lobes of the Cerebral Hemispheres

Frontal lobe syndrome is characterized by the following manifestations, in variable severity, depending on the extent and precise location of the causative lesion:

- *abnormalities of personality and behavior* (loss of drive and initiative, apathy, indifference; if only the orbitofrontal cortex is affected, there may be disinhibition, absent-mindedness, and socially inappropriate behavior);
- *primitive reflexes*, e. g., grasp reflex and brisk palmomental reflex;
- *motor phenomena*, e. g., spontaneous, compulsive grasping of objects, copying of other people's gestures (echopraxia), motor perseveration, and sometimes contralateral gaze paresis;
- *lateralized deficits*: motor aphasia in lesions of the language-dominant hemisphere, anosognosia (nonrecognition of one's own illness, e. g., hemiparesis) and contralateral apraxia (p. 42) in lesions of the nondominant hemisphere;
- *akinetic mutism*, usually caused by extensive, bilateral lesions (the patient is awake, but does not re-

spond to environmental stimuli and does not speak; see above):
- in lesions affecting the frontal eye fields: *déviation conjuguée* to the side of the lesion, because voluntary gaze to the opposite side is impossible;
- *irritative signs*: adversive seizures (epileptic seizures in which the head and trunk are involuntarily turned to the side opposite the lesion; the contralateral arm is sometimes raised as well).

Syndrome of lesions of the precentral and postcentral gyri. Each of these gyri contains a somatotopic cortical representation of the entire body, as described in detail 50 years ago by the neurosurgeon Wilder Penfield (Fig. 5.4 shows the classic "*Penfield homunculus*"). Lesions involving these paracentral gyri thus impair the function of specific parts of the body, with the specific site and extent of bodily dysfunction depending on the site and extent of the brain lesion. This can be most impressively observed in lesions of the precentral gyrus:
- There are *focal motor deficits*, e. g., monoplegia of a limb; if the lesion is restricted to the precentral gyrus itself, the weakness may be flaccid, but this is rarely the case. Simultaneous dysfunction of the premotor cortex usually causes spastic weakness.
- *Sensory deficits* are less frequently observed in such patients and cannot be clinically distinguished from those caused by thalamic lesions.
- The *intrinsic muscle reflexes* are generally increased on the contralateral side of the body and there are accompanying *pyramidal tract signs.*
- *Irritative phenomena* may appear in the form of Jacksonian epilepsy of focal onset (motor and/or somatosensory) or Kozhevnikov's epilepsia partialis continua (p. 166).

Temporal lobe syndrome takes different forms depending on the precise location of the lesion:
- *impairment of memory* (e. g., in lesions affecting the hippocampus on both sides);
- *sensory aphasia* (Wernicke aphasia, p. 41) in lesions involving the language-dominant (usually left) hemisphere;

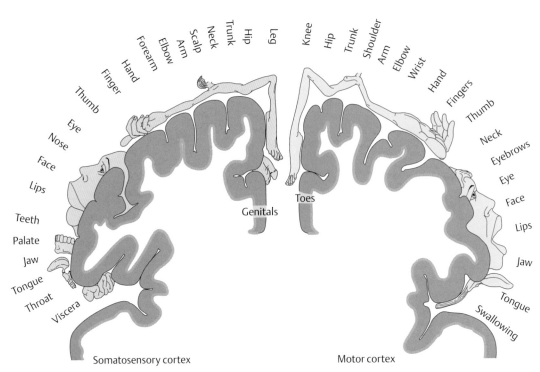

Fig. 5.4 The cortical representation of different parts of the body in the primary somatosensory cortex of the postcentral gyrus (left) and the primary motor cortex of the precentral gyrus (right) in the human being. (After Penfield, W., H. Jasper: *Epilepsy and the Functional Anatomy of the Human Brain.* Little, Brown, Boston 1954.)

- *possible disturbance of spatial orientation* in lesions involving the non-language-dominant (usually right) hemisphere;
- in deep-seated lesions, a visual disturbance taking the form of *contralateral homonymous upper quadrantanopsia*;
- *irritative phenomena*: complex partial seizures (temporal lobe seizures, p. 166), sometimes with ictal olfactory or gustatory hallucinations (uncinate fits)—these are usually reported as unpleasant;
- *mental abnormalities*: irritability, depression.

Parietal lobe syndrome manifests itself in somatosensory deficits and a variety of neuropsychological abnormalities:
- The most prominent sign is usually a *hemisensory deficit.*
- Lesions of the language-dominant hemisphere (usually left) can cause left/right confusion, finger agnosia, acalculia, and agraphia (*Gerstmann syndrome*), and/or *astereognosia.*
- Lesions of the nondominant hemisphere (usually right) can cause *anosognosia* (see above).
- With regard to motor function, there are often poorly coordinated, *ataxic hand and foot movements* on the side opposite the lesion.
- With regard to somatic sensation, there may be *neglect* for the contralateral half of the body (so-called extinction phenomenon: raw sensation is intact bilaterally, but if the examiner touches the patient simultaneously and equally intensely at mirror-

image sites on the two sides, the patient will report having felt something on one side only).
- Deep-seated lesions may produce *contralateral homonymous lower quadrantanopsia* or *hemianopsia*, or else only *visual neglect* for the contralateral hemifield.

Occipital lobe syndrome is mainly characterized by:
- a contralateral visual field defect (*homonymous hemianopsia*; cf. Fig. 3.6, p. 19);
- possible *cortical blindness* (in the case of bilateral occipital lobe lesions), in which elementary or formed visual hallucinations, or seeing gray, may be present; patients often deny being blind (anosognosia);
- *visual agnosia*, i. e., the inability to recognize colors or shapes, despite normal visual acuity;
- *irritative phenomena*: visual hallucinations, perhaps as the initial symptom of an epileptic seizure.

Syndromes of the Extrapyramidal Motor System

Function. The extrapyramidal motor system plays an important role in the smooth and purposeful execution of all motor processes, both voluntary and involuntary. One of its functions is to efficiently *combine individual motor components into complex patterns of movement* and to enable their largely *automatic execution.* Further ones are to give the signals for the initiation and termination of a movement and to *regulate muscle tone*.

Anatomical substrate. The main nuclei of the extrapyramidal motor system are the *basal ganglia* (caudate nucleus, putamen, and globus pallidus). Further components are the *subthalamic nucleus* (in the diencephalon) as well as the *substantia nigra* and the *red nucleus* (both in the midbrain). Extensive fiber connections link these nuclei to each other and to higher motor cortical areas (by way of the thalamus). They influence the activity of spinal motor neurons through a number of afferent and efferent spinal pathways.

Deficits. Lesions of individual components of the extrapyramidal motor system produce various types of disturbance, corresponding to the precise location of the lesion. Because the functions of the extrapyramidal system are essentially as described above, functional impairments can manifest themselves as an *excess or deficiency of movement-initiating impulses, automatic movement, and/or muscle tone*:

- There may be diminished spontaneity of movement, i. e., *hypokinesia* (e. g., in Parkinson disease) usually combined with elevated muscle tone, i. e., *rigidity* → **hypertonic–hyperkinetic syndrome**, p. 127.
- On the other hand, there may be *hyperkinesia* of a wide variety of types, which may be thought of as the uncontrolled expression of complex motor programs resulting from a removal of their normal inhibition by the extrapyramidal motor system. These involuntary, repetitive movements include *chorea, athetosis, ballism*, and *dystonia*, all of which are described in detail on p. 131. Choreatic syndromes are often associated with *diminished muscle tone* → **hypotonic–hyperkinetic syndrome**.
- Acute basal ganglionic lesions can also cause transient *hemiparesis*.

Thalamic Syndromes

Function. The thalamus is the *synaptic relay station for many somatosensory and special sensory pathways*; it transmits afferent impulses from peripheral extero- and proprioceptors, as well as from the higher sensory organs (eye, ear), to higher centers. In the thalamus, impulses pertaining to the body's various senses are *integrated, affectively colored, and then passed on to the cortex* (conscious perception appears to be possible only if the impulses reach the cortex). The thalamus also receives neural input from the extrapyramidal motor system and participates in the *regulation of attention and drive* as a component of the ascending reticular activating system (see below). Finally, certain components of the thalamus play a role in *memory*.

Deficits. Because the functions of the thalamus are as we have just described, lesions affecting it can produce the following deficits:

- *Somatosensory deficits*: these mainly consist of impaired proprioception on the side opposite the lesion. There may also be painful, burning sensations that either arise spontaneously (*dysesthesia*) or are

induced by, and outlast, a tactile stimulus delivered to the skin (*hyperpathia*).
- *Deficits of movement and coordination*: there may be contralateral hemiparesis (which is usually transient) or hemiataxia.
- *Contralateral hemianopsia* may be present.
- *Abnormal posture*, particularly of the hands, may be present. In the "*thalamic hand*," the metacarpophalangeal joints are flexed, while the interphalangeal joints are hyperextended.

Brainstem Syndromes

Function. The brainstem is a "*throughway*" *for many fiber pathways of the nervous system*, which lie adjacent to one another here in a very tightly confined space. All of the motor and somatosensory projections to and from the periphery pass through the brainstem; some of them cross here (decussate) to the other side and some undergo a synaptic relay. In addition, the brainstem contains *many nuclei*: all of the somatic and visceral motor and sensory nuclei of cranial nerves III through XII are located within it. Two brainstem nuclei, the red nucleus and substantia nigra, belong to the extrapyramidal motor system. Finally, among the nuclei of the reticular formation are found the *vital autonomic regulatory centers* controlling cardiovascular and respiratory function, as well as nuclei of the *ascending reticular activating system* that send activating impulses to the cerebral cortex and are essential for the maintenance of consciousness.

Deficits. As one would expect from the very large number of important neural structures located within the brainstem and fiber tracts passing through it, a correspondingly wide variety of deficits can be produced by lesions of different sizes and at different locations in the brainstem. The pattern of clinical manifestations usually enables the clinician to localize the *level* of the lesion to one of the three brainstem segments (midbrain, pons, or medulla). One can also clinically distinguish **focal lesions** from partial or complete **cross-sectional lesions** of the brainstem:

Unilateral focal lesions are usually of vascular origin (lacunar infarct). The typical clinical picture is the so-called **alternating hemiplegia syndrome**, in which a cranial nerve deficit on the side of the lesion appears together with a motor and/or sensory deficit on the contralateral half of the body. There are different alternating hemiplegia syndromes depending on the level of the lesion; some of these are described further in Table 6.**4**, p. 86.

Focal *diencephalic lesions* can produce diabetes insipidus as well as disturbances of thermoregulation, the sleep–wake cycle, eating behavior, and other instinctual behaviors.

Bilateral partial cross-sectional lesions of the brainstem. The classic example of a disturbance produced by this type of lesion is the **locked-in syndrome**, which is due to an *extensive lesion of the ventral portion of the pons* (e. g., an infarct secondary to thrombosis of the basilar a.). *The corticobulbar and corticospinal pathways*

Table 5.**7**   **Findings in deep brainstem lesions**

Site of lesion or functional disturbance	Pupils: appearance and reactivity to light	Corneal reflexes	Vertical VOR (see p. 186)	Horizontal VOR (see p. 186)	Respiration
Cerebral hemispheres (bilateral)	equal, reactive	bilaterally present	present	present (elicitable in both directions)	Cheyne–Stokes respiration, continual hyperventilation
Midbrain	unilaterally or bilaterally fixed and dilated	present	absent	present	may be irregular, with pauses
Pons	small, equal, fixed	unilaterally or bilaterally absent	may be absent	absent	may be irregular, with pauses
Medulla	equal, reactive	present	may be absent	may be absent	irregular, apneustic
Extensive brainstem lesion	unilaterally or bilaterally fixed and dilated	unilaterally or bilaterally absent	absent	absent	irregular, apneustic

of the basis pontis are totally interrupted and part of the pontine reticular formation may be as well. All four limbs are paralyzed (quadriplegia), and the caudal cranial nerves are dysfunctional: the patient cannot swallow, speak, or, usually, produce facial expressions. Vertical eye movements and lid closure, both of which are midbrain functions, are preserved, but horizontal eye movements, which are a function of the pons, are abolished. Consciousness remains intact because the reticular formation is largely spared. The patient can communicate through vertical eye movements and lid closure.

Bulbar palsy and pseudobulbar palsy are two further syndromes caused by bilateral partial cross-sectional lesions of the brainstem. (True) **bulbar palsy** is produced by *system atrophy of the motor cranial nerve nuclei of the medulla* and therefore manifests itself as bulbar dysarthria, dysphagia, and tongue atrophy, with fasciculations. In **pseudobulbar palsy**, the causative lesion does not involve the cranial nerve nuclei themselves, but rather their innervating *corticonuclear pathways* bilaterally, or else the *cortical areas* from which these pathways arise. The clinical picture resembles that of bulbar palsy, but tongue atrophy and fasciculations are absent because the peripheral motor neuron is intact.

Complete cross-sectional lesions of the brainstem (brainstem transection) are due either to a pathological process in the posterior fossa or the brainstem itself (*infratentorial lesion*), or to acute *intracranial hypertension in the supratentorial compartment*, with secondary herniation and brainstem compression. Systemic processes (prolonged hypoxia or cardiorespiratory arrest; see above) can also cause extensive damage to the brainstem, as well as to the cerebral hemispheres. Midbrain lesions cause severe **impairment of consciousness**, ranging to deep coma, and characteristic **motor** and **oculomotor signs**. The same is true of pontine lesions. The most prominent sign of medullary transection is **loss of all autonomic function**. The level of brainstem injury can almost always be correctly deduced from the pattern of clinical deficits and the findings of a few special tests (particularly of the brain stem reflexes), as described in Table 5.**7**. A patient who survives acute, extensive damage to the midbrain will probably be quadri-

plegic and suffer from akinetic mutism (see above).

Cerebellar Syndromes

Function. The tasks of the cerebellum are to *optimize the amplitude, speed, and precision of voluntary movement* and simultaneously to regulate the motor control of balance and adapt muscle tone to the demands placed on the body's movement apparatus. The cerebellum also plays a role in the *regulation of gaze-related movements of the eyes* and in ensuring the *smooth complementary functioning of agonist and antagonist muscle groups*.

In order to perform these coordinating tasks, the cerebellum requires information from various different parts of the nervous system. These different types of information are processed separately in three parts of the cerebellum that are distinct from one another both functionally and phylogenetically:

- **Impulses from the cerebral cortex** for the initiation and planning of voluntary movement travel in the corticopontocerebellar pathway, by way of the brachium pontis (middle cerebellar peduncle), to the **neocerebellum** (located in the cerebellar hemispheres). This phylogenetically youngest part of the cerebellum is mainly responsible for the fine control of very precise movements, particularly of the limbs (especially the hands and fingers) and of the motor apparatus of speech.
- **Information regarding joint position and muscle tone** from peripheral proprioceptors (muscle spindles and Golgi tendon organs) travels, by way of the anterior and posterior spinocerebellar tracts, through the restiform body and brachium conjunctivum (inferior and superior cerebellar peduncles) to the **paleocerebellum** (located in part of the vermis and the paraflocculus). This part of the cerebellum is mainly responsible for the smooth, synergistic functioning of the muscles when the individual stands or walks (see above).
- **Impulses from the vestibular system** travel by way of the restiform body (inferior cerebellar peduncle) to the **archicerebellum** (nodulus and flocculus). This phylogenetically oldest part of the cerebellum

mainly serves to keep the upright body in balance during standing and walking.

The cerebellum integrates the various types of afferent impulses it receives and then influences the motor regulatory functions of the brain and spinal cord in the manner of a feedback system. Efferent impulses travel:

- from the cerebellar cortex to the dentate nucleus, where further processing takes place, and then through the superior cerebellar peduncle to the lateral nucleus of the thalamus, and onward to the *cerebral cortex* (Fig. 5.**5**),
- while other efferent impulses travel from the dentate nucleus via the red nucleus to the thalamus, or via the red nucleus to the olive, and then back to the cerebellum. These two neuronal loops give off descending fibers to the rubrospinal and reticulospinal tracts, which terminate in the *motor nuclei of the spinal cord* (Fig. 5.**5**).

The integration of the cerebellum in the complex functional system controlling voluntary movement is shown in Fig. 5.**6**.

Deficits. In accordance with the functions of the cerebellum described above, cerebellar lesions produce *disturbances of muscle tone and movement*:

- basal lesions near the midline (mainly affecting the archicerebellum) produce *disturbances of truncal posture and the maintenance of balance,* which are particularly evident when the patient tries to sit;
- vermian lesions (mainly affecting the paleocerebellum) produce *impaired coordination of stance and gait*;
- lesions of the cerebellar hemispheres (mainly affecting the neocerebellum) produce *impaired coordination of (fine) movements of the limbs on the side of the lesion.*

A detailed list of clinical manifestations of cerebellar disease is provided in Table 5.**8**.

Fig. 5.**5 Anatomical connections of the cerebellum.** The connections to the cerebral cortex, brainstem, vestibular system, and spinal cord are illustrated. For details, see text.

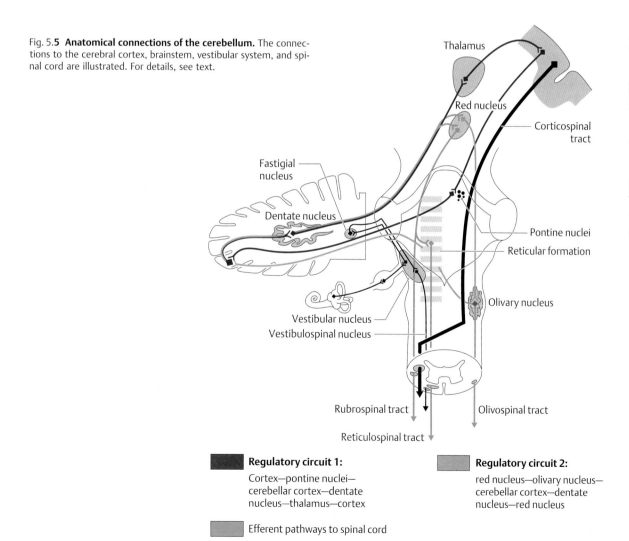

Thalamus

Red nucleus

Corticospinal tract

Fastigial nucleus

Dentate nucleus

Pontine nuclei

Reticular formation

Olivary nucleus

Vestibular nucleus

Vestibulospinal nucleus

Rubrospinal tract

Olivospinal tract

Reticulospinal tract

Regulatory circuit 1:
Cortex—pontine nuclei—cerebellar cortex—dentate nucleus—thalamus—cortex

Regulatory circuit 2:
red nucleus—olivary nucleus—cerebellar cortex—dentate nucleus—red nucleus

Efferent pathways to spinal cord

5

Topical Diagnosis and Differential Diagnosis

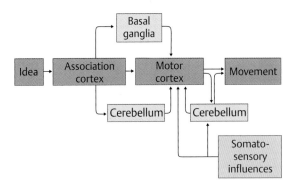

Fig. 5.**6 Functional relations of the cerebellum to other motor centers.** To keep the diagram simple, the sensory feedback to the cerebellum and basal ganglia is not shown (modified from Ellen and Tsukahara 1974).

Table 5.**8   Clinical manifestations of cerebellar disease**

Clinical manifestation	Definition/description	Remarks
Diminished muscle tone	can be felt by the examiner during repeated passive movement, e. g., pronation and supination of the forearm	
Dyssynergia	lack of coordination of the various muscle groups participating in a single movement	e. g., when walking on all fours, lack of precise alternation of limbs (each arm with opposite leg)
Dysmetria	poor control of the force, speed, and amplitude of voluntary movement	e. g., opening fingers too wide when trying to grasp a small object
Intention tremor	alternating, progressively severe deviation from the ideal course of a directed movement as the limb approaches the target	cf. Fig. 3.20
Pathological rebound phenomenon	when a muscle is actively contracted against resistance and the resistance is suddenly released, the antagonist muscles fail to contract within a normally brief interval after the release	cf. Fig. 3.21
Dysdiadochokinesia	the alternating contraction of agonists and antagonists cannot be performed as rapidly and smoothly as normal	cf. Fig. 3.17
Sinking of a limb in postural testing	the tonic muscle contraction needed to keep the limb in a particular antigravity posture cannot be sustained as long as normal on the affected side	the sinking limb is ipsilateral to the cerebellar lesion
Truncal ataxia	the patient is unable to stay sitting up	indicates a vermian lesion
Unsteady stance	observable in the Romberg test	cf. Fig. 3.1e
Cerebellar gait	wide-based, unsteady, ataxic gait	indicates involvement of the vermis
Past-pointing in the Bárány pointing test	slowly lowering the extended arm onto a previously demonstrated target, with eyes closed; deviation to the side of the affected cerebellar hemisphere	also positive in ipsilateral vestibular lesions, cf. p. 26
Nystagmus	coarse nystagmus toward the side of the lesion, increasing with gaze toward the side of the lesion, decreasing on closure of the eyes	cf. Fig. 11.1
Pathological nystagmus suppression test	the patient stands up, stretches out his or her arms forwards, stares at his or her own extended thumbs, and keeps on doing so while the examiner rapidly rotates the patient around the bodily axis; staring at the thumbs completely suppresses the induced vestibular nystagmus in normal persons, but not in persons with cerebellar disease	cf. Fig. 11.5
Cerebellar dysarthria	choppy, explosive speech ("scanning dysarthria")	patients with degenerative cerebellar diseases are said to develop a "lion's voice"

6 Diseases of the Brain and Meninges

Congenital and Perinatally Acquired Diseases of the Brain

Fundamentals

The developing brain is vulnerable to damage by a number of different pathological mechanisms. The variably severe neurological deficits that result are known collectively as cerebral movement disorders or infantile cerebral palsy (CP). In general, this term implies the presence of deficits of multiple types:

- **Disturbances of movement** of many different kinds; the more common ones are summarized in Table 6.1. These are usually accompanied by a variably severe delay of motor development.
- **Mental retardation** (sometimes designated "childhood psycho-organic syndrome") is common and is characterized by the delayed acqui-

Table 6.1 The most important cerebral movement disorders

Name of disorder	Clinical features	Pathoanatomical substrate	Causes
infantile spastic diplegia (Little disease)	spasticity, predominantly in the legs; pes equinus, scissor gait, mentally often normal	pachymicrogyria (abnormally hard, small gyri)	perinatal injury (disturbance of cerebral development, embryopathy, severe neonatal jaundice)
congenital cerebral monoparesis	usually, paresis of arm and face	porencephaly (cavities in the brain parenchyma), localized atrophy	birth trauma (asphyxia, hemorrhage)
congenital hemiparesis	arms more severely affected than legs, seizures in ca. 50%, usually mentally impaired	porencephaly	birth trauma (asphyxia, hemorrhage)
congenital quadri-paresis (bilateral hemiparesis)	arms more severely affected than legs, occasionally bulbar signs, seizures; severe mental impairment	porencephaly, bilateral; often hydrocephalus	birth trauma (asphyxia, hemorrhage), also prenatal injury
congenital pseudo-bulbar palsy	dysphagia to liquids, dysarthria, usually not mentally impaired	bilateral lesions of the corticobulbar pathways	prenatal injury or birth trauma, congenital malformation (syringobulbia)
atonic–astatic syndrome (Foerster)	generalized flaccid weakness, inability to stand, impaired coordination, severe mental impairment	frontal lobe atrophy cerebellar defects	
bilateral athetosis (athétose double) **and congenital chorea** (choreoathetosis)	athetotic or other involuntary movements, often combined with spastic paresis	basal ganglionic defects, status marmoratus (multiple confluent gliotic areas in the basal ganglia); status dysmyelinisatus (Vogt) in cases of later onset	disturbances of cerebral development, perinatal injury, esp. severe neonatal jaundice
congenital rigor	rigor without involuntary movements, postural abnormalities, no pyramidal tract signs, severe mental impairment, seizures	status marmoratus	disturbances of cerebral development, perinatal injury, esp. severe neonatal jaundice
congenital cerebellar ataxia	gait ataxia, intention tremor and impaired coordination, motor developmental retardation, dysarthria, possibly in combination with other motor syndromes	cerebellar developmental anomalies	disturbances of cerebellar development

sition of mental abilities, by impaired attention, and often also by hyperactivity and inability to concentrate. The term **psychomotor retardation** refers to a combination of movement disturbances and mental retardation.
- **Epileptic seizures** often arise later on.

Common types and their causes. Tables 6.**1**, 6.**2** provide an overview of the major types of brain damage that are present at birth, or acquired in early childhood, and their causes. These include genetic disorders, cerebral hypoxia during the birth process, birth trauma, intrauterine infections (rubella embryopathy, toxoplasmosis, cytomegalovirus, syphilis, HIV), and chronic intoxications (alcohol embryopathy). Prematurity and difficult delivery are the most important risk factors.

Possible indications of brain damage in the newborn include cyanosis at birth, a weak cry, and hypotonia. In the early prenatal period, there may be further abnormalities of muscle tone, as well as pathological reflexes (cf. p. 43 ff.). Later on, a squint or left-handedness may be a sign of brain damage.

Treatment consists of physical therapy (e. g., of the Bobath or Vojta type), which should be begun as early as possible, making use of the child's reflex behavior, as well as special education and rehabilitation. The goal of treatment is maximal independence.

Prognosis. Although the neurological deficits of cerebral palsy do not progress over time, certain manifestations may not appear until later in life (e. g., epileptic

seizures), and certain symptoms may worsen over the course of the individual's life.

Special Clinical Forms

Some of the more important etiological types of early childhood brain damage will now be discussed individually:

Hydrocephalus is a pathological dilatation of the inner (and sometimes also the outer) cerebrospinal fluid spaces. Various types of hydrocephalus are listed in Table 6.**3**. In terms of **pathogenesis**, the most common type of hydrocephalus in childhood is *occlusive hydrocephalus* (gliosis, stenosis, or malformation of the aque-

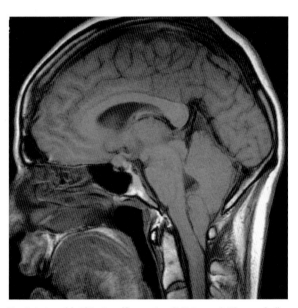

Fig. 6.1 Arnold–Chiari malformation (MR image). The cerebellar tonsils are caudally displaced below the arch of the atlas deep into the cervical spinal canal (courtesy of Dr. D. Huber, Radiological Institute, Hirslanden–Klinik, Zurich).

Table 6.**2** **Important causes of congenital and perinatally acquired brain damage**

Perinatal asphyxia

(Genetically determined) **structural anomalies of the brain**, e.g.:
- microcephaly
- meningoencephalocele
- meningomyelocele
- micropolygyria
- Arnold–Chiari malformation, with or without hydrocephalus

Phakomatoses
- tuberous sclerosis (Bourneville disease)
- encephalofacial angiomatosis (Sturge–Weber disease)
- neurofibromatosis (von Recklinghausen disease)
- von Hippel–Lindau disease

Brain damage acquired in utero
- rubella embryopathy
- congenital toxoplasmosis
- congenital cytomegaly
- congenital syphilis
- congenital HIV infection
- alcohol embryopathy

Severe neonatal jaundice (due to Rh incompatibility)

Synostosis and craniostenosis

Traumatic intracranial hemorrhage during delivery
- subdural hematoma
- intracerebral hemorrhage
- intraventricular hemorrhage

Table 6.**3** **Types and terminology of hydrocephalus**

Internal hydrocephalus	enlargement of the ventricles:
● obstructive	due to obstruction of CSF flow within the ventricular system (e. g., aqueductal stenosis) or at its exits (e. g., obstruction of foramina of Magendie and Luschka)
● communicating	nonobstructive internal hydrocephalus
● malabsorptive	a subtype of communicating hydrocephalus due to impaired CSF resorption (e. g., cisternal adhesions or dysfunction of the pacchionian granulations)
External hydrocephalus	enlargement of the subarachnoid space over the cerebral convexities and/or in the cisterns
External and internal hydrocephalus	combination of the above
Hydrocephalus ex vacuo	internal and external hydrocephalus secondary to brain atrophy

duct, Arnold–Chiari malformation [Fig. 6.1] with impaired outflow through the foramina of Luschka and Magendie). In the Arnold–Chiari malformation, part of the medulla and the cerebellar tonsils are displaced below the foramen magnum into the cervical spinal canal. This anomaly may be combined with internal hydrocephalus and syringomyelia.

There may also be communicating hydrocephalus, whose etiology and pathogenesis are often unclear.

The chief **clinical sign** of hydrocephalus in childhood is *abnormal enlargement of the head*, which may already be noted in a prenatal ultrasound study or at birth, and which progresses over time. Protrusion of the frontal bone and depression of the orbital plate make the upper part of the sclera visible and cause the lower part of the iris to sink below the lower lid, in the so-called "setting-sun sign." The essential **diagnostic tests** are CT and/or MRI. The treatment, if required, is neurosurgical, usually the implantation of a ventriculoperitoneal or ventriculoatrial **shunt**. The **prognosis** of isolated hydrocephalus, in the absence of other neurological abnormalities, is good: once the hydrocephalus is treated, two-thirds of children go on to have a normal physical and mental development.

Microcephaly is usually due to *prenatal toxic influences* (e. g., alcohol) or *infections* (e. g., cytomegalovirus), or to genetic factors. Affected persons are generally of lower than normal intelligence.

Dysraphic malformations. The most common type is **spina bifida with meningomyelocele**: in this disorder, there is a *closure defect of the posterior arches of multiple vertebrae*, usually in the lumbosacral region, accompanied by a *prolapse of the meninges and spinal cord* through the defect. The level and extent of spinal cord involvement determine whether paralysis of the lower limbs will be manifest at birth. Even if the defect is surgically repaired in the first few hours after birth, major sensorimotor impairment and urinary disturbances generally persist. This type of malformation may be accompanied by internal hydrocephalus and by anomalies of the craniocervical junction, which often require treatment. Other dysraphic syndromes include **acrania** (partial or total absence of the skull), **anencephaly** (absence or degeneration of most of the brain, with acrania—practically always a fatal condition), and **encephalocele** (prolapse of the meninges and brain tissue through a defect in the bony skull).

Areas of neuronal heterotopia (i. e., islands of gray matter anomalously lying outside the cerebral cortex) may be found in the periventricular zones or in a subcortical layer (lamina) that creates the appearance of a "double cortex" on MRI. *Subcortical laminar heterotopia* (SCLH) is a genetic disorder of dominant inheritance caused by a mutation of the doublecortin gene on the X chromosome. The disorder is more severe, and often lethal, in males, because they lack a normal copy of the gene. In surviving males, SCLH is often combined with lissencephaly ("smooth brain," i. e., absence of the cerebral gyri and sulci). Heterotopia is a common cause of epilepsy.

Ulegyria is a type of early childhood brain damage characterized by scarring and abnormally small gyri (microgyria). These structural abnormalities can be seen on MRI.

Phakomatoses are genetic disorders that cause complex malformations and tumors predominantly affecting the *ectodermally derived structures* of the body, i. e., the brain, peripheral nervous system, and skin. They are also called *neurocutaneous disorders*. The internal organs may also be affected. An overview is provided in Table 6.**4**.

The main types of brain disorder acquired in utero are the following:

- **Rubella embryopathy** occurs in 10 % of infants that have been exposed by maternal infection in the first trimester of pregnancy. The associated anomalies include cataracts, deafness, microcephaly, and heart defects.
- **Congenital toxoplasmosis** occurs when the fetus is infected in the second half of gestation by maternal infection in a mother without previous exposure to *Toxoplasma gondii.* Its manifestations include psychomotor retardation, convulsions, progressive hydrocephalus, and visual disturbances due to chorioretinitis. Plain radiographs and CT reveal intracerebral calcifications.
- **Congenital cytomegalovirus infection** causes premature birth and low birth weight, microcephaly, hydrocephalus, convulsions, periventricular calcifications, and abnormalities in organs outside the nervous system as well.
- **Congenital HIV infection** occurs in one-quarter of all babies born to HIV-positive mothers. It causes encephalopathy with psychomotor retardation, as well as immune deficiency, with later complications.
- **Congenital syphilis** is now rare. Its typical stigmata include a saddle nose, cutaneous fissures at the corners of the mouth, and later crescentic defects of the teeth (Hutchinson teeth), interstitial keratitis, and hearing loss.
- Malformations of the skull come in many different forms: there are *dysraphic malformations* characterized by faulty closure of the cranial vault (*cranioschisis*), premature closure of the cranial sutures (*craniostenosis*), and *anomalies of the craniocervical junction* including basilar impression, platybasia, Arnold–Chiari syndrome (p. 84), and Dandy–Walker syndrome (malformation of the posterior fossa with aplasia of the inferior portion of the cerebellar vermis, cystic enlargement of the fourth ventricle, and occlusive hydrocephalus). The more common types of craniosynostosis are listed and illustrated in Table 6.**5**.

6

Diseases of the Brain and Meninges

Table 6.**4**   **The most important phakomatoses**

Disease	Neuropathology and clinical neurological manifestations	Further features	Age of onset and other remarks
tuberous sclerosis (Bourneville disease)	**glial tumors** (giant cell astrocytomas, "tubers") in the ventricular walls and surface of the brain, often calcified; as a result, thickening and sclerosis of the gyri of the cerebral and cerebellar cortex. Clinical manifestations: **mental retardation, epileptic seizures**	multiple (fibro-)adenomas in the face (typically butterfly-shaped, **adenoma sebaceum**) as well as on the gums and nails; adenomas in the heart, kidney, and retina	salaam seizures often appear as early as infancy; autosomal dominant inheritance
encephalofacial angiomatosis (Sturge–Weber disease)	calcified, mixed capillary and venous **angioma of the leptomeninges**, usually unilateral, with reactive atrophy and gliosis of the neighboring brain parenchyma; serpentine intracranial calcification is a typical radiograph finding. Possible clinical manifestations: **epileptic seizures, mental retardation**, and sometimes **hemiparesis**	**choroidal hemangioma** and angioma of the face **(nevus flammeus)** on the same side as the intracranial lesion	onset in early childhood; sporadic or dominant inheritance pattern, with variable penetrance
von Hippel–Lindau disease	cystic hemangioblastoma, usually in a cerebellar hemisphere, causing progressive cerebellar signs and signs of intracranial hypertension	**retinal angiomatosis;** less commonly, cystic changes of other internal organs (esp. kidney, pancreas, epididymis)	onset in middle age; autosomal dominant inheritance
neurofibromatosis (von Recklinghausen disease)	**multiple neurofibromas** of peripheral nerves, nerve roots (particularly in the cauda equina) and cranial nerves; intracranially, in some cases, **bilateral acoustic neuroma** and/or **meningioma** (in neurofibromatosis type II), or **optic glioma** and/or **astrocytoma** (type I); clinically, progressive **radicular or peripheral nerve deficits** (flaccid paresis, sensory deficits), signs and symptoms of a cerebellopontine angle tumor (esp. hearing loss, tinnitus), visual impairment with optic glioma	variable number and density of nodular skin lesions, which may be either broad-based or pedunculated **(cutaneous neurofibroma)**; café-au-lait spots	the cutaneous changes are often present at birth or become apparent in early childhood; they typically become very prominent in puberty. Malignant degeneration is possible. Autosomal dominant inheritance, with frequent new mutations

Table 6.**5**   **Types of craniosynostosis**

Type	Fused suture	Shape of head	Remarks
scaphocephaly (=dolichocephaly)	sagittal suture	long, narrow ("boat-shaped")	most common form
acrocephaly	coronal suture	high, broad on top; flat forehead	
oxycephaly	sagittal, coronal, and lambdoid sutures	pointed	second most common form
brachycephaly	coronal and lambdoid sutures	short, broad	

Continued →

Table 6.**5** **Types of craniosynostosis** (Continued)

Type	Fused suture	Shape of head	Remarks
plagiocephaly	premature fusion (or incomplete fusion) of a coronal suture	asymmetrical (e.g., flattened on one side)	often due to asymmetrical muscle tone in cerebral palsy
Crouzon disease (craniofacial dysostosis)	mainly the coronal suture, and maxillary sutures in the face	broad skull and face, jutting forehead, exophtalmos, hypertelorism, hook nose, prognathism	the airway may be compromised
trigonocephaly	metopic suture	pointed forehead	
platycephaly	lambdoid suture	broad occiput	

Traumatic Brain injury

Fundamentals

Traumatic injuries of the bony skull and the underlying brain can be of different types and varying severity, depending on the nature and intensity of the causative event. There may be a **skull fracture** affecting the cranial vault or the base of the skull, a **brain contusion**, an injury to larger sized blood vessels producing a **traumatic hematoma**, or any combination of these types of injury.

- Brain injuries are either **closed** (i. e., with the dura mater intact) or **open** (with a wound extending into the subdural compartment or deeper into the brain parenchyma). Open brain injuries are associated with the risk of early or late intracranial infection.
- The **scale of clinical severity** of traumatic brain injury extends from a simple *contusion of the bony skull* to the *concussion syndrome* and the *brain contusion syndrome*. The leading clinical manifestation of a traumatic parenchymal injury is *impairment or loss of consciousness*, usually accompanied by *memory impairment* (retrograde and anterograde amnesia). A neurological deficit or epileptic seizures may also be present.
- Large traumatic hematomas, or extensive damage to the brain parenchyma with accompanying edema, may lead to a rapid rise of intracranial pressure, caus-

ing **brain compression** and possibly **brainstem herniation**.
- Traumatic hematomas may be located within the brain parenchyma (*traumatic intracerebral hematoma*) or in the adjacent meningeal compartments (*subdural* and *epidural hematoma*). Traumatic subarachnoid hemorrhage is less common.
- Frequent **late complications** of severe traumatic brain injury include *neuropsychological deficits, personality changes*, and *symptomatic epilepsy*.

Relevant Aspects of the Clinical History and Neurological Examination

In the initial phase after trauma, the *severity of injury* is assessed, with particular attention to the following aspects of the **history**:
- the duration of unconsciousness (as reported by eyewitnesses);
- the duration of amnesia for events that occurred before the injury (*retrograde amnesia*);
- the duration of amnesia for events that have occurred since the injury (*anterograde amnesia*, perhaps accompanied by confusion);
- the duration of the entire period of amnesia, which is the sum of the durations of retro- and anterograde amnesia;

- early epileptic seizures;
- bleeding from the ear or nose (indicating a basilar skull fracture).

The depth of impaired consciousness or coma in a brain-injured patient is graded numerically on the Glasgow Coma Scale (Table 6.**6**).

Important aspects of the **initial physical examination** are:

- the patient's *level of consciousness* (see above);
- *externally visible injuries*, especially of the head;
- *bleeding* and possibly *flow of cerebrospinal fluid* from the nose or ears, or in the pharynx (a CSF leak is conclusive evidence of an open brain injury, while bleeding is not);
- *injuries of the cervical spine*;
- *periorbital hematoma*; *neurological findings* (pupillary reflexes, visual impairment, nystagmus, deafness, weakness, pyramidal tract signs), general state of health, and, in particular, circulatory status.

Ancillary tests, to be performed as indicated by the clinical situation, include cervical spine radiographs and a CT and/or MRI scan of the head. Skull radiographs are hardly ever indicated.

! *Traumatic brain injuries are often accompanied by cervical spine injuries.*

Grades of Severity of Traumatic Brain Injury

The clinical grade of severity of traumatic brain injury is closely correlated with the initially evident extent of structural damage to the skull and brain, but the correlation is not absolute. For example, a patient may have an

Table 6.**6** **The Glasgow Coma Scale**

Category	Points
Best verbal response:	
none	1
unintelligible sounds	2
inappropriate words	3
disoriented	4
oriented	5
Eye opening:	
none	1
to painful stimuli	2
to auditory stimuli	3
spontaneous	4
Best motor response:	
none	1
abnormal extension	2
abnormal flexion	3
withdraws (pulls away from pain)	4
localizes (fends off painful stimulus)	5
follows commands	6
Patient's overall score	...

The overall score is the sum of the scores in the three categories.

extensive skull fracture, but no neurological deficit; another patient may sustain a relatively minor blow to the head that ruptures a bridging vein and produces a slowly growing subdural hematoma, which can compress the brain and ultimately cause coma and death. The clinical state of the patient after traumatic brain injury can be classified as follows (in order of increasing severity):

Skull contusion. Patients with the simple skull contusion syndrome have no evidence of a brain injury, i. e., no loss of consciousness or amnesia, a normal neurological examination, and normal intracranial findings on CT or MRI (if performed). Some patients with this syndrome have scalp lacerations, or even skull fractures, and headache may be present. Adequate therapy consists of a temporary restriction of activity and symptomatic medication, as required (analgesics, antiemetics).

Concussion (= mild traumatic brain injury) is characterized by a *brief, transient loss of consciousness*, usually lasting no more than a few minutes and sometimes followed by a period of confusion. The periods of retro- and anterograde amnesia are very brief. *Headache, dizziness, nausea*, and (sometimes) *vomiting* are common accompaniments of concussion in the early phase. A standard neurological examination reveals no deficit. In the past, it was generally assumed that concussion produced no structural damage to the brain, but T2-weighted MR images do, in fact, reveal diffuse axonal injury in some patients. Moreover, neuropsychological testing reveals that some patients said to have sustained no more than a concussion actually have deficits of certain characteristic types, collectively designated *minimal brain injury*. Occasional patients suffer from persistent *posttraumatic headaches*. The clinical distinction between concussion and brain contusion (see below) is not always easy to draw.

Treatment of concussion. As in the skull contusion syndrome, transient restriction of activity suffices (e. g., a few days of bed rest), combined with symptomatic medication as required (see above). The patient should on no account be immobilized any longer than necessary: as long as there is no contraindication (such as hemodynamic instability), the patient should stand up and walk with assistance on the day of injury, or within the next few days at latest. Rapidly mobilized patients tend to have less severe postconcussive symptoms with a lesser tendency toward chronification.

Brain contusion and penetrating injuries. By definition, these types of injury involve *damage to the brain parenchyma*. Compared with concussion, they produce considerably longer periods of unconsciousness and retro- and anterograde *amnesia*; indeed, the patient may not remember anything for a period of several days surrounding the time of the injury. Examination in the acute phase often reveals *neurological deficits*, which may persist. Residual anosmia is common (p. 180). CT or MRI reveals foci of contusion (Fig. 6.**2**) or intracranial hemorrhage, e. g., an acute epidural hematoma. Parenchymal injuries can be found both directly underlying the site of the external blow ("**coup**" injuries) and at the diametrically opposite location in the brain ("**contrecoup**" injuries). Injuries of the latter type are due to the violent, tissue-distorting force transmitted across the brain to the other side at the moment of injury. The Pathoanatomical findings in foci of brain contusion include ischemic and hemorrhagic tissue necrosis, small hemorrhages, tears of brain tissue and blood vessels, and secondary brain edema. Lumbar puncture, if performed (generally contraindicated!), yields bloody or xanthochromic cereobrospinal fluid.

Large brain contusions and extensive traumatic hematomas (see below), combined with the associated secondary brain edema, can cause very rapid and pronounced increases in intracranial pressure, leading to brain compression and **herniation** of the midbrain and diencephalon through the tentorial notch, and/or of the medulla through the foramen magnum. The clinical signs of brainstem herniation are: progressive impairment of consciousness leading to coma; a dilated pupil, initially only on the side of the expansive lesion; flexor and, later, extensor spasms; and, finally, a loss of autonomic regulatory functions (breathing, temperature, cardiac activity, vascular tone), bilaterally fixed and dilated pupils, and death.

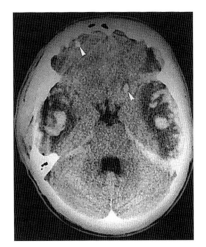

Fig. 6.**2 Brain contusion (CT scan).** There are extensive hemorrhagic contusions in both temporal lobes and smaller ones in both frontal lobes (arrowheads).

> ! *All patients with traumatic brain injury must be carefully clinically observed for signs of increasing intracranial pressure. In patients with a diminished level of consciousness, or coma, the width and reactivity of the pupils and other brainstem reflexes should be checked regularly, so that intracranial hypertension can be detected at the earliest possible moment. In some patients, pressure-measuring devices will be implanted intracranially for continuous, invasive ICP monitoring.*

Treatment of the brain contusion syndrome. Depending on his or her clinical state, the patient may need to be observed in an *intensive care unit* or dedicated neurotrauma unit, with frequent checking of the vital signs and neurological functions, and possibly with invasive ICP monitoring. Extensive parenchymal injuries and the associated brain edema usually elevate the intracranial pressure; thus, *ICP-reducing measures* may need to be taken, including elevation of the patient's head, hyperventilation (in some patients), osmotherapy, or even craniectomy to relieve brain compression (p. 93). Recent studies have shown a positive effect of *therapeutic hypothermia*, in which the patient is cooled to ca. 34 °C.

If the patient survives, MRI may reveal a permanent injury to the brain parenchyma (Fig. 6.**3**). The late posttraumatic symptoms resemble those of concussion, but they are more intense and usually persist longer. For further details, see p. 91.

Traumatic Hematomas

Traumatic hematomas come about when the traumatic injury tears a larger artery or vein (Fig. 6.**4**). They are classified as follows:

Intracerebral hematomas are usually found in the frontal or temporal lobe. They may exert considerable mass effect; combined with the surrounding edema,

Fig. 6.**3 Parenchymal defects 6 years after brain contusion.** The T2-weighted MR images reveal cortical defects in the left temporal (**a**) and frontal lobes (**b**), accompanied by signal changes in the underlying white matter.

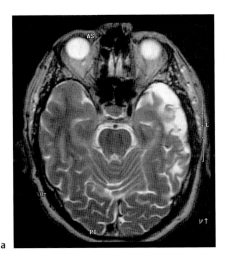

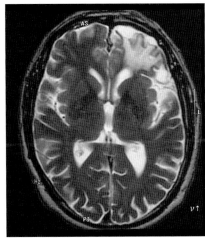

a   b

they may cause sufficient pressure on the brain to produce a *progressive decline of consciousness* and *increasingly severe neurological deficits.* In such patients, neurosurgical evacuation of the hematoma should be considered, depending on its size and location.

Epidural hematomas (Fig. 6.5) are generally produced by traumatic tearing of a dural artery, usually the middle meningeal a. The tear itself is usually the result of a temporoparietal skull fracture, but sometimes occurs in the absence of a skull fracture. The blood collection lies between the periosteum and the dura mater. The arterial hemorrhage can compress the brain very rapidly: a patient who is initially comatose because of a coexisting brain contusion may fail to emerge from coma because of the development of an epidural hematoma in the minutes or hours after injury. On the other hand, an initially awake or only transiently unconscious patient may lapse into coma after a so-called "*lucid interval*" lasting minutes or hours. The side of the hematoma can often be ascertained by clinical examination: incipient uncal herniation compresses the ipsilateral oculomotor n. and causes dilation of the ipsilateral pupil, while the *hemiparesis* is contralateral to the hematoma. When an acute epidural hematoma is suspected, a CT scan should be performed immediately to confirm the diagnosis (*not*

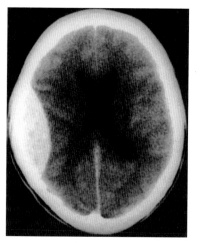

Fig. 6.**5 Epidural hematoma (CT scan).**

plain films or MRI; see note, below). The hematoma is usually seen as a *hyperdense, biconvex zone* that is sharply demarcated from the adjacent brain tissue. Once diagnosed, it must be neurosurgically evacuated immediately to prevent brainstem herniation and death. Patients often make an excellent recovery if they

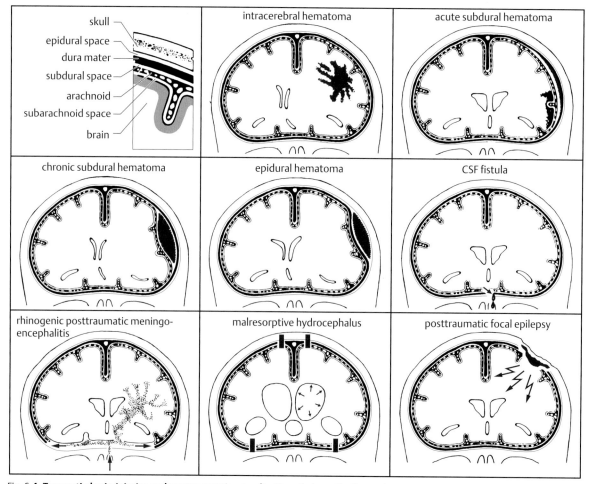

Fig. 6.**4 Traumatic brain injuries and posttraumatic complications** (schematic diagram).

have no other accompanying brain injuries and if the hematoma has been removed early enough.

Note: when an epidural hematoma is suspected, plain radiographs of the skull and MRI are both contraindicated. The former might reveal a fracture, but cannot reveal the hematoma; the latter will show the hematoma, but takes longer than CT, and time is of the essence.

Subdural hematomas can be *acute, subacute,* or *chronic.* The blood collection lies between the dura mater and the arachnoid and comes about because of a tear in a bridging vein.

Acute subdural hematoma is usually a component of severe traumatic brain injury with extensive intra-parenchymal contusional hemorrhages. Clinical examination alone does not enable a clear-cut distinction between subdural and epidural hematomas: subdural hematoma, too, is characterized by a *rapidly progressive decline of consciousness, ipsilateral pupillary dilatation,* and *contralateral hemiparesis.* The diagnosis is established by CT: a subdural hematoma is typically seen as a hyperdense or isodense area (depending on the time elapsed since the traumatic event), either crescent shaped or closely applied to the skull; unlike an epidural hematoma, a subdural hematoma is poorly demarcated from the underlying brain tissue. Subdural hematomas, too, are treated by immediate neurosurgical evacuation.

Chronic subdural hematoma may arise in the aftermath of a mild traumatic brain injury or even after a relatively trivial blow to the head, of which the patient may no longer have any recollection. A few weeks or (rarely) months after the causative event, the patient begins to suffer from *increasingly severe headache,* fluctuating disturbances of consciousness, *confusion,* and ultimately *progressive somnolence.* Hemiparesis, if present, is usually mild and signs of intracranial hypertension are usually absent. The diagnosis is established by CT or MRI. The treatment is by *neurosurgical evacuation* through one or two burr holes (this is a relatively brief and uncomplicated procedure and can be performed under local anesthesia in cooperative patients). Therapeutic anticoagulation is a risk factor for the development of a chronic subdural hematoma.

Complications of Traumatic Brain Injury

Early Complications

Early posttraumatic infection. Any open or penetrating brain injury (e. g., depressed skull fractures, gunshot wounds) provides a route of access for bacterial contamination of the meningeal spaces and the brain. *Early posttraumatic meningitis, subdural empyema, cerebritis,* or a *brain abscess* may appear a few days or weeks after the traumatic event.

Later Complications

Late infection. A skull base fracture associated with a dural tear may create a **cerebrospinal fluid fistula,** manifesting clinically as leakage of clear fluid out the nose or ear (CSF rhino- or otorrhea) or into the pharynx. Leaking CSF fistulae are sometimes accompanied by *orthostatic headache* due to intracranial hypotension. If the fistula remains undiscovered or untreated, it can serve as a portal for bacterial infection. The patient may present with **meningitis** and/or a **brain abscess,** perhaps years after the initial trauma. The presence and exact location of a CSF fistula can be demonstrated by isotope cisternography (Fig. 4.**12**, p. 53); other useful studies include MRI and thin-section CT, which may reveal a bony defect or fracture. CSF fistulae should be surgically repaired.

Posttraumatic neurological deficits. The commonest *cranial nerve* deficit after traumatic brain injury is anosmia (p. 180), which is permanent in two-thirds of patients, followed by optic nerve injuries and palsies of the nerves to the eye muscles. Optic nerve dysfunction only rarely improves, but palsies of cranial nerves III, IV, and VI usually resolve in two to three months. Fractures of the petrous pyramid(s) may cause facial nerve palsy as well as deafness, due to injury either to the vestibulo-cochlear nerve or to the cochlea itself; when caused by a transverse fracture, deafness is usually permanent. A fracture extending into the jugular foramen may cause a combined palsy of the glossopharyngeal, vagus, and accessory nerves (Siebenmann syndrome). *Focal brain lesions* cause deficits according to their localization. *Diencephalic lesions* often cause diabetes insipidus. Spasticity may be uni- or bilateral. Cerebellar lesions are characterized by ataxia, which does not always resolve.

Posttraumatic epilepsy is seen within two years in 80 % of the patients who develop it, but it can also arise many years after the initial trauma in rare cases. The seizures may be focal, secondarily generalized, or primarily generalized (cf. p. 164).

Neuropsychological deficits and personality changes. Posttraumatic neuropsychological deficits (variously designated focal organic brain syndrome, psycho-organic syndrome, or posttraumatic encephalopathy) and personality changes are often the most disabling sequelae of traumatic brain injury for the patient and his or her family. The severity of these problems is positively correlated with the length of the initial loss of consciousness and with the duration of retrograde and anterograde amnesia around the time of the injury. Both short- and long-term memory are impaired and the attention span is shorter than normal. The patient has difficulty coping with complex tasks and situations and is easily fatigued. Impatience, irritability, diminished initiative, poor concentration, and lack of interest ranging to apathy characterize the patient's behavior. The adverse psychosocial effects in personal and professional life are often very serious.

Rarer posttraumatic phenomena include a *persistent Lhermitte sign* (p. 157) or *malresorptive hydrocephalus.*

Malresorptive hydrocephalus most commonly arises after a traumatic subarachnoid hemorrhage and consists of an *impairment of CSF flow and resorption due to adhesions of the arachnoid and of the arachnoid granulations.* It can also arise in the aftermath of aneurysmal subarachnoid hemorrhage (p. 108), meningitis, or venous sinus thrombosis, or spontaneously, i. e., without any known risk factor. Impaired CSF (out-)flow causes ventricular dilatation. The clinical findings include:

- a progressively severe gait disturbance with spastic paraparesis,
- urinary incontinence,
- fluctuating neuropsychological abnormalities,
- and sometimes also headache.

CT reveals enlarged and rounded lateral ventricles, while the subarachnoid space appears tight or of normal dimensions, but never widened. The CSF pressure measured at lumbar puncture is within normal limits (hence the alternative name of this condition, "normal pressure hydrocephalus"). If 20–50 mL of CSF are removed, the symptoms listed above all improve, particularly the gait disturbance: the originally "sticky" and small-stepped gait suddenly becomes much more fluid.

Intracranial Pressure and Brain Tumors

Intracranial Pressure

Intracranial masses rapidly elevate the intracranial pressure because the skull is a closed compartment. Intracranial hypertension is most commonly caused by **tumor, hemorrhage, extensive stroke, trauma** (and the edema accompanying these conditions), and **hydrocephalus**. It can also be caused by a variety of other conditions (cf. Table 6.**7**). Intracranial hypertension **impairs cerebral perfusion and CSF circulation** and may also result in **compression of intracranial structures** (e. g., compression of cranial nerves against the base of the skull, occlusive compression of the posterior cerebral a.) and to **shifting of large portions of the brain** within the skull (e. g., herniation of the medial portion of the temporal lobe into the tentorial notch, or of the cerebellar tonsils into the foramen magnum). Intracranial hypertension may arise **acutely**, i. e., in a few minutes or hours (especially in brain hemorrhage), or **chronically** (for example, when caused by a slowly growing brain tumor). Its clinical manifestations vary accordingly (Table 6.**8**). Its treatment consists of general measures to lower intracranial pressure as well as specific treatment of the underlying cause.

Intracranial hypertension is diagnosed from its characteristic clinical manifestations and ancillary test

Table 6.**7** **Causes of intracranial hypertension**

Category	Particular entities	Clinical features	Remarks
intracranial mass	brain tumor, subdural hematoma, intracerebral hematoma, extensive infarction (esp. middle cerebral a. territorial infarction)	focal neurological and neuropsychological deficits, headache	
infection	encephalitis, meningitis	fever, meningism	e. g., neurobrucellosis, syphilis
traumatic brain injury	contusion, brain edema, intracerebral hematoma	progressively severe manifestations due to brain edema; focal seizures	
impairment of cerebrospinal fluid flow or resorption	intraventricular tumors aqueductal stenosis malresorptive hydrocephalus	headache (possibly ictal), vomiting diagnosis by CT spasticity of legs, urinary incontinence, psycho-organic syndrome.	intermittent intracranial hypertension with history of prior subarachnoid hemorrhage or meningitis
elevation of cerebrospinal fluid protein concentration	e. g., in polyradiculitis, spinal tumors (esp. schwannoma)	lumbar puncture yields cerebrospinal fluid with elevated protein	
toxic processes	lead poisoning, insecticide poisoning	psycho-organic syndrome, anemia, lead line (on gums), sometimes other neurological and systemic signs and symptoms	
iatrogenic	steroids, oral contraceptives, tetracycline		
altitude sickness	rapid ascent	headache, pulmonary edema, retinal hemorrhage, angina pectoris	descend immediately!
pseudotumor cerebri		usually affects obese young women; slit ventricles, sometimes papilledema	a diagnosis of exclusion
empty sella syndrome		CT shows an apparently empty sella turcica containing air	may be associated with visual disturbances

Table 6.**8**   **Signs of intracranial hypertension**

subjective	headache (diffuse and persistent, most severe in the morning); *with acute or rapidly progressive elevation of intracranial pressure*, nausea and vomiting (typically in the morning–paroxysmal dry heaves), hiccups; *with chronic elevation of intracranial pressure*, progressive lack of motivation, apathy
signs of impending herniation	*with acute or rapidly progressive elevation of intracranial pressure*, confusion, respiratory disturbance, bradycardia, hypertension, cerebellar fits (opisthotonus and extensor spasms of arms and legs), dilated pupils
ocular findings	papilledema (present in ca. two-thirds of cases, may appear within hours), occas. retinal hemorrhage; enlarged blind spot, attacks of amblyopia with transient blindness; occas. oculomotor nerve palsy or abducens nerve palsy (the abducens n. has the longest course in the subarachnoid space of any of the cranial nerves)
skull radiograph	the plain skull radiograph is abnormal only in *chronic intracranial hypertension*–increased digitate markings, enlarged sella turcica with demineralized dorsum sellae, diastasis of one or more cranial sutures in children and adolescents
CT/MRI	slit ventricles (when elevation of ICP is due to cerebral edema), compressed gyri, periventricular signal change; CT and MRI may reveal the causative lesion for intracranial hypertension (e. g., tumor, hemorrhage)
EEG	diffusely abnormal, nonspecific
lumbar puncture	*contraindicated when a dangerous elevation of ICP is suspected!* If LP is nonetheless performed in the face of intracranial hypertension, the opening pressure is generally over 200 mm CSF; may be normal, however, if CSF flow is blocked at the occipitocervical or spinal level

results, as listed in Table 6.**8**. Lumbar puncture for direct measurement of the CSF pressure is nearly always *contraindicated*.

> **!** *A lumbar puncture should, in general, not be performed if there is clinical evidence of intracranial hypertension. It may be performed only if the imaging studies and ophthalmoscopic examination have yielded no evidence of acutely elevated ICP with impending brain herniation.*

Treatment of intracranial hypertension includes the following general measures to lower the intracranial pressure:

- elevation of the head of the patient to 30°;
- hyperventilation (if the patient is intubated);
- osmotic diuretics, such as mannitol, given intravenously, in fractionated daily doses; rapid infusion is important for the generation of an effective osmotic gradient; saluretics, too, can transiently lower the intracranial pressure (caution: excessive use of diuretics can lead to dehydration and impairment of cerebral perfusion);
- corticosteroids (e. g., dexamethasone, given intravenously) are used to counteract cerebral edema, particularly of the vasogenic type; they are mainly effective against peritumoral and inflammatory brain edema, less so against ischemic and traumatic brain edema, which are predominantly of the cytotoxic type.

Brain Tumors

Fundamentals

The prevalence of brain tumors is roughly one per 10 000 to 20 000 individuals. Brain tumors are one of the more common causes of intracranial hypertension. They are subdivided into **primary brain tumors** arising from the brain tissue itself (either the neuroepithelial tissue or the neighboring mesenchymal tissues, e. g., the meninges) and **brain metastases**. Brain tumors produce **focal brain signs** of different types depending on the location of the tumor, as well as **signs of intracranial hypertension** that may be more or less rapidly progressive depending on the rate of tumor growth.

General clinical manifestations of brain tumors include the following:

- *epileptic seizures* (focal or generalized);
- *mental changes* (irritability, fatigability, impairment of memory and concentration);
- *focal neurological* and/or *neuropsychological deficits* depending on the location and type of the tumor;
- less commonly, *headache* (diffuse, at night as well as in the daytime) and occasionally *nausea and vomiting*;
- in some patients, *further signs of intracranial hypertension* (as listed in Table 6.**8**).

The clinical manifestations of a brain tumor progress more or less rapidly depending on the type and growth rate of the tumor. Malignant tumors typically present with a **"crescendo" course**, in which overt signs and symptoms arise soon after the onset of the illness, then progress steadily and rapidly. The manifestations of benign tumors, on the other hand, often progress slowly and insidiously, perhaps over many years. Indeed, the tumor may be present for years before it becomes clinically evident.

Diagnosis. Neuroimaging studies are essential (contrast-enhanced CT or, better, *MRI*; cf. Table 6.**9**) but cannot always unequivocally identify the type of tumor. A definitive determination is often not possible until the tumor has been at least partly removed and the tumor tissue can be histopathologically examined. If a brain tumor is inoperable because of its location, or if primary resection is contraindicated by the patient's general condition or other illnesses, then a **stereotactic brain bi-**

opsy can be performed to obtain tissue for diagnosis. This should, in general, be done before any nonsurgical treatment is undertaken, such as chemotherapy or radiotherapy, so that the form of treatment can be chosen for maximum effectiveness. A further reason for doing so is that a small percentage of suspected "brain tumors" will turn out, on biopsy, to be brain abscesses. These can often be effectively treated with antibiotics (and, in some patients, resection).

Treatment. Complete resection of the tumor is indicated whenever it is possible. The operability of brain tumors, however, depends largely on their size, location, histological grade, and relation to the surrounding brain tissue (infiltration vs. displacement). Not every tumor is neurosurgically accessible or fully resectable. Depending on the type of tumor, radiotherapy and/or chemotherapy may have to be used, either as the primary form of treatment, or as adjuvant therapy after a complete or incomplete surgical removal.

The brain edema that usually accompanies malignant tumors is treated with corticosteroids (usually dexamethasone).

Individual Types of Brain Tumor

The WHO classification of brain tumors (1993) is summarized in Table 6.**9**, which also includes figures concerning the relative frequency of tumor types. The characteristic locations, clinical manifestations, and course of brain tumors all depend on the type of tumor.

Astrocytoma, the most common category of neuroepithelial tumor, has the following histological subtypes:

Glioblastoma multiforme is the most malignant grade of astrocytoma (grade IV astrocytoma). This *most common and most malignant tumor of the cerebral hemispheres* usually arises *between the ages of 40 and 60.* It grows by infiltration into brain tissue and is thus nearly impossible to resect totally, as nests of tumor cells nearly always remain beyond the margins of resection even if all macroscopically evident tumor tissue is removed. Though it generally arises in a single hemisphere, it can infiltrate across the corpus callosum into the opposite hemisphere, creating a so-called butterfly tumor. Glioblas-

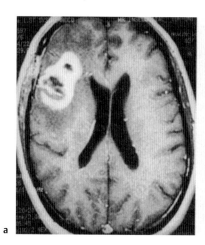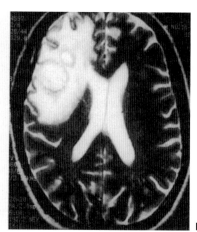

Fig. 6.**6 Glioblastoma multiforme in the right frontal lobe.** The T1- and T2-weighted spin-echo images (**a** and **b**, respectively) reveal a polycystic tumor surrounded by marked edema.

a   b

Table 6.**9   Classification and diagnosis of brain tumors**

WHO Classification (1993)	WHO grade *
Neuroepithelial tumors	
● astrocytic tumors	
○ fibrillary, protoplasmic, mixed	II
○ anaplastic (malignant) astrocytoma	III
○ glioblastoma multiforme	IV
○ pilocytic astrocytoma	I
○ pleomorphic xanthoastrocytoma	I
○ subependymal giant cell astrocytoma (in tuberous sclerosis)	I
● oligodendroglial tumors	
○ oligodendroglioma	II
○ anaplastic (malignant) oligodendroglioma	III
● ependymal cell tumors	
○ ependymoma	II
○ anaplastic (malignant) ependymoma	III
○ myxopapillary ependymoma, subependymoma	I
● mixed gliomas	
○ oligoastrocytoma	II
○ anaplastic (malignant) oligoastrocytoma	III

* Grading, on a scale of increasing malignancy from I to IV, is based on histologic criteria (mitoses, etc.).

Continued →

Table 6.**9** **Classification and diagnosis of brain tumors** (continued)

WHO Classification (1993)	WHO grade *
• choroid plexus tumors	
• choroid plexus papilloma	I
• choroid plexus carcinoma	III, IV
• neuroepithelial tumors of uncertain origin	variable
• neuronal and mixed neuronal–glial tumors	I–III
• pineal parenchymal tumors	
• pineocytoma	II
• mixed pineocytoma/pineoblastoma	III, IV
• pineoblastoma	IV
• embryonal tumors	
• medulloepithelioma; neuroblastoma; ependymoblastoma	IV
• primitive neuroectodermal tumors (PNETs)	IV
• medulloblastoma and variants	IV
Tumors of the cranial and spinal nerves	
• schwannoma (neurilemmoma, neurinoma)	I
• neurofibroma	I
• malignant peripheral nerve sheath tumor (MPNST), neurogenic sarcoma, neurofibrosarcoma, anaplastic neurofibroma, "malignant schwannoma"	III, IV
Tumors of the meninges	
• meningothelial tumors	
• meningioma and its variants	I
• atypical meningioma	II
• papillary meningioma	II, III
• anaplastic (malignant) meningioma	III
• mesenchymal, nonmenigothelial tumors (benign, e. g., lipoma; malignant, e. g., meningeal sarcoma)	
• primary melanocytic lesions	
• diffuse melanosis, melanocytoma, malignant melanoma	
• tumors of uncertain histogenesis	
• hemangioblastoma	
Lymphoma and neoplasms of the hematopoietic system	"Kiel classification"
• malignant lymphoma	
• plasmacytoma	
• others	
Germ cell tumors	
• germinoma, embryonal sarcoma, choriocarcinoma	III, IV
• teratoma	I
• mixed germ cell tumors	
Cysts and tumorlike lesions	
Tumors of the sellar region	
• pituitary adenoma	I
• pituitary carcinoma	III, IV
• craniopharyngioma	I
Local extensions of regional tumors	
Metastases	
Unclassified tumors	

* Grading, on a scale of increasing malignancy from I to IV, is based on histologic criteria (mitoses, etc.).

Relative frequency of primary brain tumors: pilocytic astrocytoma 1 %, low-grade astrocytoma 27 %, anaplastic astrocytoma 3 %, glioblastoma 28 %, oligodendroglioma 2 %, ependymoma 1 %, medulloblastoma 2 %, meningioma 22 %, neurinoma 4 %, primary CNS lymphoma 1 %

Ancillary diagnostic tests
Imaging studies:
- reveal the site and extent of the tumor before surgery (biopsy or resection)
- CT with contrast: often the method by which a mass is first diagnosed, but of limited diagnostic value:
  - advantages: good at displaying tumor calcification and the relation of certain types of tumor (e. g., meningioma) to adjacent bony structures
  - disadvantages: even with contrast, some tumors such as low-grade astrocytomas are revealed poorly or not at all; poor distinction between tumor tissue and surrounding brain edema; artifact impairs visibility at the skull base and in the posterior fossa
- MRI with contrast: the imaging method of choice for all intracranial tumors:
  - advantages: highly sensitive (reveals clinically "silent" metastases), clear visualization of the site and borders of the tumor in multiple imaging planes
  - disadvantage: calcification not reliably seen
- angiography: preoperative visualization of blood vessels is useful for certain types of tumor (e. g., medial sphenoid wing meningiomas impinging on the internal carotid a.); reveals possible infiltration or occlusion of the venous sinuses; provides access for intravascular treatment ("embolization") of meningiomas; enables diagnosis and precise anatomical characterization of vascular malformations and aneurysms

6

Diseases of the Brain and Meninges

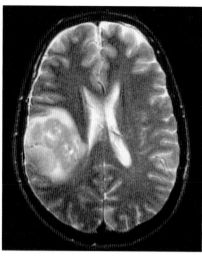

Fig. 6.**7 Grade III astrocytoma** (partly cystic) in the right parieto-temporal region, as revealed by MRI.

tomas grow rapidly, causing rapidly progressive clinical manifestations; they are, therefore, usually diagnosed within a few weeks or (at most) months of the onset of symptoms. *Focal neurological* and/or *neuropsychological deficits* arise first, sometimes accompanied by *epileptic seizures*, soon followed by *general manifestations of intracranial hypertension* (see above). The diagnosis can be made with a fair degree of confidence from the typical appearance in neuroimaging studies (Fig. 6.**6**), though this does not obviate the need for histological examination of tumor tissue. CT characteristically reveals a central hypodense area, corresponding to necrosis in the interior of the tumor. There may be hyperdense areas indicating intratumoral hemorrhage. Peritumoral brain edema is often extensive, causing mass effect and midline shift. Ringlike enhancement is seen after the administration of contrast medium.

Even with the best currently available treatment, i. e., gross total resection of the tumor with or without adjuvant radio- or chemotherapy, patients with glioblastoma survive only a few months, or a few years at most, because of the nearly inevitable recurrences. Grade III astrocytoma (Fig. 6.**7**) is another type of histologically malignant astrocytoma. The prognosis of patients with this type of tumor, though marginally better than that of glioblastoma patients, is still poor.

Grade I and II astrocytomas (so-called "benign" astrocytomas) are *less malignant* than grades III and IV. **Astrocytomas of the cerebral hemisphere(s)** generally affect *adults aged 30 to 40.* Though these tumors displace and infiltrate the surrounding brain tissue, they are better demarcated from it than glioblastoma; they often grow quite slowly, sometimes over many years. Their clinical manifestations include *behavioral and neuropsychological changes*, increasingly severe *focal neurological deficits* (e. g., hemiparesis), focal or secondarily generalized *epileptic seizures*, and signs of *intracranial hypertension.* If epileptic seizures are the only manifestation, tumor resection may be useful for seizure control, if the location of the tumor permits. After a tumor is totally resected, it may not recur until years later.

Cerebellar astrocytoma is *considerably more benign* than the other varieties, usually affects *children aged 5 to 15*, and is *well demarcated* from the surrounding brain tissue. It is usually found in the cerebellar hemispheres or vermis and may extend into the pons. Its main clinical manifestations are thus *ataxia, disequilibrium, nystagmus,* and, often, signs of *intracranial hypertension* (esp. papilledema) secondary to occlusive hydrocephalus. Total resection often results in permanent cure.

Brainstem astrocytoma is usually inoperable, though tumors of this type are sometimes at least partly resectable in special cases.

Ependymoma is a *benign tumor* usually seen in *children and adolescents.* On pathological examination, these tumors are often cystic and partly calcified. They develop from the neuroepithelium of the walls of the cerebral ventricles and the central canal of the spinal cord; as they grow, they displace, but do not invade, the adjacent neural tissue. Ependymomas usually arise in the posterior fossa, most commonly near the fourth ventricle, and in the conus medullaris of the spinal cord (Fig. 7.**7**, p. 147). Their main clinical manifestations are *focal (often cerebellar) neurological deficits* and signs of *intracranial hypertension*, secondary to compression of the CSF pathways and occlusive hydrocephalus. An unusually persistent, continuous *headache* in children should arouse suspicion of an ependymoma or other mass in the posterior fossa. The treatment is by resection, followed by radiotherapy of the entire neuraxis. Seventy percent of treated patients survive for 10 years or longer.

Medulloblastoma also mainly affects children (in three-quarters of cases). This is an *undifferentiated, highly malignant* tumor characterized by rapid growth and *rapidly progressive clinical manifestations.* Medulloblastomas usually arise from the roof of the fourth ventricle, sometimes filling the entire ventricle, and grow into the inferior portion of the vermis. They grow by infiltration and often metastasize via the CSF into the spinal canal (*drop metastases*). The signs and symptoms resemble those of cerebellar astrocytoma (*headache, nausea, truncal ataxia*—see above), possibly combined with manifestations referable to the *spinal cord and cauda equina.* Medulloblastoma is treated by resection followed by radiotherapy or chemotherapy. The prognosis after radical removal is not unfavorable, but often no more than an incomplete removal can be achieved, in which case tumor recurrence is the rule.

Oligodendroglioma is usually found in the cerebral hemispheres, particularly the frontal lobes. It tends to arise *between the ages of 40 and 50* and is usually a *relatively well-differentiated tumor* that grows slowly over the years and often becomes calcified. It usually presents with *epileptic seizures*; recurrent seizures affect 70% of patients with this type of tumor. Oligodendroglioma is mostly radioresistant and is best treated by radical resection. If this can be achieved, radiotherapy is usually not given. Nonetheless, apparently radical resection can be followed by tumor recurrence, which may not take place until years after surgery.

Table 6.**10**   **Common sites of meningiomas, and associated clinical features**

Site	Most common initial manifestations	Course	Special features
olfactory groove	anosmia	epileptic seizures, headache, frontal-type personality change, possible involvement of optic nerve	the frontal branch of the temporal artery may be enlarged
convexity	epileptic seizures	hemiparesis	
parasagittal and falx	lower extremity paresis, (sometimes) bilateral Babinski sign	epileptic seizures	rarely causes paraparesis
sphenoid wing	visual disturbances (when medially located, adjacent to optic nerve)	exophthalmos, hemiparesis	lateral tumors may be externally evident as temporal hyperostosis
tuberculum sellae	visual disturbances, pale optic discs	progressive visual field defect	
cerebellopontine angle	deafness, vertigo	facial and trigeminal nerve deficits, brainstem compression	differential diagnosis: acoustic neuroma
foramen magnum	spastic quadriparesis, dysphagia, dysarthria	lower cranial nerve deficits	
intraventricular	intermittent headaches and vomiting	progressive hydrocephalus	often found in trigone
intraspinal	progressive paraparesis	paraparesis/paraplegia	

Gliomas of the optic nerve and chiasm are found almost exclusively in children, often in the setting of neurofibromatosis.

Meningiomas arise from the dura mater and are nearly always *benign*, well-demarcated lesions that displace rather than invade the adjacent neural tissue as they grow. These mesodermal tumors most often become clinically evident *between the ages of 40 and 50*. They are diagnosed by MRI or CT scanning (Fig. 6.**8**), which reveals marked, homogeneous contrast enhancement. Meningiomas tend to appear in certain *classic locations* with corresponding typical neurological manifestations, as listed in Table 6.**10**. They often grow very slowly and are not uncommonly discovered as an incidental radiological finding. The indications for treatment must then be carefully considered: resection may be desirable in younger patients, but unnecessary in older ones.

Pituitary tumors usually arise from the cells of the anterior pituitary lobe. Depending on their cells origin, they can produce hormones in excess or cause hormone deficiency. Thus, they present clinically with *endocrine disturbances* and/or *compressive effects* on the adjacent neural tissue (see below). They most commonly present *between the ages of 30 and 50*. The rare **eosinophil adenomas** produce excessive growth hormone, causing *acromegaly*, while **basophil adenomas** produce excessive ACTH, causing *Cushing syndrome* (which, when caused by a pituitary tumor, constitutes *Cushing disease*). **Prolactinomas** produce *galactorrhea* and *secondary amenorrhea* in women and impotence in men. Although basophil adenomas and prolactinomas rarely cause mass effect, eosinophil adenomas and, above all, the hormonally inactive **chromophobe adenomas** tend to grow quite large, causing compression and dysfunction of the normal pituitary tissue, clinically evident as *hypopituitarism* (multiple pituitary hormone deficiencies, including hypothyroidism and secondary hypogonadism). Chromophobe adenomas can also compress the optic chiasm, causing a *visual field defect*, usually bitemporal upper

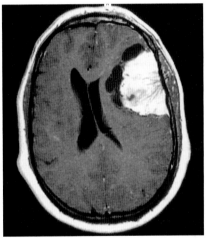

Fig. 6.**8 Meningioma of the left cerebral convexity** as seen by MRI after the intravenous administration of gadolinium. Marked mass effect deforms the ventricles and shifts the midline structures rightward. There are cystic cavities at the tumor–brain interface. Blood vessels supplying the tumor are seen entering it from its "navel" on the outer surface.

quadrantanopsia or bitemporal hemianopsia. Compression of the optic nerves themselves may impair visual acuity. Prompt neurosurgical removal of the tumor can often reverse these visual difficulties if they are still incomplete at the time of surgery. Most pituitary tumors do not present with signs of mass effect (only one in 10 enlarges the sella turcica visibly on plain films of the skull). Tumors that do cause mass effect should be neurosurgically removed, preferably by the transsphenoidal route. Hormonally active microadenomas can sometimes be treated with medication alone (e. g., prolactinoma can be treated with inhibitors of prolactin secretion, such as bromocriptine and lisuride).

Malformations and hamartomatous tumors include craniopharyngioma, dermoid and epidermoid tumors, and cavernoma. **Craniopharyngioma** arises in or above the pituitary fossa, often growing upward toward the diencephalon and third ventricle. This is a cystic tumor derived from epithelial remnants in Rathke's pouch, generally containing calcifications as well as cholesterol crystals. It presents with *hypopituitarism* (see above), *diencephalic manifestations* (diabetes insipidus), and *visual disturbances.* Like a pituitary tumor, it can cause hemi- or quadrantanopsia and impair visual acuity; it can also cause *occlusive hydrocephalus.* Craniopharyngioma is the most common suprasellar tumor in *children and adolescents.* It is best treated by complete resection.

Cavernoma (also called cavernous angioma or cavernous malformation) consists of a well-demarcated agglomeration of blood vessels. Cavernomas can be multiple and familial (genetic locus on chromosome 7). They present with *epileptic seizures and hemorrhage.*

Epidermoid tumors are found at the base of the brain, are often calcified, and cause *focal deficits* or *epileptic seizures.* Their peak incidence is *between the ages of 25 and 45.*

Neurinomas (schwannomas) are benign neoplasms arising from Schwann cells. The most common type affects the eighth cranial nerve and is usually (though incorrectly) designated **acoustic neuroma**. This tumor of the cerebellopontine angle presents initially with *eighth nerve dysfunction*: progressive hearing loss, tinnitus, and disequilibrium. As it grows, it impinges on the other cranial nerves of the cerebellopontine angle, causing *facial palsy* and *trigeminal sensory deficits.* Further growth leads to compression of the cerebellum and brainstem, causing *cerebellar signs* (esp. ataxia) and possibly *pyramidal tract signs.* Acoustic neuroma typically *markedly elevates the CSF protein concentration.* Until recently, the optimal treatment in all patients was complete resection of the tumor. Now many smaller acoustic neuromas can be treated safely and effectively with stereotactic radiosurgery.

Brain metastases account for about 15 % of malignant brain tumors. The most common source of a brain metastasis is *bronchial carcinoma* in men and *carcinoma of the breast* in women, followed in both sexes by *melanoma* and *renal cell carcinoma.* Brain metastases sometimes produce symptoms before the primary tumor does; in such cases, multiple brain metastases are usually already present, even if only a single one is apparent on the neuroimaging study. Generally speaking, surgical resection makes sense only for solitary metastases and the surgical indication should always be carefully considered in the light of the extent of disease. Only about 20 % of patients so treated live more than five years after the operation and postoperative radiotherapy, if they have not already died of the effects of their primary tumor. Brain metastases usually produce extensive peritumoral edema and often cause epileptic seizures; thus, corticosteroids and antiepileptic drugs can be given for palliation. This usually brings a substantial, if only temporary, clinical improvement.

Circulatory Disorders of the Brain and Nontraumatic Intracranial Hemorrhage

The term "stroke" encompasses both ischemic and hemorrhagic disturbances of the cerebral circulation producing central neurological deficits of acute or subacute onset. Ischemia accounts for 80 to 85 % of stroke, hemorrhage for 15 to 20 %.

Cerebral Ischemia

Ischemia causes **critical hypoperfusion** in an area of the brain. Depending on its extent and duration, hypoperfusion can induce neurological deficits that may be either **transient** (TIA, RIND) or **permanent** (completed stroke, infarction). The more common causes of ischemia are **blockage of the arterial blood supply** by arteriosclerotic processes of both larger and smaller blood vessels (**macroangiopathic and microangiopathic processes**) and **embolic events** (arterio-arterial and cardiogenic embolization). A less common cause is obstruction of **venous outflow** (e. g., venous sinus thrombosis). Every ischemic event should prompt thorough diagnostic evaluation to identify its etiology, so that effective measures can be taken to prevent a recurrence.

Nontraumatic Intracranial Hemorrhage

Regulation of cerebral perfusion. *Glucose* is the brain's nearly exclusive source of energy. The brain accounts for only about 2 % of body weight, but it receives about 15 % of the cardiac output. *Regulatory mechanisms* ensure that the cerebral perfusion remains constant despite fluctuations in the arterial blood pressure, as long as the latter remains within a certain range. Thus, if the arterial blood pressure should fall, a compensatory dilatation of the cerebral arteries occurs to maintain cerebral perfusion, which is significantly reduced only when the systolic blood pressure falls below 70 mmHg (or below 70 % of the baseline value in hypertensive individuals). Hyperventilation and elevated intracranial pressure reduce cerebral perfusion, while hypoventilation (i. e., an elevated partial pressure of CO_2) increases it.

Consequences of ischemia. Normal *cerebral perfusion* is ca. 58 mL per 100 g brain tissue per minute. Signs and symptoms of ischemia begin to appear when perfusion falls below 22 mL per 100 g per min. In this stage of **relative ischemia**, the functional metabolism of the affected brain tissue is impaired, but the *infarction threshold* has not yet been reached and the tissue can regain its normal function as soon as the perfusion renormalizes. The longer relative ischemia lasts, however, the less likely it is that normal function will be regained. The zone of tissue in which the local cerebral perfusion lies between the functional threshold and the infarction threshold is called the **ischemic penumbra** ("partial shadow").

Total ischemia causes irreversible structural damage of the affected region of the brain. If the blood supply of the entire brain is cut off, unconsciousness ensues in 10 to 12 seconds and cerebral electrical activity, as demonstrated by EEG, ceases in 30 to 40 seconds (Fig. 6.9). Cellular metabolism collapses, the sodium/potassium pump ceases to function, and interstitial fluid—i.e., sodium and water—flows into the cells. The resulting cellular swelling is called **cytotoxic cerebral edema**. Later, when the blood–CSF barrier collapses, further plasma components, including osmotically active substances, enter the brain tissue; a net flow of fluid from the intravascular space into the intercellular and intracellular spaces then produces **vasogenic cerebral edema**. In a vicious circle, these two varieties of edema lead to additional compression of brain tissue, thereby impairing the cerebral perfusion still further.

Dynamic time course of cerebral ischemia. Cerebral perfusion can cause a wide variety of clinical manifestations. In clinical practice, these are often classified by their temporal course and their degree of reversibility or irreversibility (Table 6.11). Although classification in this way is useful, it says nothing about the underlying etiology of the ischemic events. Moreover, the boundaries between the listed entities (e. g., TIA and RIND) are not sharp.

Arterial blood supply of the brain. To understand how the localization and extent of cerebral infarcts depends on the particular artery that is occluded, one must know the anatomy of the territories of the individual vessels, as well as their numerous anastomoses. The anastomotic arterial *circle of Willis*, at the base of the brain, provides a connection between the carotid and verte-

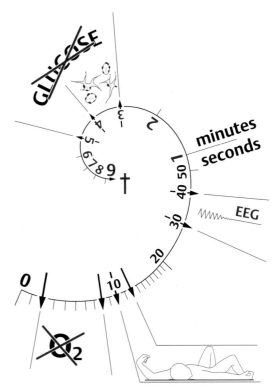

Fig. 6.**9** **Time course of cerebral ischemia.** Diagram of the effect of sudden total deprivation of blood supply to the brain on tissue metabolism, consciousness, the EEG, neuronal morphology, and tissue glucose concentration.

bral circulations and between the blood supplies of the right and left cerebral hemispheres (Fig. 6.10). The territories of the major cerebral arteries are shown in Fig. 6.11.

Table 6.**11** **Classification of cerebral ischemia by temporal course**

Designation	Duration of deficits	Remarks
TIA = **t**ransient **i**schemic **a**ttack	usually 2–15 minutes, sometimes as long as 24 hours	transient focal neurological and/or neuropsychological deficit (e. g., aphasia); a TIA in the distribution of the ophthalmic a. presents as amaurosis fugax
RIND = **r**eversible **i**schemic **n**eurological **d**eficit	up to 7 days	mostly minor neurological deficits
stroke in evolution, progressive stroke	stroke with neurological deficits that continue to worsen for hours or days after onset	
completed stroke	established neurological deficit that is irreversible or only partly reversible	

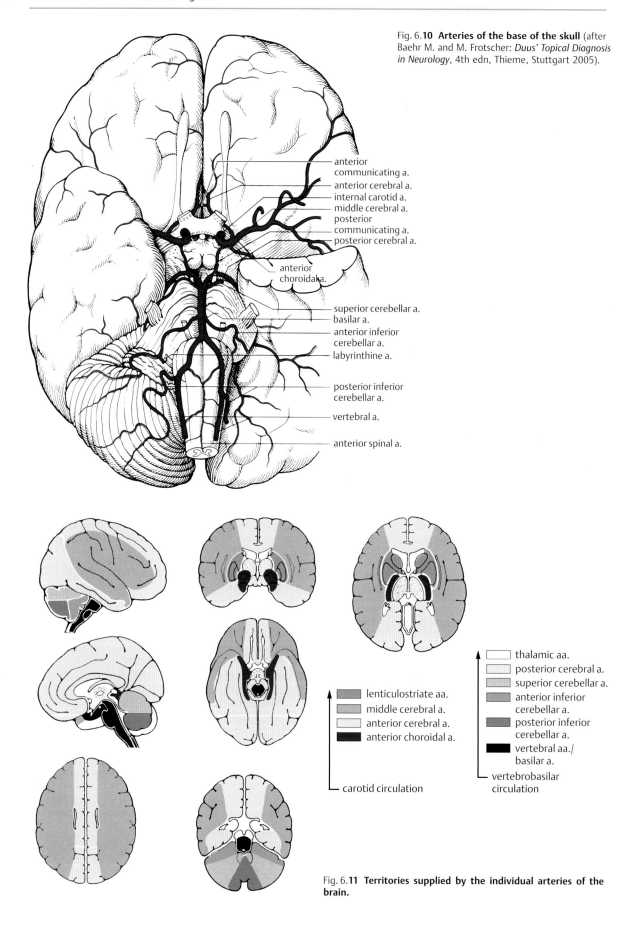

Fig. 6.**10 Arteries of the base of the skull** (after Baehr M. and M. Frotscher: *Duus' Topical Diagnosis in Neurology*, 4th edn, Thieme, Stuttgart 2005).

anterior communicating a.
anterior cerebral a.
internal carotid a.
middle cerebral a.
posterior communicating a.
posterior cerebral a.

anterior choroidal a.

superior cerebellar a.
basilar a.
anterior inferior cerebellar a.
labyrinthine a.

posterior inferior cerebellar a.

vertebral a.

anterior spinal a.

lenticulostriate aa.
middle cerebral a.
anterior cerebral a.
anterior choroidal a.

carotid circulation

thalamic aa.
posterior cerebral a.
superior cerebellar a.
anterior inferior cerebellar a.
posterior inferior cerebellar a.
vertebral aa./ basilar a.

vertebrobasilar circulation

Fig. 6.**11 Territories supplied by the individual arteries of the brain.**

Ischemic Stroke

> Ischemic stroke occurs when persistent ischemia or a complete interruption of the blood supply to a particular area of the brain produces **irreversible destruction of brain tissue**. The resulting neurological deficits usually arise quite suddenly (whence the term "stroke") but can sometimes progress over a longer period of time ("stroke in evolution"). They are irreversible, or at most only partly reversible.

Etiology. Ischemic stroke has many causes. **Embolic events** and **vascular stenosis due to atherosclerosis** play important roles, as do hypertensive atherosclerotic changes of medium-caliber or small cerebral arteries.

> ! The most important risk factor for stroke is arterial hypertension.

The major etiologies of ischemic stroke are summarized in Table 6.**12**. The acute symptoms are sometimes produced by a sudden drop in blood pressure. The major risk factors for atherosclerosis and ischemic stroke are listed in Table 6.**13**.

Types of infarct. There are *three basic types of brain infarct*, distinguished from each other by the caliber of the occluded arteries:

Territorial infarcts are mainly produced by *occlusions of the main trunks or major branches of cerebral arteries* (cerebral macroangiopathy), which may be due to thrombosis, embolism, or other causes. The infarct includes both cortex and subcortical white matter and sometimes the basal ganglia and thalamus (Fig. 6.**12**). It is usually possible to infer which vessel has been occluded from the pattern of neurological deficits that are produced.

Table 6.**12** Classification of ischemic stroke by etiology

I.	**Atherosclerosis of large extra- and intracranial vessels**, leading to: ● thrombosis in the region of an atherosclerotic plaque, ● hemodynamic insufficiency in the poststenotic circulation, or ● arterio-arterial embolism
II.	**Cardiogenic and aortogenic embolism**
III.	**Cerebral small vessel disease/arteriolosclerosis**, usually due to hypertension
IV.	**Other etiologies**, e. g.: ● vasculopathies ● coagulopathies
V.	**Undetermined etiology**

Table 6.**13** Risk factors for atherosclerosis and ischemic stroke

Positive family history of early onset of atherosclerotic disease (< 55 years of age)

Arterial hypertension

Cigarette smoking

Truncal obesity, hypercholesterolemia

Diabetes mellitus

Sleep apnea syndrome

Past history of cardio- or cerebrovascular disease or occlusive peripheral vascular disease

Watershed infarcts (border zone infarcts) are infarcts of hemodynamic origin that are likewise due to microangiopathic processes. Narrowing of small vessels *impairs perfusion in the vulnerable regions at the borders between the territories of two or more arteries* (Fig. 6.**13**). If the perfusion pressure is inadequate, infarction ensues.

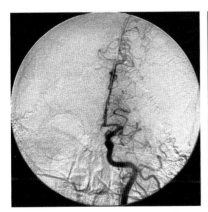 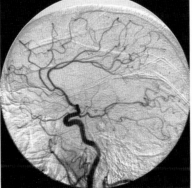 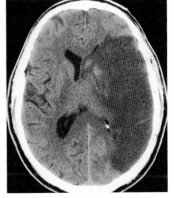

a   b   c

Fig. 6.**12** **Infarct in the territory of the left middle cerebral a.** in a 60-year-old man with acute right hemiplegia. **a** The left carotid angiogram (a–p view) reveals occlusion of the main stem of the middle cerebral a. at its origin. Only the anterior cerebral artery is visualized. **b** The lateral view shows only the pericallosal artery, with its branches, and the posterior cerebral a., while the middle cerebral a. and its branches are not seen (cf. normal carotid angiogram, p. 51). **c** A CT scan obtained 2 days after the onset of symptoms reveals massive infarction in the territory of the middle cerebral a., extending from the cortex to the basal ganglia.

6

Diseases of the Brain and Meninges

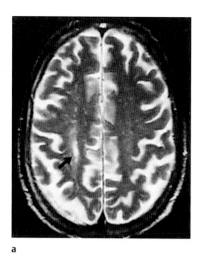

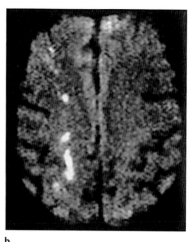

a b

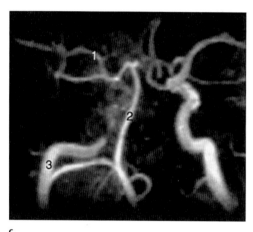

c

Fig. 6.**13 Watershed infarct.** A 58-year-old man with an infarct in the watershed zone between the right anterior and middle cerebral a. territories, caused by occlusion of the right internal carotid a. The vascular territories are shown in Fig. 6.**10** (p. 100). The infarct is well seen in the T2-weighted spin-echo-image (arrow in **a**), and still better in the diffusion-weighted image (**b**), as a longitudinal signal abnormality in the watershed zone between the two arterial territories. The internal cerebral a. is occluded below the siphon, as the MR angiogram shows (**c**). 1, middle cerebral a.; 2, basilar a.; 3, right internal carotid a.

Lacunar infarcts are caused by microangiopathy (usually atherosclerosis of small vessels due to hypertension). The infarcts (lacunes) are less than 1.5 cm in diameter and often multiple. They are found mainly in the basal ganglia, thalamus, and brainstem, and sometimes in the cerebral cortex and subcortical white matter (Fig. 6.**13**). Their clinical presentation depends on their number and localization. Multiple subcortical infarcts due to hypertension are the hallmark of *subcortical arteriosclerotic encephalopathy*, also called Binswanger disease (Fig. 6.**14**).

Signs and Symptoms of Ischemic Stroke. The neurological deficits produced by ischemic stroke depend on the area of the brain that is ischemic or infarcted. We will now briefly summarize the clinical manifestations of the major cerebrovascular syndromes and the typical deficits produced by ischemia in circumscribed areas of the brain.

Ophthalmic a. Transient ischemia in the territory of this vessel produces **amaurosis fugax** (transient monocular blindness), while longer-lasting ischemia causes **retinal infarction**. Retinal ischemia is often due to embolism of cholesterol crystals from ulcerating plaques in

the internal carotid a. into the ophthalmic a. Embolized crystals within the arteries of the retina can occasionally be seen by ophthalmoscopy.

Internal carotid a. Stenosis or occlusion of this vessel can cause simultaneous ischemia of the eye with monocular visual loss (see above) and contralateral hemiparesis, in combination with neuropsychological deficits. This **oculocerebral syndrome** is rare, however, as ischemia in the territory of the internal carotid a. usually presents with *either* monocular visual loss *or* variably severe hemiparesis and neuropsychological deficits.

Middle cerebral a. (MCA). The site of occlusion (main trunk vs. branch of the middle cerebral a.) determines the clinical manifestations. As a rule, a mainly **brachiofacial hemiparesis and hemisensory deficit** are found, often accompanied by *homonymous hemi- or quadrantanopsia* and, in the initial phase, a *horizontal gaze palsy* toward the side of the hemiparesis. An MCA occlusion on the language-dominant (usually left) side additionally produces *aphasia* and *apraxia*, while one on the nondominant side produces *impairment of spatial orientation*. An occlusion of the main stem of the MCA causes ischemia not only of the cortex, but also of the basal

Fig. 6.**14 Binswanger disease (cerebral microangiopathy)** with lacunar infarct (arrowhead) and severe white matter changes. MR images in a 70-year-old man. The microangiopathic lesions are seen on the T2-weighted images as multifocal signal abnormalities in the white matter. The most severe changes are typically found in the periventricular zones abutting the frontal and occipital horns of the lateral ventricles.

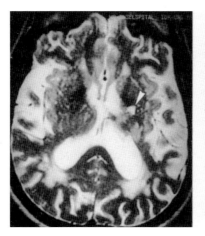
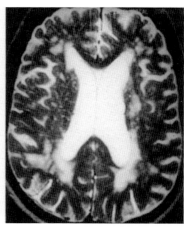

ganglia and internal capsule, producing a more severe contralateral hemiparesis. If the hemiparesis fails to improve over time, or does so only partially, a typical, permanent impairment of gait results: circumduction of the spastically extended lower limb, flexion of the paretic upper limb at the wrist and elbow, and absence of arm swing on the affected side (*Wernicke–Mann gait*) (Fig. 6.**15**).

Anterior choroidal a. Ischemia in the territory of this vessel causes a **homonymous visual field defect**, a **hemisensory deficit**, and, less commonly, **hemiparesis**. The clinical manifestations resemble those of occlusion of the lenticulostriate aa. (branches of the middle cerebral a. supplying the basal ganglia and internal capsule). There may also be extrapyramidal motor signs, such as hemiballism.

Anterior cerebral a. An infarct in the territory of this artery causes **contralateral hemiparesis mainly affecting the lower limb**, sometimes accompanied by contralateral ataxia and, if the lesion is left-sided, by apraxia. Occasionally there may be apathy, abulia (pathological lack of drive and motivation), and urinary incontinence.

Posterior cerebral a. Occlusion of this artery can produce infarction in the cerebral peduncle, the thalamus, mediobasal portions of the temporal lobe, and the occipital lobe. The most prominent clinical sign of a distal occlusion (beyond the origin of the posterior communicating a.) is **contralateral homonymous hemianopsia**, possibly combined with neuropsychological deficits.

Basilar a. Occlusion of the main stem or of a branch of the basilar a. causes **brainstem**, **cerebellar**, and **thalamic** signs (see below). Main stem thrombosis can produce *locked-in syndrome* and is often fatal (p. 77).

Thalamic infarction results from occlusion of one of the arteries supplying the thalamus. It usually presents with a **contralateral hemisensory deficit**, in addition to mild paresis and hemiataxia. The patient's memory, too, is often impaired.

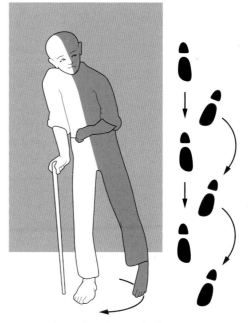

Fig. 6.**15 Typical gait disturbance of a hemiplegic patient.** Circumduction of the spastically paretic leg with predominant extensor tone, and flexion of the spastically paretic arm at the elbow because of predominant flexor tone.

Brainstem infarcts are usually lacunar. They arise in the territory of one or more small perforating arteries that branch off the basilar trunk. Their clinical presentation depends on the particular brainstem nuclei and fiber tracts that they affect. Brainstem stroke therefore takes many different clinical forms, corresponding to the wide variety of functions served by brainstem structures. As a rule, brainstem stroke causes **ipsilateral cranial nerve deficits** and a **contralateral hemisensory defect** and/or **hemiparesis** (cf. Table 6.**14**).

The large number of brainstem vascular syndromes that have been described and given eponymous names are only rarely seen in "pure" form in clinical practice.

6

Diseases of the Brain and Meninges

Table 6.**14**   **Selected brainstem syndromes**

Name	Localization	Ipsilateral signs	Contralateral signs	Special features
Benedikt syndrome (upper red nucleus syndrome)	midbrain, red nucleus	oculomotor palsy, sometimes gaze palsy toward the side of the lesion	hemiataxia (sometimes), intention tremor, hemiparesis (often without Babinski sign)	staggering gait
Weber syndrome	midbrain, cerebral peduncle	oculomotor nerve palsy	hemiparesis	
Millard–Gubler syndrome	posterior portion of pontine tegmentum	peripheral facial palsy	hemiparesis	
Wallenberg syndrome	dorsolateral medulla	Horner syndrome, vocal cord paresis, palatal and posterior pharyngeal paresis, trigeminal nerve deficit, hemiataxia	dissociated sensory disturbance	nystagmus (this syndrome is caused by occlusion of the posterior inferior cerebellar a.)

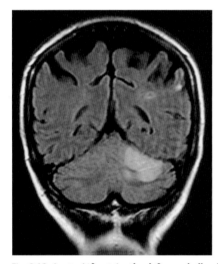

Fig. 6.**16 Acute infarct in the left cerebellar hemisphere, revealed by MRI.** The infarct involves the territory of the superior cerebellar a. There are also two small ischemic foci in the left cerebral hemisphere.

The most important among them is *Wallenberg syndrome*, which results from occlusion of the posterior inferior cerebellar a. (PICA). Some of the more common vascular syndromes affecting different parts of the brainstem are summarized in Table 6.**14**.

Cerebellar infarction presents with vertigo, nausea, unsteady gait, dysarthria, and often acute headache and progressive impairment of consciousness. The neurological examination reveals **ataxia**, **dysmetria**, and **nystagmus**. Often, simultaneous infarction of part of the brainstem produces additional brainstem signs. Not uncommonly, edema in and around the infarcted area rapidly leads to a life-threatening elevation of intracranial pressure in the posterior fossa. A typical MR image of cerebellar stroke is presented in Fig. 6.**16**.

Diagnostic Evaluation of Ischemic Stroke. Diagnostic evaluation in the acute phase is focused on the determination of the *anatomic site and extent* of cerebral ischemia and, above all, its *etiology*.

Acute diagnostic evaluation. In pursuit of these goals, the initial work-up should always begin with the following:
- *precise history taking* concerning not only the present illness, but also the past medical history, with special attention to risk factors and systemic illnesses;
- *a thorough clinical neurological examination* enabling localization of the lesion (see above); and
- *examination of the cardiovascular system* (measurement of pulse and blood pressure and auscultation of the heart, the carotid aa., and perhaps other vessels, depending on the clinical situation; particular attention should be paid to bruits and to any irregularities of the pulse that suggest arrhythmia).

Ancillary testing in the acute phase. The following ancillary tests should also be performed on all stroke patients in the acute phase:
- *Laboratory tests,* mainly for the identification of risk factors, infectious/inflammatory disorders, and coagulopathies (erythrocyte sedimentation rate, blood sugar, lipid profile, complete blood count and hemoglobin, coagulation profile, and sometimes protein C, antiphospholipid antibodies, syphilis serology, etc.).
- *Imaging studies.* Even before these are performed, any central neurological deficit of acute onset is very likely to be due to a cerebrovascular accident, of which ischemic stroke is the most common type; yet neuroimaging is still indicated for definitive confirmation of the diagnosis. Any patient thought to be suffering from acute ischemic stroke should undergo CT as soon as possible, as this will have important implications for the course of treatment, even though areas of ischemia usually cannot be seen by CT till several hours after the onset of symptoms. Early CT does, however, reveal acute brain hemorrhage, if present. MRI can also be performed, if avail-

able. MRI reveals the infarct zone and perifocal edema as soon as the patient begins to experience symptoms and it displays brainstem and cerebellar infarcts more clearly than CT.

- *Doppler ultrasonography* of the extra- and in- tracranial vessels to detect vascular stenosis, occlu- sion, and vascular collateralization.
- An *electrocardiogram* (arrhythmia pointing to a likely cardioembolic event? Old or acute myocardial infarc- tion? Evidence of regional cardiac wall motion ab- normalities, creating a danger of intracardiac throm- bosis and embolism?).

> **!** *When an ischemic stroke is suspected, the most impor- tant immediate question in the differential diagnosis is whether the patient is not, in fact, suffering from an in- tracerebral hemorrhage, rather than from cerebral ischemia. The history and physical examination alone cannot provide a reliable answer; therefore, a neuro- imaging study must be performed.*

Further diagnostic tests after the acute phase. De- pending on the clinical situation, the following tests can also be performed after the acute phase:

- *angio-MRI* to reveal stenosis of the carotid or verte- bral a. (Fig. 6.**17**);
- transthoracic or transesophageal *echocardiography* to reveal potential sources of emboli in the heart and aortic arch, as well as any dysfunction of the heart valves;
- *cerebral angiography* to reveal stenosis or occlusion of the cerebral blood vessels (also performed in the acute phase as a part of thrombolytic treatment); and
- *SPECT* to demonstrate impaired perfusion (cf. Fig. 4.**13**, p. ■■).

Treatment of Ischemic Stroke. Once the diagnosis of ischemic stroke has been made and an intracerebral hemorrhage has been excluded, the initial goal of treat- ment is to minimize the amount of brain tissue that will be irreversibly damaged. Brain tissue in the zone of rela- tive ischemia (the ischemic penumbra, p. 99) can be "salvaged" by prompt restoration of its obstructed blood supply.

> **!** *Patients with suspected stroke should be immediately transported to an acute care hospital and admitted. In- patient treatment markedly improves prognosis.*

In parallel with the acute measures already discussed, a further treatment strategy should also be settled upon for long-term prevention of recurrent stroke. The appro- priate strategy depends on the etiology of the infarct.

General treatment strategies for ischemic stroke are as follows:

- *keeping the blood pressure relatively high* (values up to 200–220 mmHg systolic and 110 mmHg diastolic are tolerable);
- *stabilization of cardiovascular function* (adequate hy- dration, treatment of heart failure and/or arrhyth- mia, if present);

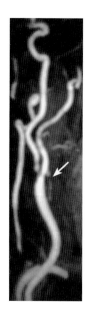

Fig. 6.17 High-grade stenosis of the right common carotid a. in a 72-year-old woman. The MR angiogram, obtained after the injec- tion of contrast medium, reveals high-grade narrowing at the carotid bifurcation (arrow).

- *treatment of cerebral edema*, if present (p. 93); and
- in some patients, *intravenous thrombolysis* within three hours of the onset of symptoms, or *intra-arte- rial thrombolysis* within six hours; if thrombolysis is contraindicated, aspirin is the drug of choice.

Optimization of oxygen and substrate delivery to the ischemic zone:

- *monitoring of respiratory function* (with blood gas analyses, if necessary, and prophylaxis and treatment of pneumonia);
- *treatment of pathological metabolic processes that ele- vate the demand for oxygen and energy* (e.g., treat- ment of fever, suppression of epileptic seizures); and
- *optimal blood sugar management*, with prevention and, if necessary, treatment of hyper- or hypogly- cemia.

Further therapeutic measures include rehabilitation and prophylactic measures against recurrent stroke:

- Early rehabilitation: mobilization (decubitus pro- phylaxis), physical and occupational therapy, and, if needed, speech therapy.

Prevention of recurrent stroke:

- *General medical treatment*: minimization of vascular risk profile (optimal treatment of hypertension, dia- betes mellitus, hypercholesterolemia, or sleep apnea syndrome, if present, and cessation of smoking); treatment of heart failure and/or arrhythmia.
- *Antithrombotic therapy*: the type to be given depends on the etiology of the initial stroke. The following op- tions are available:
  - *inhibition of platelet aggregation* (mainly aspirin, but also clopidogrel or aspirin with dipy- ridamole);
  - *full heparinization* and *oral anticoagulation* (mainly after cardio- or aortoembolic stroke,

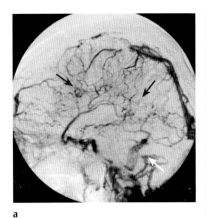
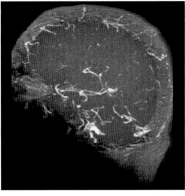
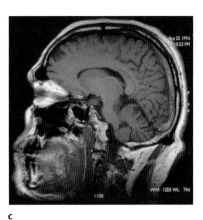

a   b   c

Fig. 6.**18 Thrombosis of the superior sagittal sinus. a** In this angiogram (venous phase) of a 43-year-old male patient, only the posterior portion of the sinus is filled with contrast medium, while the anterior segment (black arrows) and the veins draining into it are not seen. The cavernous sinus is well visualized (white arrow). **b** Another patient with superior sagittal sinus thrombosis: a number of cerebral cortical veins and bridging veins are seen in this angio-MRI, but the superior sagittal sinus is not seen, as it contains no flowing blood. **c** The thrombus is revealed in the sagittal section as an irregular, crescent-shaped structure lying between the dura mater and the arachnoid.

basilar artery thrombosis, stroke in evolution, venous thrombosis, or venous sinus thrombosis (see below); there is no consensus on other potential indications);

- *surgical therapy*: endarterectomy for high-grade carotid stenosis, or insertion of an intravascular stent.

Venous Thrombosis and Venous Sinus Thrombosis

Besides the much more common arterial disorders just discussed, obstruction to *venous* flow can also cause cerebral ischemia. Venous obstruction is usually due to thrombosis of the large venous channels draining the brain (venous sinus thrombosis) and of the veins that empty into them (cerebral venous thrombosis). Damming of blood behind a venous obstruction leads to a secondary reduction of arterial inflow and thus to hypoperfusion and infarction. Smaller or larger diapedetic hemorrhages can also occur in the infarcted area (hemorrhagic infarction).

Etiology and frequency. Thromboses of the cerebral veins and venous sinuses are somewhat more common in women than in men; they account for no more than 1% of all cerebral ischemic events. The *superior sagittal sinus* is most commonly affected, the other sinuses and the cortical veins less commonly. These thromboses are usually *bland*, i. e., no specific etiology can be identified. A minority of cases are due to infection, either systemic or in the immediate vicinity of the sinus (e. g., chronic otitis); other causes include hypercoagulability states and systemic diseases (e. g., Behçet disease).

Clinical manifestations. The common signs and symptoms are *headache*, *focal* or *generalized epileptic seizures*, *papilledema*, and *sensory* and *motor deficits*, depending on the site of the thrombosis.

Diagnostic evaluation. Imaging studies reveal unilateral or bilateral hemorrhagic infarction; the thrombosis itself can usually be seen by MRI, or by CT after the administration of contrast medium. In a minority of cases, it is revealed only by angiography (Fig. 6.**18**). The diagnostic method of choice is *MRI*.

Treatment consists of anticoagulation (heparin followed by oral anticoagulation), usually for a few months.

Nontraumatic Intracranial Hemorrhage

Nontraumatic intracranial hemorrhage is defined as a spontaneous hemorrhage into the brain parenchyma (**intracerebral hemorrhage**) or the cerebrospinal fluid space (**subarachnoid hemorrhage**). Intracerebral hemorrhages cause acute signs and symptoms resembling those of cerebral ischemia and account for about 10% of strokes. One of the more common forms of intracerebral hemorrhage is hypertensive hemorrhage. The main symptom of subarachnoid hemorrhage is headache; its most common source is a ruptured aneurysm.

General manifestations of intracranial hemorrhage. Though the manifestations of intracranial hemorrhage and cerebral ischemia are similar, generally speaking (sudden onset of focal neurological deficits), there are a number of clinical signs and symptoms that are more characteristic of hemorrhage than of ischemia. These include:

- acute *headache*, often accompanied by *vomiting*;
- rapidly or very rapidly *progressive neurological deficits* (whose type depends on the site of hemorrhage);
- progressive *impairment of consciousness*, perhaps leading to coma;
- in many patients, *epileptic seizures*.

If these manifestations are present, an intracranial hemorrhage is the probable cause. The definitive diagnosis, however, can only be made with neuroradiological methods.

Intracerebral Hemorrhage

Etiology. Most cases of intracerebral hemorrhage are due to the rupture of *vascular lesions of hypertensive origin* ("rhexis hemorrhages" of pseudoaneurysms of lipohyalinotic arterioles), aneurysms, or arteriovenous malformations (Figs. 6.**19**, 6.**20**). Intracerebral hemorrhage may also be a complication of therapeutic (over-) anticoagulation. Smaller hemorrhages, particularly those that are near the cortical surface, are often due to amyloid angiopathy. There can also be bleeding into an infarct, a primary brain tumor, a metastasis, or a cavernoma. The more common etiologies of intracerebral hemorrhage are listed in Table 6.**15**.

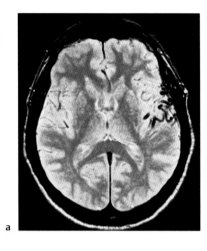
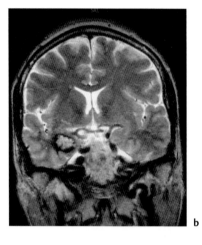

Fig. 6.**19 a Arteriovenous malformation** in the left temporal lobe of a 68-year-old man with epileptic seizures. **b Cavernoma** in the right hippocampus of another patient (T2-weighted image).

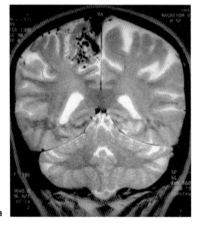
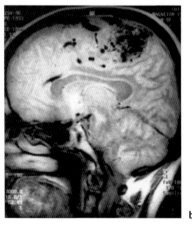

Fig. 6.**20 Arteriovenous malformation.**
a The T2-weighted spin-echo image reveals the feeding and draining vessels as signal-free areas ("flow voids").
b Analogous finding in a sagittal image.
c The right carotid angiogram shows that the malformation is fed by branches of the right middle cerebral and pericallosal aa. **d** The left carotid angiogram shows that it also derives part of its blood supply across the midline from the *left* pericallosal a.

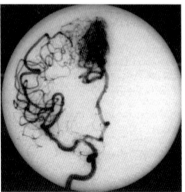
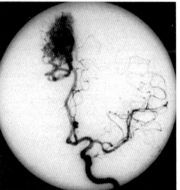

6

Diseases of the Brain and Meninges

Table 6.15 Causes of nontraumatic cerebral hemorrhage

Chronic arterial hypertension

Aneurysm rupture

Hemorrhage into a preexisting lesion (infarct, tumor)

Vascular malformation (cavernoma, arteriovenous malformation)

Vascular fragility due to vasculopathy, e. g., cranial arteritis, amyloid angiopathy

Bleeding diathesis due to hematologic disease or therapeutic anticoagulation

Cerebral venous thrombosis and venous sinus thrombosis

Rarely, in the setting of a hypertensive crisis or drug abuse (e. g., cocaine)

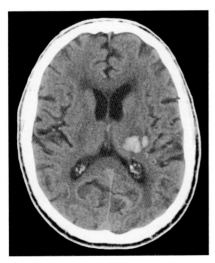

Fig. 6.21 Acute left thalamic hemorrhage as seen by CT in a 76-year-old man with a right-sided hemisensory deficit of acute onset.

Clinical manifestations. The clinical picture mainly depends on the site and extent of the hemorrhage and to a much lesser extent on etiological factors. Certain aspects of the clinical course can, however, suggest that one etiology is more likely than another:

- Chronic arterial hypertension and advanced age (typically 60–70) make a rhexis hemorrhage more likely. These hemorrhages are ultimately caused by hypertension and are usually very large. Common sites are the pallidum, the putamen, and the internal capsule, with the corresponding clinical manifestations: *contralateral, usually dense, hemiparesis* or hemiplegia, *horizontal gaze palsy*, and initially, in many cases, *déviation conjuguée and deviation of the head to the side of the lesion.* Less common sites are the subcortical white matter, brainstem, thalamus (Fig. 6.21), and cerebellum. Very large hemorrhages, particularly if located in the posterior fossa, can rapidly elevate the intracranial pressure, causing brainstem compression and, in turn, impairment of consciousness and coma.
- *Acute worsening* of more or less severe, *preexisting signs and symptoms,* perhaps accompanied by *addi-*

tional impairment of consciousness, suggests hemorrhage into an infarct or tumor.
- *Focal or generalized epileptic seizures* preceding the onset of the acute event point toward a tumor, vascular malformation, or other structural lesion of the brain as the likely cause of hemorrhage.

Diagnostic evaluation. The diagnosis of intracranial hemorrhage is suggested by the characteristic clinical findings (p. 106) and then definitively confirmed by the demonstration of blood on *CT* or *MRI.* When performed in the acute phase, these studies may fail to reveal an underlying vascular malformation, if present, which may be obscured by the hemorrhage; *angiography* may be necessary to complete the diagnostic work-up. The obtaining of a complete *coagulation profile* is indicated in some patients.

Treatment and prognosis. Patients suffering from an acute intracerebral hemorrhage require *close clinical observation*; in particular, signs of intracranial hypertension (vomiting, progressive impairment of consciousness, and sometimes anisocoria and papilledema) must be vigilantly watched for. Intracranial hypertension may be due to recurrent hemorrhage or to progressive brain swelling; in either case, it must be promptly detected and treated (for treatment measures, cf. p. 93). In addition, *stabilization of vital functions* and the *treatment of epileptic seizures,* if present, are essential. In each case, the possible indication for *neurosurgical removal of the hematoma* should be carefully considered, in light of the neurological manifestations, site of the hemorrhage, and age and general condition of the patient. Cerebellar hemorrhage with mass effect generally confers a risk of impending brainstem compression and death and is often an indication for life-saving emergency surgery.

Although about one-third of all patients with an intracerebral hemorrhage will die of it, while others go on to enjoy a more or less complete spontaneous recovery.

Subarachnoid Hemorrhage (SAH)

Nontraumatic subarachnoid hemorrhage, defined as spontaneous hemorrhage into the subarachnoid space, accounts for about 7 % of all "strokes." It can occur at any age, with peak incidence around age 50. Children are very rarely affected.

Etiology. Subarachnoid hemorrhage is usually due to the *spontaneous rupture of a saccular aneurysm on an artery at the base of the brain,* usually one of the arteries forming the circle of Willis. Common sites of saccular aneurysms are shown in Fig. 6.22. Less frequent causes of subarachnoid hemorrhage include arteriovenous malformations, vasculopathies, coagulopathies, and preceding trauma.

Clinical manifestations of subarachnoid hemorrhage are:
- sudden, extremely intense **headache**, often described as the "worst headache of my life;" the headache may have been preceded by an earlier, transient episode of headache or other minor symptoms ("*pre-*

Fig. 6.22 Common locations of saccular aneurysms and their relations to the cranial nerves. Aneurysms are typically found at vascular bifurcations.

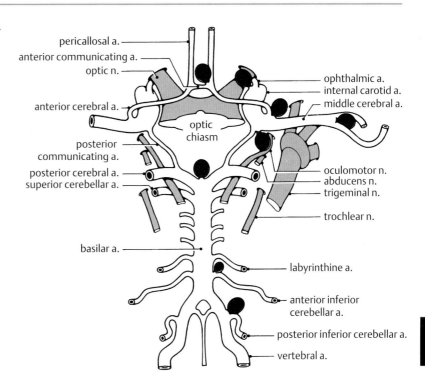

pericallosal a.
anterior communicating a.
optic n.
anterior cerebral a.
posterior communicating a.
posterior cerebral a.
superior cerebellar a.
basilar a.

ophthalmic a.
internal carotid a.
middle cerebral a.
optic chiasm
oculomotor n.
abducens n.
trigeminal n.
trochlear n.
labyrinthine a.
anterior inferior cerebellar a.
posterior inferior cerebellar a.
vertebral a.

monitory headache," "*warning leak*"); it is most commonly diffuse or bioccipital;

- often, at first, a brief and transient **impairment of consciousness**, which may be followed, at some point in the following hours or days, by a recurrent impairment of consciousness or coma;
- often, **nausea and vomiting**;
- rarely, **cranial nerve palsies** (caused by aneurysms at particular sites) or other **focal neurological deficits**, caused, e. g., by additional hemorrhage into the brain parenchyma (see below).

Diagnostic evaluation. Physical evaluation reveals:
- as the most prominent physical finding, *meningism*;

and sometimes other clinical signs that may be useful for the localization of the lesion, e. g.:

- *oculomotor nerve palsy* with aneurysms of the terminal segment of the internal carotid a. or the posterior communicating a.;
- *abulia* with an aneurysm of the anterior communicating a.;
- *hemiplegia* with an aneurysm of the middle cerebral a.;
- *brainstem and cerebellar signs* with aneurysms of the basilar a.

Whenever subarachnoid hemorrhage is suspected on clinical grounds, **neuroimaging studies** should be per-

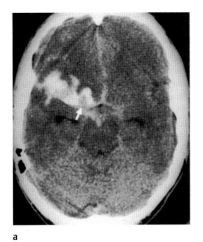

a

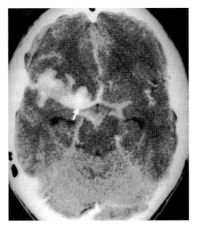

b

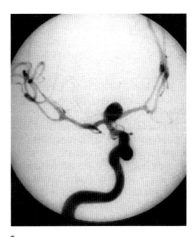

c

Fig. 6.23 Aneurysmal subarachnoid hemorrhage. a The nonenhanced CT reveals blood in the subarachnoid space, particularly along the course of the middle cerebral a. The aneurysm (arrow) is also seen. **b** The lumen of the aneurysm, dark in **a**, turns bright after the administration of intravascular contrast (arrow). **c** Carotid angiography shows the aneurysm at the bifurcation of the internal carotid a. into the anterior and middle cerebral aa.

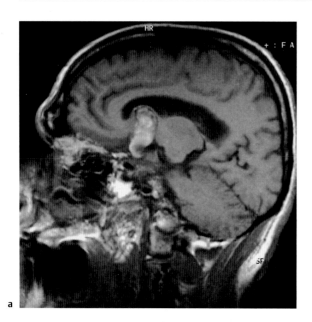

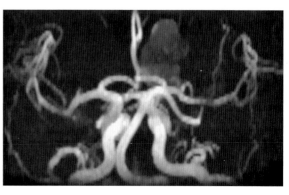

Fig. 6.24 Aneurysm of the internal carotid a. a The sagittal image shows a large, blood-filled aneurysm in the region of the terminal segment of the internal carotid a. The dome of the aneurysm protrudes upward into the frontobasal cortex. This was an incidental finding in a patient with no apparent neurological deficit. **b** The angio-MRI reveals the aneurysm of the terminal ICA segment; it is the size of a fingertip.

formed immediately. *CT or MRI with FLAIR sequences* can often demonstrate the presence of blood in the cerebrospinal fluid spaces on the day of the hemorrhage (Fig. 6.23). These studies can sometimes also reveal the source of hemorrhage (aneurysm or other), though they often will not. If CT and MRI fail to demonstrate any hemorrhage in the face of clinical suspicion, a **lumbar puncture** must be performed. Bloody CSF is found in patients with acute subarachnoid hemorrhage, xanthochromic CSF in patients whose hemorrhage occurred a few hours of more before the LP (Fig. 6.24).

> ! *A negative CT or MRI does not rule out subarachnoid hemorrhage. If clinical suspicion remains, a lumbar puncture must be performed.*

Once the diagnosis of subarachnoid hemorrhage is confirmed by imaging or lumbar puncture, **cerebral angiography** should be performed as soon as possible to determine the source of the hemorrhage, usually an aneurysm. Angiography is only indicated, however, if the patient is clinically stable enough to undergo an operation (unless interventional neuroradiological treatment is available—see below).

Blood coming into contact with the outer walls of arteries that course through the subarachnoid space causes vasospasm, which can be detected with **transcranial Doppler or duplex ultrasonography**.

Treatment. Patients with aneurysmal subarachnoid hemorrhage must be immediately admitted or transferred to a hospital with a neurosurgical department.

The goal of treatment is exclusion of the aneurysm from the circulation as soon as possible to prevent a potentially fatal recurrent hemorrhage. This is done either with neurosurgical clipping or, less often, with interventional neuroradiological techniques ("coiling" and others).

In addition, **general measures** including strict bed rest, stabilization of cardiovascular functions, fluid and electrolyte administration, analgesia, sedation, and the administration of a calcium-channel blocker (nimodipine) to prevent vasospasm (see above) are indicated. The performance of transcranial ultrasonography at regular intervals enables prompt detection of vasospasm, which may require treatment.

Clinical course and long-term prognosis. The clinical course of subarachnoid hemorrhage is often dramatic. **Recurrent hemorrhage** after the initial bleed is particularly worrisome and often fatal. Without treatment, about 25% of patients die in the first 24 hours and 40% in the first three months. The course is often further complicated by vasospasm arising three to 14 days after the initial hemorrhage (usually in the first three to five days). This may cause transient ischemia or infarction in the distribution of the spastic artery. Vasospasm may not resolve until three or four weeks later. Another potential complication is **malresorptive hydrocephalus** (p. 92), presumably caused by adhesions of the arachnoid villi obstructing the outflow of CSF. Patients who survive an initial aneurysmal subarachnoid hemorrhage without further treatment of the aneurysm have a long-term risk of recurrent hemorrhage of about 3% per year.

Infectious Diseases of the Brain and Meninges

The intracranial structures, like the rest of the body, can be infected by bacteria, viruses, parasites, and other microorganisms. Different organisms tend to infect either the meninges or the brain substance itself. Thus, there are two main forms of intracranial infection, **meningitis** and **encephalitis** (cf. Fig. 6.25). Mixed forms also occur: a meningeal infection can spread to the brain (and/or spinal cord), or vice versa, causing **meningo-(myelo)encephalitis**. The latter term is only used if the patient unequivocally manifests clinical signs of *both* meningeal *and* cerebral involvement.

Infectious diseases of the central nervous system can be classified, broadly speaking, into three basic clinical situations: a predominantly meningitic syndrome, which can be either acute or subacute to chronic, and a predominantly encephalitic syndrome. These three syndromes, and the organisms that cause each, will be discussed individually in this section.

In addition, **focal infections** of the brain parenchyma can lead to the formation of brain abscesses, which will also be discussed below.

6

Diseases of the Brain and Meninges

Fig. 6.**25 Sites and nomenclature of intracranial (a) and spinal (b) infections.**

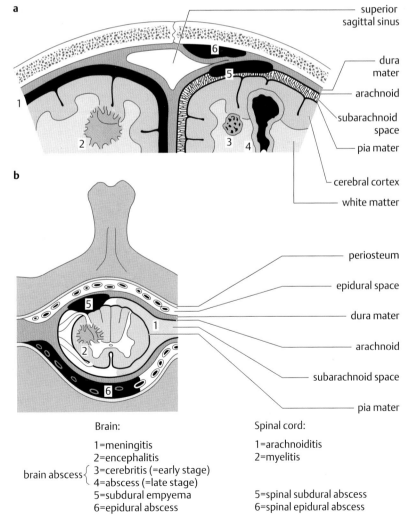

a

superior sagittal sinus

dura mater

arachnoid

subarachnoid space

pia mater

cerebral cortex

white matter

b

periosteum

epidural space

dura mater

arachnoid

subarachnoid space

pia mater

Brain:
1=meningitis
2=encephalitis
brain abscess { 3=cerebritis (=early stage)
4=abscess (=late stage)
5=subdural empyema
6=epidural abscess

Spinal cord:
1=arachnoiditis
2=myelitis

5=spinal subdural abscess
6=spinal epidural abscess

Infections Mainly Involving the Meninges

General manifestations of a meningitic syndrome
● reheadache;
● fever (though elderly and immune-deficient patients are often afebrile);
● nausea and vomiting due to intracranial hypertension;
● meningism, which, in severe cases, may be evident as a spontaneous extended posture of the neck, or opisthotonus;
● positive meningeal signs with neck extension, i.e., the Lasègue, Brudzinski, and Kernig signs (p. 16).

The clinical aspects of individual types of meningitis depend on the inciting organism and the immune state of the host.

Acute Meningitis

Acute Bacterial Meningitis

Acute bacterial meningitis is caused by bacteria that can reach the meninges by any of three routes: **hematogenous spread** (e. g., from a focus of infection in the nasopharynx), **continuous extension** (e. g., from the middle ear or paranasal sinuses), or **direct contamination** (through an open wound or CSF fistula). The clinical onset of purulent meningitis is usually **acute or subacute** and patients very quickly become severely ill. The initiation of antibiotic therapy as rapidly as possible is essential for a good outcome.

Etiology. The organisms that most commonly cause acute, purulent meningitis are:
● in **neonates**, *Escherichia coli*, group B streptococci, and *Listeria monocytogenes*;
● in **children**, *Hemophilus influenzae*, pneumococci, and meningococci (*Neisseria meningitidis*);
● in **adults**, pneumococci, meningococci, and, less commonly, staphylococci and gram-negative enterobacteria.

Clinical manifestations. The course of purulent meningitis is characterized by the meningitic signs and symptoms listed above, as well as by:
● myalgia, back pain;
● photophobia;
● if the infection is mainly located over the cerebral convexity, with irritation of the underlying brain parenchyma, epileptic seizures (40%);
● cranial nerve deficits (10 to 20%, sometimes permanent deafness, particularly after pneumococcal infection);
● variably severe impairment of consciousness;
● in infection with *Neisseria meningitidis*, there may be petechial cutaneous hemorrhages and hemorrhagic necrosis of the adrenal cortex due to endotoxic shock (Waterhouse–Friderichsen syndrome).

Diagnostic evaluation. The most important and most urgent component of the diagnostic evaluation is *lumbar puncture*. Whenever acute meningitis is suspected, a lumbar puncture should be performed at once, as soon as papilledema (a sign of intracranial hypertension) has been ruled out by ophthalmoscopy. The CSF is typically turbid, with 1000 to several thousand cells/mm³ (mainly granulocytes), the protein concentration markedly elevated (positive Pandy test), and the glucose concentration diminished. CSF examination enables confirmation of the diagnosis of meningitis and, in two-thirds of patients, demonstration of bacteria by Gram stain and identification of the causative organism by CSF culture.

Treatment begins with *antibiotic therapy*, with a single drug, or multiple drugs, chosen for their effectiveness against the most likely causative organisms in the given clinical setting. Once the organism has been identified by CSF culture and its antibiotic sensitivity spectrum has been determined, the antibiotic treatment can be tailored for maximum effectiveness against this organism.

> **!** *The antibiotic treatment of bacterial meningitis must be started immediately after the lumbar puncture, without waiting, e. g., for a CT or MRI to be performed (if these or other tests are planned). The elapsed time between the clinical presentation and the beginning of treatment is the most important prognostic factor!*

Acute Viral Meningitis

A number of viruses can cause so-called **aseptic** or **lymphocytic meningitis**, which usually presents acutely (less commonly, subacutely) after a nonspecific prodromal stage with flulike or gastrointestinal symptoms. The more common causative viruses are *enteroviruses* (polio- and Coxsackie viruses), *arboviruses*, and *HIV*; other, rarer ones include *lymphocytic choriomeningitis virus (LCV)*, *cytomegalovirus*, *type II herpesvirus*, and the *mumps*, *Epstein–Barr*, and *influenza viruses*. The main clinical manifestations are headache, fever, meningism (often mild), and general symptoms such as fatigue and myalgia. The causative virus is identified by serologic testing. The natural course of aseptic meningitis is usually favorable, provided the brain is not involved (i. e., provided there is no encephalitic component). Antiviral treatment is given if the causative virus is found to be one for which an effective treatment exists. Residual neurological deficits, such as deafness, are rare.

Chronic Meningitis

Chronic meningitis is caused by different organisms from the pus-forming bacteria that cause acute meningitis and therefore takes a **less acute and dramatic course**, at least initially: the **meningitic symptoms** arise gradually, often fluctuate, and, depending on the causative organism, may progressively worsen over a long period of time. **Fever** and other clinical and laboratory **signs of infection** (elevated ESR and CRP, blood count abnormalities, general symptoms such as fatigue and myalgia) are common but may be absent. There may be variably severe neurological deficits. The spectrum of causative organisms is very wide.

Fig. 6.**26 Tuberculous meningitis. a** Typical contrast enhancement surrounding the brainstem. **b** This T1-weighted MR image shows the typical meningeal contrast enhancement along the course of the middle cerebral a. (arrows).

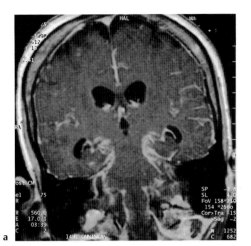
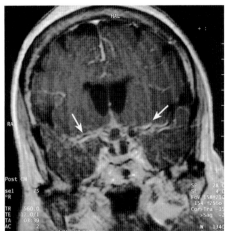

Tuberculous Meningitis

Etiology. *Mycobacterium tuberculosis* bacilli reach the meninges by hematogenous spread, either directly from a primary complex (*early generalization*), or else from a focus of tuberculosis in an internal organ (*late generalization*). The site of origin may be clinically silent.

Clinical manifestations. *Meningitic symptoms* usually develop gradually. Febrile bouts and general symptoms (see above) are often but not always present. Because the infectious process typically centers on the base of the brain (so-called *basal meningitis* [Fig. 6.**26**], in contrast to bacterial meningitis, which is typically located around the cerebral convexities), *cranial nerve palsies* are common, particularly of the nerves of eye movement and the facial n. Moreover, *arteritis of the cerebral vasculature* may result in focal brain infarction. The protein concentration in CSF is typically markedly elevated and gelatinous exudates in the subarachnoid space, including the basal cisterns, cause progressive hardening of the meninges and *malresorptive hydrocephalus.*

Diagnostic evaluation. The most important part of the evaluation is the *detection of the causative organism* in the CSF or other bodily fluids (sputum, tracheal secretions, gastric juice, urine). In the past, the detection of mycobacteria in the CSF often required weeks of culture; at present, it can be done relatively quickly with *PCR*. Occasionally, a Ziehl–Neelsen stain of the CSF will directly and immediately reveal acid-fast bacilli (mycobacteria).

Treatment generally begins with a **combination of four tuberculostatic drugs** (*isoniazid, rifampicin, pyrazinamide, and myambutol*), followed by a combination of three drugs, and then of two, for at least 12 months. Untreated tuberculous meningitis is lethal.

Other Causes of Chronic Meningitis. A number of other organisms can rarely cause chronic meningitis, usually accompanied by variably severe encephalitis.

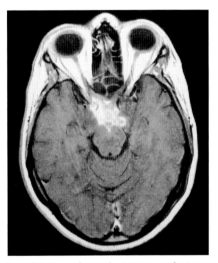

Fig. 6.**27 Sarcoidosis.** This MR image of a 31-year-old woman with sarcoidosis shows infiltration of the basal meninges. There is marked signal abnormality in the basal ambient cistern.

Fungal meningitis mainly affects immune-deficient patients, though not exclusively; the causative species include *Cryptococcus neoformans, Candida albicans,* and aspergilli. Further causative organisms include **protozoa** (*Toxoplasma gondii*) and **parasites** (cysticerci, echinococci).

The noninfectious causes of the chronic meningitic syndrome include **sarcoidosis**, which, like tuberculous meningitis, is mainly found around the base of the brain (Fig. 6.**27**), and **seeding of the meninges with metastatic carcinoma or sarcoma** (carcinomatous or sarcomatous meningitis).

6

Diseases of the Brain and Meninges

Infections Mainly Involving the Brain

Infections with a predominantly encephalitic, rather than meningitic, syndrome typically cause **focal neurological and neuropsychological deficits** as well as a variably severe impairment of consciousness. Encephalitis, like meningitis, can be of **viral**, **bacterial**, **fungal**, **protozoal**, or **parasitic origin**. **Prion diseases** are a special category of encephalitis.

These infectious processes often involve other structures in the nervous system simultaneously with the brain (e.g., the peripheral nerves and plexuses, nerve roots, spinal cord, and meninges). In particular, the three important clinical varieties of spirochetal infection (syphilis, borreliosis, and leptospirosis) often present initially with meningitic or polyradiculitic and polyneuritic manifestations.

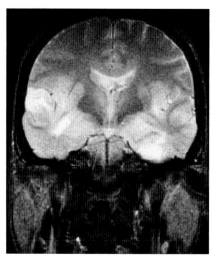

Fig. 6.**28** **Herpes simplex encephalitis** affecting both temporal lobes.

General signs and symptoms of an encephalitic syndrome are:
- fever,
- headache,
- impairment of consciousness,
- personality changes and neuropsychological abnormalities,
- epileptic seizures,
- focal neurological deficits.

Viral Encephalitis

Herpes Simplex Encephalitis

Herpes simplex encephalitis is a serious infectious condition caused by the herpes simplex virus, type I.

Pathogenesis. This viral disease is characterized by hemorrhagic–necrotic inflammation of the basal portions of the frontal and temporal lobes, combined with severe cerebral edema. The inflammatory foci are found in both hemispheres, but one is usually more strongly affected than the other.

Clinical manifestations. After a *nonspecific prodromal phase* with fever, headache, and other general symptoms, the disease presents with *progressive impairment of consciousness*, *epileptic seizures* (usually of complex partial type, with or without secondary generalization, because of the temporal localization of the disease), and *focal neurological* and *neuropsychological deficits*, particularly impairment of memory and orientation. *Aphasia* and *hemiplegia* may ensue.

Diagnostic evaluation. *CSF examination* reveals up to 500 cells/mm3, mainly lymphocytes but also granulocytes; the CSF is sometimes bloody or xanthochromic. Viral DNA can be identified in the CSF by the polymerase chain reaction (PCR) in the first few days of illness and, two weeks later, IgG specific for herpes simplex virus can be identified in the CSF as well. The *EEG*, in addition to nonspecific changes, may reveal characteristic focal findings over one or both temporal lobes. The *CT scan* is usually normal at first but, within a few days, reveals temporal or frontal hypodense areas, which may contain foci of hemorrhage (Fig. 6.**28**). *MRI* may reveal corresponding signal changes even earlier.

Treatment. *Acyclovir* is given intravenously. *Corticosteroids* are given to combat cerebral edema and *antiepileptic drugs* to prevent seizures.

! *If there is good reason to suspect herpes simplex encephalitis (progressive impairment of consciousness, aphasia, epileptic seizures [particularly of the complex partial type], an inflammatory CSF profile, focal EEG abnormalities), intravenous acyclovir therapy must be started immediately.*

Early Summer Meningoencephalitis (ESME)

This disease is caused by an *arbovirus* and transmitted by tick bites. In endemic areas (e.g., Austria and southern Germany), it affects one in every 100 to 1000 tick-bite victims. After an incubation period of one to four weeks, in which there are nonspecific prodromal manifestations such as fever and flulike or gastrointestinal symptoms, about 20% of patients develop *headache*, *meningism*, and *focal neurological deficits* referable to the brain and spinal cord. *Peripheral nerve deficits* may also appear some time later. When the patient has recovered from the acute illness, residual paresis and, less commonly, neuropsychological deficits may remain. The essential diagnostic test is the demonstration of virus-specific IgM antibodies. ESME can be effectively prevented by exposure prophylaxis (adequate clothing in endemic forest areas) and active immunization. Immune serum given within 48 hours of a tick bite is protective.

HIV Encephalitis and Opportunistic Infections in HIV-positive Persons

Nearly 50% of persons infected with HIV have a clinically evident infection of the brain or other parts of the nervous system at some point in the course of their illness. The nervous system can be infected with HIV itself, other, opportunistic pathogens, or both. In severe cases, patients may suffer from *encephalitis*, *myelopathy*, *mono-* and *polyneuropathy*, and/or *myopathy*. Encephalitis presents with *neuropsychological abnormalities* including delirium, personality change, and dementia.

Other Types of Viral Encephalitis

Herpes zoster encephalitis is accompanied by a segmental vesicular rash in the territory of a peripheral nerve (cranial nerve). CSF examination reveals lymphocytic pleocytosis up to 200 cells/mm^3. The disease may appear in particularly severe form after a generalized herpes zoster infection.

Rarer types. Other, rarer viruses causing meningoencephalitis, some of which are specific to particular regions, are listed in Table 6.**16** in addition to those already discussed. Fig. 6.**29** concerns one such virus (papovavirus encephalitis in an HIV-positive man).

Table 6.**16** **Viruses that cause meningoencephalitis**

Virus	Route of infection	Season of peak incidence	Persons at risk	Clinical features	Special aspects of diagnostic evaluation
Echovirus	fecal–oral	summer/fall	children and family members living with them	*M*, rash, gastrointestinal symptoms	virology
Coxsackie virus A	fecal–oral	summer/fall	children and family members living with them	*M*, rash, gastrointestinal symptoms	virology
Coxsackie virus B	fecal–oral	summer/fall	children and family members living with them	*M*, rash, pleuritis, pericarditis, myocarditis, orchitis, gastrointestinal symptoms	virology
Mumps virus	inhalation	late winter/ spring	children, mainly boys	*M*, parotitis, orchitis, oophoritis, pancreatitis	elevated amylase, CSF cell count, and CSF glucose
Adenovirus	inhalation		infants and children	*M*, pharyngitis, pneumonia	
Lymphocytic choriomeningitis virus	mice	late winter/ spring	laboratory personnel	*M*, pharyngitis, pneumonia	
Hepatitis viruses	fecal–oral, sexual intercourse, blood transfusion		mainly intravenous drug abusers, homo- and bisexuals, recipients of blood transfusions	*M*, jaundice, arthritis	hepatic dysfunction
Epstein–Barr virus (infectious mononucleosis)	oral		teenagers and young adults	*M*, lymphadenopathy, pharyngitis, rash, splenomegaly	atypical lymphocytes, Paul–Bunnell reaction, hepatic dysfunction
Echovirus				*M*, enanthem and exanthem	
ESME virus (early summer meningoencephalitis)	tick bite, cutaneous	early summer, fall	persons who go into a forest in an endemic area	*M*, *E*, myelitis, meningoradiculitis	serology
Varicella-zoster virus	inhalation		children and persons who come in contact with them	*M*, radiculitis; *M*, *E*, and myelitis: pain, vesicular eruption	demonstration of intrathecal antibodies, PCR
Cytomegalovirus (CMV)			HIV-positive persons	*E*, epileptic seizures, radiculitis	detection of HIV in the CSF or urine, PCR of CSF or EDTA blood, CMV-specific intrathecal IgG synthase, CMV retinitis

Continued →

*M = predominantly meningitic manifestations, *E* = predominantly encephalitic manifestations

Diseases of the Brain and Meninges

6

Table 6.16   **Viruses that cause meningoencephalitis** (Continued)

Virus	Route of infection	Season of peak incidence	Persons at risk	Clinical features	Special aspects of diagnostic evaluation
Herpes simplex virus type I	person-to-person	all year	all persons	*E*, focal neurological deficits, epileptic seizures, impairment of consciousness	MRI, virus detection, PCR of the CSF, EEG with periodic steep waves, intrathecal HSV-specific IgG synthesis
Herpes simplex virus type II	person-to-person	all year	neonates and children, rarely adults	*E* (in neonates); *M* in others	
Arboviruses (Eastern equine, Western equine, Venezuelan equine)	mosquitoes		children and adults in the Americas	*E*, rash	virology
Human immunodeficiency virus (HIV)	sexual intercourse, blood transfusion	all year	sexual partners of HIV-positive persons, mother–child, intravenous drug abusers, homosexuals	*E*, AIDS dementia, myelopathy, polyneuropathy, myopathy, opportunistic infections	serology
Papovaviruses		all year	immunocompromised persons (AIDS, lymphoma)	*E*, myelitis, clinical picture of progressive multifocal leukoencephalopathy	MRI with subcortical T2-hyperintensities, virology

*M = predominantly meningitic manifestations, *E* = predominantly encephalitic manifestations

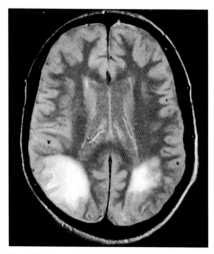

Fig. 6.**29 Asymmetrical encephalitis, probably due to papovavirus,** in a 42-year-old, HIV-positive man. MRI reveals involvement of the occipital lobes bilaterally.

Fungal, Parasitic, and Protozoal Encephalitis

Some of the **fungi** mentioned above as causes of meningitis can also cause encephalitis. In persons with normal immune competence, encephalitis can be caused by *Cryptococcus neoformans, Coccidioides immitis, Histoplasma capsulatum,* and *Blastomyces dermatitidis.* Persons with reduced immune competence due to disease or pharmacotherapy may develop encephalitis due to any of these or to *Candida, Aspergillus,* or *Zygomycetes.* **Parasites**, particularly *Toxoplasma gon-*

dii, and **protozoa** (amebae, plasmodia, trypanosomes, cysticerci, and echinococci) can also infect the brain.

Spirochetal (Meningo-)encephalitis

Neurosyphilis

Etiology. Syphilis is caused by the sexually transmitted spirochete, *Treponema pallidum.*

Clinical manifestations. Hematogenous spread of treponemes in the **secondary phase** of syphilis may lead to *meningeal irritation* or *early syphilitic meningitis* with cranial nerve palsies (basal meningitis).

In the **tertiary phase** (usually one or two years after the primary infection and secondary seeding of treponemes), *cerebrospinal syphilis* mainly affects the mesenchymal structures (blood vessels, meninges) of the brain and, often, the spinal cord. Inflammatory changes of vascular walls, particularly in the arteries of the skull base and the middle cerebral a., cause stenoses and *multiple ischemic strokes. Meningitis*, mainly in the region of the skull base, presents with fluctuating headache and cranial nerve palsies. Occasionally, tertiary syphilis gives rise to polyneuropathic and polyradicular manifestations. In the rare gummous variant of tertiary syphilis, large granulomatous masses may form within the cranial cavity, producing mass effect and intracranial hypertension.

In the **quaternary phase** of syphilis, the inflammatory process extends into the parenchyma of the brain and spinal cord, producing tabes dorsalis (spinal cord involvement) and/or progressive paralysis (chronic meningoencephalitis).

Tabes dorsalis appears in 7% of untreated syphilitics eight to 12 years after the primary infection. It is characterized, above all, by *progressive degeneration of the posterior columns and posterior roots*. Its clinical manifestations include progressively severe ataxia, lancinating pains, bladder dysfunction, diminished reflexes, loss of pupillary reactivity (p. 193), diminished sensitivity to pain, hypotonia of the musculature, and joint deformities.

Progressive paralysis appears 10–15 years after the primary infection and is caused by *parenchymal meningoencephalitis* with formation of caseating granulomas. Its major clinical sign is *progressive dementia*, with typical features including impaired judgment, lack of social inhibition, and, in some patients, expansive agitation (megalomania, nonsensical and delusional ideas). In other cases, patients may develop flattening of drive and affect, become depressed, or manifest schizophreniform phenomena (hallucinations, paranoia).

The two late forms of neurosyphilis can also be present in combination.

Diagnostic evaluation. The diagnosis of neurosyphilis is established by various *serologic tests*: the TPHA and FTA–ABS tests for the demonstration of previous contact with *Treponema pallidum*, the VDRL test for the assessment of current disease activity (though this test is not specific for *Treponema pallidum*), and the 19-S-IgM–FTA–ABS test for the demonstration of treponeme-specific IgM antibodies, which indicate an active or florid infection. Neurosyphilis also causes an *inflammatory CSF picture* with elevated leukocyte count and protein concentration, a positive VDRL test in the CSF, and an elevated CSF concentration of treponeme-specific IgG.

Treatment. All forms of neurosyphilis are treated with *penicillin G*; if the patient is allergic to penicillin, tetracycline or erythromycin can be given instead. The success of treatment depends on the time at which it is begun: improvement is less likely if the brain and spinal cord parenchyma have already sustained considerable damage.

Prognosis. The prognosis of early syphilitic meningitis is good. In the other phases of neurosyphilis, progression can be prevented by appropriate treatment, but residual deficits are common.

Neuroborreliosis

Etiology. Borreliosis is caused by *Borrelia burgdorferi*, a spirochete transmitted by bites of the tick *Ixodes ricinus*.

Clinical manifestations. *Borrelia burgdorferi* can attack the nervous system, joints, cardiovascular system, liver, and skin. Its clinical manifestations are equally varied: after transfer of the organism by a tick bite, one-quarter of patients locally develop *erythema chronicum migrans*, a red, annular rash that expands centrifugally around the site of the tick bite, clearing in the central area as it grows outward. If the spirochetes are then disseminated systemically, headache, fever, arthralgia, and sometimes generalized lymphadenopathy will follow.

Fifteen percent of patients who reach this stage without treatment go on to develop neurological manifestations, typically *lymphocytic meningitis* combined with *radiculoneuritis*, causing weakness, very unpleasant, often burning, dysesthesia, and severe pain in the distribution of the affected nerve roots (**Bannwarth syndrome**). Cranial nerve involvement is also common and may cause *facial diplegia*, a condition that should always arouse suspicion of borreliosis. Less commonly, plexus neuritis, encephalitis, or myelitis can develop at this stage or later.

Other possible complications of advanced borreliosis are *vasculitis of the cerebral vessels* and, outside the central nervous system, myopericarditis, acrodermatitis chronica atrophicans, arthralgia, and liver involvement.

In the United States, borreliosis is commonly known as "Lyme disease," after the town of Lyme, Connecticut, in which an outbreak was described.

Diagnostic evaluation. A clinical suspicion of neuroborreliosis can be supported, though not definitively confirmed, by the *demonstration of specific IgG and, above all, IgM antibodies in the serum and cerebrospinal fluid*.

> **!** Serologic testing for Borrelia is positive in at least 10% of asymptomatic individuals. Thus, the demonstration of antibodies against Borrelia is no reason to ascribe an unclear neurological condition to florid borreliosis.

The diagnosis of neuroborreliosis can only be made if there is an *inflammatory CSF profile* (elevated cell count and protein concentration, positive *Borrelia* titer in the CSF). A normal CSF profile makes the diagnosis questionable, even if the serologic tests are positive.

Treatment. If a borrelial infection is suspected after a tick bite (overt erythema chronicum migrans, flulike symptoms), *doxycycline* is given orally. In all later stages of the disease, *third-generation cephalosporins* (ceftriaxone, cefotaxime) are given intravenously.

Leptospirosis

Leptospirosis in its initial stage often causes acute *lymphocytic meningitis*. In a more advanced stage, there may be signs of *encephalitis* (epileptic seizures, delirious psychosis) or *myelitis*. The brain can also be damaged by vasculitis of the cerebral vessels. Outside the nervous system, leptospirosis can affect the liver (causing jaundice) and kidneys and cause a bleeding diathesis.

Encephalitis in Prion Diseases

Prions are infectious particles composed of protein that replicate within the body's cells even though they possess no genetic material (nucleic acids) of their own. They can arise in situ by mutation of the host's genetic material or reach the body from outside and incorporate themselves into its cells, where they replicate.

Neurons in the brain that have been infected by prions may die after a latency period of years or even decades. The typical pathological findings in prion infection are

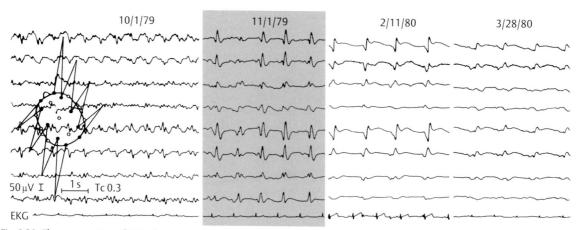

10/1/79   11/1/79   2/11/80   3/28/80

50 µV I   1 s   Tc 0.3

EKG

Fig. 6.**30 The progression of EEG changes over time in Creutz-feldt–Jakob disease.** The diagnosis of CJD in this 57-year-old woman was later confirmed by autopsy. 6 weeks after the onset of the prodromal phase (10.1.79), only a hint of periodic activity is seen. It is fully developed 1 month later (11.1.79) and slowly declines in amplitude in the ensuing months.

vacuolization and the formation of amyloid plaques (*spongiform encephalopathy, SEP*). The main prion diseases are *Creutzfeldt–Jakob disease, kuru, Gerstmann–Sträussler–Scheinker syndrome, familial progressive subcortical gliosis,* and *familial fatal insomnia.*

Creutzfeldt–Jakob disease , the most common prion disease in Europe and North America, is nevertheless rare, with an incidence of about one case per million individuals per year. It presents initially with *mental abnormalities, insomnia,* and *fatigability.* Soon, progressive *dementia* develops, along with *pyramidal tract signs, cerebellar signs, abnormalities of muscle tone, fasciculations,* and *myoclonus.* In about two-thirds of patients, the EEG reveals characteristic, periodic triphasic and tetraphasic theta and delta waves (Fig. 6.**30**). The disease progresses rapidly, leading to a decorticate state and death within months of onset. A *variant of Creutzfeldt–Jakob disease* has attracted considerable attention in the past decade, particularly in the United Kingdom, because it is contracted by eating beef derived from cows with *bovine spongiform encephalopathy* (BSE, "mad cow disease").

Slow virus diseases

The slow virus diseases are characterized by *extremely long incubation periods, a protracted, chronically progressive course,* and little or no response to treatment. SSPE is the most common slow virus disease.

Subacute sclerosing panencephalitis (SSPE) usually arises in children who had measles in their infancy. The virus persists in the central nervous system and, years later, gives rise to a disease of insidious onset and chronically progressive course, leading to death in two to three years. The initial presentation is with *mental abnormalities* such as irritability, fatigability, and impaired cognitive performance. *Involuntary movements* and *noise-induced myoclonus* appear a few weeks later. Finally, the child develops *generalized spasticity* and

severe, progressive dementia. The EEG reveals periodic, high-amplitude slow waves. The illness is always fatal.

Other illnesses whose pathogenetic mechanisms are probably similar are *progressive rubella panencephalitis* and the various types of encephalitis arising a few days or weeks after an infectious illness (measles, mumps, chickenpox, rubella).

Postvaccinal encephalitis. It has been hypothesized, but never proved, that encephalitis can rarely arise as a complication of vaccination against measles, rubella, or smallpox.

Intracranial Abscesses

Brain abscesses are produced by **focal infection of the brain parenchyma** leading to tissue destruction and pus formation. They can be solitary or multiple. A special form is **focal encephalitis,** in which systemic sepsis or the embolization of infectious material into the central nervous system gives rise to **multilocular, disseminated microabscesses.**

Brain Abscess

Etiology. Brain abscesses are caused by one or more pathogens, mainly streptococci and staphylococci and, less commonly, *Pseudomonas, Actinomyces,* and fungi. Like the organisms that cause bacterial meningitis, these pathogens can reach the brain through **local extension of infection** (especially mastoiditis, sinusitis, and otitis), **hematogenous dissemination** from a distant infectious focus (usually pulmonary infections or endocarditis), or **direct contamination** (open brain injury). Immunocompromised patients are at increased risk.

Clinical manifestations. A large **brain abscess** exerts mass effect and typically causes fever, leukocytosis, and rapidly progressive intracranial hypertension. Marked perifocal edema generally adds to the mass effect.

Alternatively, there may be a **subdural empyema** between the dura mater and the arachnoid, or an **epidural abscess** between the dura mater and the inner table of the skull. These processes usually arise as a complication of sinusitis or otitis, less commonly after trauma. Fever, headache, and meningism, accompanied by neurological deficits, are their clinical hallmarks. The course of subdural empyema is often fulminant and life-threatening, that of epidural abscess usually more protracted.

Diagnostic evaluation. The diagnosis is suspected on the basis of the *typical clinical findings* (intracranial hypertension with papilledema, impaired consciousness, sometimes hemiparesis or other focal neurological deficits), *accompanying signs of infection* (fever, elevated laboratory parameters of inflammation), and *relevant aspects of the past medical history* (such as traumatic brain injuries, known lung or heart disease, and immune suppression or diseases of the immune system). *CSF examination* may reveal inflammatory changes (predominantly granulocytic pleocytosis, elevation of total protein), and the *CT or MRI scan* shows a ring-shaped area of contrast enhancement (abscess wall) surrounding the hypodense interior of the abscess.

Treatment. *Operative removal of the abscess* is the preferred form of treatment in most patients, accompanied by *antibiotic therapy*, which is initiated before surgery and continued thereafter for at least six weeks.

Focal Encephalitis

Etiology. Focal encephalitis consists of *multilocular foci of infection in the brain parenchyma* (Fig. 6.**31**), produced either by the seeding of the brain with bacteria in generalized sepsis (*metastatic focal encephalitis*) or by the embolization of multiple infectious microthrombi into the cerebral vasculature (*embolic focal encephalitis*). The latter is usually a complication of subacute bacterial endocarditis, which, in turn, is most often caused by *Streptococcus viridans*. In contrast, the septic form may be secondary to purulent infection in practically any area of the body. Streptococcal and staphylococcal infections are the usual causes.

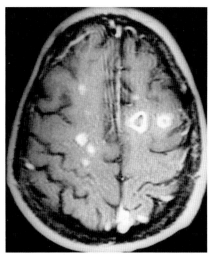

Fig. 6.**31 Embolic focal encephalitis and brain abscesses** (T1-weighted MRI after the administration of contrast medium).

Clinical manifestations. The typical findings include *signs of a generalized septic illness* (high fever, rigors) combined with *focal brain signs, impaired consciousness,* and, not uncommonly, *psychosis.* The neurological and psycho-organic signs *fluctuate* in severity. They manifest themselves in bouts, with remissions in between.

! *A septic illness accompanied by fluctuating mental status on neurological abnormalities should raise suspicion of focal encephalitis.*

Diagnostic evaluation. The diagnosis is suspected from the *clinical findings* and, possibly, *inflammatory CSF changes,* and confirmed by a *CT and/or MRI scan demonstrating multiple small lesions in the brain.* A heart murmur should always be listened for. Blood should be drawn for culture during the upward phase of the fever curve, and during rigors; blood culture may reveal the responsible pathogen.

Treatment. *Antibiotic therapy* is indicated and should be tailored to the sensitivity profile of the responsible organism, if it can be identified.

6

Diseases of the Brain and Meninges

Metabolic Disorders and Systemic Illnesses Affecting the Nervous System

The intense metabolic activity of the nervous system (both central and peripheral) makes it vulnerable to damage by a wide variety of metabolic disorders, both **congenital** (inborn errors of metabolism, i. e., metabolic diseases in the narrower sense of the term) and **acquired** (e. g., toxic). These disorders manifest themselves clinically as metabolic encephalopathy and metabolic neuropathy, of which there are many different types. Involvement of the nervous system by general medical illnesses (e. g., endocrinopathy or vasculitis) and paraneoplastic syndromes affecting the nervous system can present in similar ways.

Congenital Metabolic Disorders

Metabolic diseases are caused by **hereditary enzyme defects**. They usually present in early childhood but sometimes not until many years later. They can be roughly divided into **disorders of lipid**, **amino acid**, and **carbohydrate metabolism**. Wilson disease is due to a disturbance of copper metabolism.

General clinical manifestations. The following findings in children and adolescents suggest the presence of a metabolic disease:
- delayed motor and cognitive development,
- a slowly worsening course,
- progressive spasticity,
- progressive dementia,
- optic nerve involvement,
- epileptic seizures,
- accompanying polyneuropathy and myopathy,
- a positive family history of similar manifestations.

Diagnostic evaluation. In general, the diagnostic workup includes:
- the taking of a comprehensive family and personal history,
- a clinical neurological (neuropediatric) examination,
- amino acid screening of the urine,
- measurement of the serum concentration of glucose, ammonia, lactate, and pyruvate and screening for the lysosomal enzymes arylsulfatase A, hexosaminidase, and α-galactosidase,
- light- and electron-microscopic examination of biopsied tissue samples, with routine and special stains,
- radiologic examination of the skeleton,
- MRI of the brain.

Disorders of Lipid Metabolism

Lipid storage diseases are caused by faulty enzymatic degradation of individual lipid substances, leading to deposition of the intermediate products of lipid metabolism in various internal organs (liver, spleen, bone marrow) and in the nervous system. Disorders in which these nondegradable metabolites accumulate mainly in the *neurons* of the brain are characterized by degeneration of the cerebral cortex or of the subcortical nuclear areas (**lipidoses**); disorders in which they accumulate mainly in *white matter* are characterized by demyelination of the cerebral white matter and/or peripheral nerve sheaths (**leukodystrophies**). The lipid storage diseases affecting the nervous system are listed in Table 6.**17**. Two examples of the radiologic appearance of the brain in the leukodystrophies are shown in Fig. 6.**32**.

Disorders of Amino Acid and Uric Acid Metabolism

The more common disorders of these types include *phenylketonuria* (an autosomal recessive disorder of amino acid metabolism), *maple syrup urine disease*, *Hartnup disease*, and *homocysteinuria* (Table 6.**18**).

Disorders of Carbohydrate Metabolism

These disorders include the **monosaccharidoses** (e. g., galactosemia), the **glycogenoses**, and the **mucopolysaccharidoses** (Table 6.**19**). *Myoclonus epilepsy*, a type of mucopolysaccharidosis, is characterized by generalized epileptic seizures, myoclonus, and dementia.

Disorders of Copper Metabolism

A disturbance of copper metabolism causes **hepatolenticular degeneration** (Wilson disease), an autosomal recessive disorder whose genetic locus lies on the long arm of chromosome 13. The concentration of the copper transport protein ceruloplasmin is abnormally low and, as a result, the serum free copper concentration is high and an abnormally large amount of copper is eliminated in the urine. Free copper is deposited in the liver, the edge of the cornea (producing the typical Kayser–Fleischer ring), and the brain. *Hepatopathy* dominates the clinical picture in childhood and the *neurological manifestations* come later; the most impressive of these is a coarse postural and intention tremor of the extremities (recognizable on extension of the arms to both sides, for example, as a "flapping tremor"). Dysarthria, dystonia, and rigidity are common, as are mental abnormalities (depression, personality changes, or even psychotic episodes). The Kayser–Fleischer ring, a brown ring around the periphery of the cornea, helps to establish the diagnosis. MRI reveals cortical atrophy, enlarged ventricles, and signal abnormalities in the basal ganglia. This disorder is treated with D-penicillamine or zinc sulfate.

Fig. 6.**32** **Leukodystrophies** (T2-weighted MRI images). **a** MRI in an 8-year-old boy: symmetrical, diffuse signal abnormalities in the white matter of the occipital and parietal lobes. **b** MRI in a 43-year-old man: symmetrical signal abnormalities in white matter.

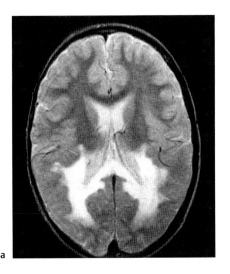
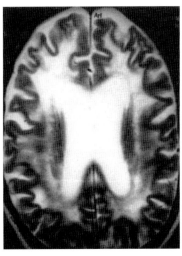

a

b

Table 6.**17** **Lipidoses and leukodystrophies affecting the nervous system**

Diseases	Clinical features	Remarks
Lipidoses		
GM1-gangliosidoses and **GM2-gangliosidoses**	infantile progressive encephalopathy, progressive myopathy in adults; possibly myoclonus, convulsions, visual impairment, progressive spasticity and dementia; muscle atrophy and progressive weakness	galactosidase deficiency in GM1-gangliosidoses; hexosaminidase deficiency in GM2-gangliosidoses, including **Tay–Sachs disease** and **Sandhoff disease**, with characteristic cherry-red spot
Fabry disease (angiokeratoma corporis diffusum)	onset of symptoms in childhood or adolescence; burning pain in the limbs, particularly in warm surroundings; deficient sweating; maculopapular, purplish-red skin changes; renal failure; frequent cerebrovascular accidents	X-linked inheritance; α-galactosidase deficiency with intracellular accumulation of trihexosylceramides
Gaucher disease juvenile and adult forms	diverse neurological manifestations, gaze paresis, bulbar signs, spasticity, polyneuropathy, psychosis, dementia, myoclonus, epileptic seizures	autosomal recessive inheritance, glucocerebrosidase deficiency; foam cells in bone marrow
Niemann–Pick disease	progressive developmental delay beginning in the first year of life; juvenile forms with encephalopathy or hepatomegaly, progressive dementia, spasticity, and ataxia as well as epileptic seizures and psychosis	autosomal recessive inheritance; genetic defect in Ashkenazi Jews
Refsum disease (heredopathia atactica polyneuritiformis)	onset of symptoms in middle age; night blindness due to retinitis pigmentosa, hearing loss, polyneuropathy with areflexia and gait ataxia; mental abnormalities	lack of phytanic acid α-dehydrogenase, accumulation of phytanic acid in the body (liver, kidneys, nervous system); a low-phytanic-acid diet and plasmapheresis are effective treatments
Cerebrotendinous xanthomatosis (cholestanol storage disease)	onset of symptoms in adolescence or later; mental retardation; juvenile cataracts, progressive spasticity and ataxia; xanthomas, particularly on extensor tendons and Achilles' tendons; polyneuropathy and muscle atrophy	autosomal recessive inheritance; impaired synthesis of bile acids; accumulation of cholestanol in plasma and brain, tendon xanthomas
Neuronal ceroid lipofuscinosis (Batten–Kufs disease)	presentation in infancy and early childhood (Spielmeyer–Vogt type) or in adulthood (Kufs disease); ataxia, myoclonus, epileptic seizures, progressive visual loss and mental deterioration	
Leukodystrophies:		
Metachromatic leukodystrophy	*late infantile type:* from the age of 1 year onward, spastic weakness progressing toward quadriplegia, loss of mental function, areflexia, bulbar and pseudobulbar signs, optic atrophy; *juvenile type:* presentation at age 2–10 years, elevated CSF protein, white matter hypodense in CT and hyperintense in T2-MRI	autosomal recessive inheritance; lack of arylsulfatase A; accumulation of sulfatide in the brain, peripheral nerves, and other tissues; demonstration of arylsulfatase A deficiency in leukocytes and urine
Globoid cell leukodystrophy (Krabbe disease)	infantile, juvenile, and adult types; spasticity, optic atrophy, and polyneuropathy	lack of galactocerebrosidase

Table 6.**18**   **Disorders of amino acid and urate metabolism**

Disease	Clinial features	Remarks
Phenylketonuria	clinical manifestations from the age of 6 months onward, if untreated: mental retardation, epileptic seizures, spasticity, tremor, hypopigmentation	autosomal recessive inheritance; lack of hydroxylation of phenylalanine to tyrosine; treated with a low-phenylalanine diet; neonatal screening (Guthrie test)
Maple syrup urine disease	presentation in the neonatal period: impaired alertness, diminished muscle tone, mental retardation	impaired degradation of branched amino acids; sweet-smelling urine (like maple syrup)
Hartnup disease	bouts of pellagralike dermatitis, accompanied by episodes of ataxia, nystagmus, and gait unsteadiness, progressive dementia, and spasticity	impaired tubular and intestinal resorption of tryptophan; aminoaciduria
Homocysteinuria	arterial and venous thromboembolism, lens ectopy, mental retardation	impairment of methionine metabolism

Table 6.**19**   **Disorders of carbohydrate metabolism**

Disease	Clinical features	Remarks
Galactosemia	onset in infancy: failure to thrive, retardation, jaundice, cataracts	impaired enzymatic degradation of galactose; accumulation of the phosphorylated form in the liver, kidneys, lenses, and brain
Glycogenoses, types I–XI	accumulation of glycogen in the liver, kidneys, muscles, and brain; clinically, hepatic dysfunction, possibly myopathy, mental retardation, epileptic seizures	impaired enzymatic degradation of glycogen
Mucopolysaccharidoses	*Pfaundler–Hurler syndrome:* onset in infancy, corneal opacification, joint swelling, dwarfism, mental retardation, possibly quadriparesis due to spinal cord compression *Scheie syndrome:* juvenile type, with slow progression *Progressive myoclonus epilepsy (Lafora type):* generalized epileptic seizures, myoclonus, progressive dementia, psychosis	deposition of acidic mucopolysaccharides in various tissues, due to hydrolase deficiency deposition of mucopolysaccharides in the form of Lafora bodies in the brain, muscles, and liver

Other Metabolic Disorders

A number of other metabolic disorders must be mentioned here for completeness, some of which are of as yet unknown causes. **Adrenoleukodystrophy** is due to an inherited defect of the X chromosome, which causes a deficiency of lignoceroyl coenzyme A synthetase. Most patients are male. In the first or second decade of life, they develop spastic gait disturbances, visual impairment, and mental changes. Affected adults may develop adrenal insufficiency. In **adrenomyeloneuropathy**, the same manifestations are present, with polyneuropathy in addition. **Reye syndrome** is probably of multifactorial origin. A few days after a viral illness, the patient becomes progressively somnolent, with nausea, delirium, and cerebral edema. In the various types of **α-lipoproteinemia**, the serum cholesterol and triglyceride levels are abnormally low. These disorders are clinically characterized by ataxia, nystagmus, disturbances of eye movement, and polyneuropathy, in combination with retinitis pigmentosa. These manifestations are often accompanied by acanthocytosis (Bassen–Kornzweig).

Acquired Metabolic Disorders

Intoxications

> **Medications, recreationally used substances, drugs of abuse, industrial toxins**, and numerous other substances can exert a toxic influence on the nervous system.

Intoxications of the nervous system are classified according to their clinical presentation in Table 6.**20**, which also includes iatrogenic intoxications.

Alcohol-induced Disorders of the Nervous System

Because of their importance in clinical practice, the effects of alcohol on the nervous system are listed in detail in a separate table (Table 6.**21**).

Table 6.**20**   **Neurological manifestations of toxic or iatrogenic origin**

Neurological signs and syndromes	Causes
Headache	nearly all headache preparations when overused; withdrawal of caffeine, ergotamine, or amphetamine; oral contraceptives and other hormone preparations (pseudotumor cerebri); nitrates, aminophylline, tetracycline, sympathomimetics, IV immunoglobulins, tamoxifen, H₂-antagonists
Ischemic stroke	oral contraceptives and other hormone preparations, antihypertensive agents, ergotamine, amphetamine, cocaine, sympathomimetics, intra-arterial methotrexate, angiography, interventional intra-arterial procedures, cardiovascular surgery, radiotherapy, fat injection ("liposculpturing"), chiropractic manipulation
Hemorrhage (intracerebral, extracerebral, spinal)	anticoagulants, fibrinolytic agents, inhibitors of platelet aggregation, amphetamine, cocaine, sympathomimetics; femoral nerve palsy due to psoas hematoma
Epileptic seizures	antibiotics (penicillin, isoniazid), general and local anaesthetics (e. g., lidocaine), insulin, radiological contrast media, withdrawal of benzodiazepines or other sedatives, anticonvulsant withdrawal, phenytoin overdose, antidepressants, aminophylline and theophylline, phenothiazines, pentazocine, tripelennamine, cocaine, meperidine, cyclosporine, antineoplastic agents, other
Coma	insulin, barbiturates, benzodiazepines and other sedatives, analgesics, other
Neurasthenic symptoms, acute and chronic **encephalopathy**	heavy metals, lithium, aluminum, heroin pyrolysate, cyclosporine, anticholinergics, dopamine agonists, benzodiazepines and other sedatives, antihistamines, antibiotics, anticonvulsants, corticosteroids, H₂-antagonists, disulfiram, methotrexate, organic solvents, hallucinogens, radiotherapy, dehydration, water intoxication, dialysis encephalopathy, other
Extrapyramidal movement disorders (acute dystonia, dyskinesia, akathisia, drug-induced parkinsonism, tardive dyskinesia)	neuroleptics (phenothiazines, thioxanthenes, butyrophenones, dibenzapines), antiemetics containing metoclopramide or phenothiazines, dopamine agonists, levodopa, antihypertensive agents (e. g., reserpine, captopril), flunarizine, cinnarizine, MPTP
Cerebellar ataxia	phenytoin, carbamazepine, barbiturates, lithium, organic solvents, heavy metals, acrylamide, 5-fluorouracil, cytosine arabinoside, procarbazine, hexamethylmelamine, vincristine, cyclosporine, ciguatera fish poisoning
Central pontine myelinolysis	too rapid correction of hyponatremia
Malignant neuroleptic syndrome	neuroleptics
Malignant hyperthermia	succinylcholine, halothane, other general anaesthetics
Polyneuropathy	see p. 176 ff.
Optic neuropathy	tobacco, ethanol, methanol, myambutol
Deafness	aminoglycosides, cytostatic agents
Disorders of neuromuscular transmission	penicillamine, muscle relaxants, procainamide, magnesium, quinine, aminoglycosides, α-interferon
Myopathy and **rhabdomyolysis**	ethanol, cocaine, heroin and other opiates, pentazocine, benzene, corticosteroids, thyroxine, antimalarial agents, colchicine, antilipid agents (fibrates and statins), zidovudine, cyclosporine, diuretics (via hypokalemia), ipecac

Table 6.**21**   **Effects of alcohol on the nervous system**

Clinical condition	Features	Remarks
Acute alcohol intoxication	euphoria, dysphoria, disinhibition, ataxia, somnolence, stupor	respiratory arrest may cause death
Alcohol withdrawal syndrome, delirium tremens	diaphoresis, tachycardia, insomnia, tremor, hallucinations, epileptic seizures, psychomotor agitation, possibly delirium	when the patient's alcohol intake is cut off, the blood alcohol level falls and the patient passes through the stages of alcohol withdrawal syndrome, from mild autonomic symptoms to predelirium and delirium; full delirium (delirium tremens) is the most severe form of the alcohol withdrawal syndrome; treated with clomethiazole
Alcoholic dementia	chronic alcohol abuse with systemic effects on the liver and peripheral nervous system	brain atrophy, visible in CT and MRI, reversible with abstinence
Wernicke encephalopathy	memory impairment, confusion, oculomotor dysfunction (abducens palsy, nystagmus, conjugate gaze palsy), ataxia, dysarthria	signal abnormalities around the cerebral aqueduct and third ventricle in T2-weighted MRI; caused by thiamine deficiency and malnutrition; often combined with Korsakoff psychosis

6

Diseases of the Brain and Meninges

Continued →

Table 6.**21**   **Effects of alcohol on the nervous system** (Continued)

Clinical condition	Features	Remarks
Korsakoff syndrome	acute amnestic syndrome with anterograde and retrograde amnesia, confabulation, reduced drive, and reckless behavior	thiamine deficiency; seen also in nonalcoholics
Marchiafava–Bignami syndrome	acute confusion, epileptic seizures, impairment of consciousness; demyelination of corpus callosum and centrum semiovale; patients who survive the acute phase are often abulic and demented	predominantly seen in Italian drinkers of red wine
Alcoholic cerebellar degeneration	progressive limb ataxia mainly affecting the lower limbs, with impairment of gait	
Central pontine myelinolysis	confusion, followed within a few days by dysphagia, dysarthria, quadriparesis with pyramidal tract signs, and oculomotor disturbances (bilateral abducens palsy or horizontal conjugate gaze palsy); progressive impairment of consciousness, later development of the locked-in syndrome	seen in malnourished chronic alcoholics, also as an iatrogenic process after excessively rapid correction of hyponatremia; also in liver disease
Alcoholic polyneuropathy	predominantly sensory polyneuropathy, often painful; distal sensory deficit in the lower limbs, loss of reflexes	
Fetal alcohol syndrome (alcohol embryopathy)	caused by maternal alcoholism; short stature, psychomotor retardation, microcephaly, facial dysmorphism (stub nose, thin lips, micrognathism)	

Endocrine Diseases

> Neurological manifestations often accompany dysfunction of the endocrine glands, particularly the **thyroid gland**, the **parathyroid glands**, the **pancreatic islet cells**, and the **adrenal gland**.

Hypothyroidism causes *cretinism* in infants, *mental retardation* and *short stature* in children. In adults, it can cause *ataxia*, *dysarthria*, and *nystagmus*, a predominantly *sensory polyneuropathy*, and *muscle weakness*, with characteristically delayed relaxation of muscle fibers after elicitation of the deep tendon reflexes. *Mental abnormalities* may also be present (apathy, depression, dementia, delirium).

Table 6.**22**   **Clinical manifestations of hypoglycemia**

Autonomic manifestations
Dizziness, diaphoresis, nausea, pallor, palpitations, precordial pressure, abdominal pain, hunger, anxiety, headache

Cerebral manifestations
- paresthesiae, blurred vision, diplopia, tremor, unusual or abnormal behavior
- epileptic seizures: simple partial, complex partial, or generalized
- impairment of consciousness ranging from somnolence to coma
- focal neurological deficits, e. g., hemiparesis, hemianopsia, aphasia, apraxia

Permanent neurological deficits (after prolonged or repeated episodes of hypoglycemia)
- cognitive deficits, dementia
- cognitive deficits of focal type, focal neurological deficits
- mainly distal muscular atrophy due to damage of anterior horn cells and axons

Hyperthyroidism can produce, in addition to its characteristic *general manifestations* (nervousness, insomnia, tremor, sweating, tachycardia, diarrhea, heat intolerance), a variety of neurological deficits:
- *cerebral manifestations*: irritability, psychotic episodes, tremor, choreoathetosis, spastic elevation of muscle tone, pyramidal tract signs;
- *ocular manifestations*: diminished frequency of blinking (Stellwag sign), ophthalmoplegia, diplopia, optic neuropathy; in Graves disease, lid retraction (Graefe sign), weakness of convergence (Möbius sign), exophthalmos;
- *muscular manifestations*: thyrotoxic myopathy with mainly proximal weakness, myasthenia gravis, and thyrotoxic periodic paralysis;
- partial and generalized *epileptic seizures*;
- rarely, *polyneuropathy*.

Hypoparathyroidism. A deficiency of parathyroid hormone causes *hypocalcemia*, leading to tetany, epileptic seizures, intracranial hypertension with headache and papilledema, hypomotor and hypermotor movement disorders, and neurastheniform mental manifestations and delirium.

Hyperparathyroidism. An excess of parathyroid hormone manifests itself clinically mainly through *behavioral disturbances* (emotional lability, agitation, fatigability, and confusional states) and *dementia-like cognitive impairment*, in addition to muscle weakness, ataxia, dysarthria, and sometimes spasticity and epileptic seizures.

Disturbances of insulin metabolism. *Hyperinsulinism* is one of the possible causes of hypoglycemia, which causes the neurological manifestations listed in Table 6.**22**. The most prominent neurological manifestation of the *insulin deficiency* of diabetes mellitus is poly-neuropathy (see p. 176); in addition, diabetic arteriopathy may secondarily harm the nervous system (ischemic stroke, mononeuropathies of peripheral or cranial nerves).

Gastrointestinal Diseases

> Gastrointestinal diseases can cause **toxic** damage to the nervous system (e. g., in hepatic dysfunction). The nervous system can also be harmed by secondary **nutritional deficiencies** and **hypovitaminoses** (e. g., in stomach diseases and intestinal resorptive disorders).

Neurological manifestations are commonly seen in **hepatic diseases**, particularly *chronic hepatopathy* with *portal hypertension*, and a *portacaval shunt.* Ammonia and other toxic substances bypass the portal circulation, enter the systemic circulation, and are transported to the brain, where they cause *hepatic encephalopathy.* This disorder is characterized at first by somnolence and apathy, later by progressive impairment of consciousness and delirium. As in renal insufficiency, *asterixis* can be seen (see below). In addition, there may be *spasticity,* with exaggerated deep tendon reflexes and pyramidal tract signs.

Other gastrointestinal diseases. In **sprue**, impaired intestinal resorption can cause malnutrition, which in turn causes polyneuropathy and cerebellar ataxia (vitamin B_{12} deficiency). The gliadin antibodies that are present in sprue are also often associated with ataxia. **Crohn disease** may be accompanied by myelopathy and muscle weakness, while ulcerative colitis may be accompanied by peripheral neuropathy.

Hematologic Diseases

> Hematologic diseases can alter the **viscosity and coagulability of the blood**, putting the patient at risk of thrombosis or hemorrhage. They can also alter its **transport properties** (quantitative and structural anomalies of the blood cells or plasma proteins). Finally, some hematologic diseases involve **malignant neoplasia** of certain types of blood cells. All of these phenomena can have damaging effects on the nervous system.

Anemia reduces the oxygen-carrying capacity of the blood and can lead to *cerebral hypoxic (ischemic) manifestations.* The vitamin B_{12} deficiency of untreated *pernicious anemia* causes funicular myelosis (p. 153) and polyneuropathy (cf. Table 10.**1**, p. 176).

Polycythemia vera is associated with headache, dizziness, and paresthesiae, as well as ischemic stroke and extrapyramidal manifestations.

Leukemia often leads to cerebrovascular complications (hemorrhage, infarct, venous sinus thrombosis). One-third of leukemia patients have a meningeal leukemic infiltrate (leukemic meningitis). Leukemic infiltrates can cause various kinds of focal deficits of the central and peripheral nervous system.

Collagen Diseases and Immune Diseases

> Collagenoses affect not only the skin, joints, and internal organs, but also the nervous system. Secondary damage of nervous tissue (ischemia and/or hemorrhage) occurs because of inflammatory changes of the blood vessels of the brain, spinal cord, and peripheral nerves (vasa nervorum). These vascular changes are mostly produced by autoimmune mechanisms.

In this section, we will merely list the neurological manifestations of the main types of collagen disease. More detailed discussions can be found in textbooks of internal medicine.

> **!** *Though collagen diseases and vasculitic conditions are only briefly discussed in this book, the clinician must keep them in mind when formulating the differential diagnosis of practically any condition with neurological manifestations.*

Collagen diseases are diagnosed by their typical clinical manifestations, the demonstration of specific (auto-)antibodies in the serum, and further evidence derived from angiography or from biopsies of tissue and/or blood vessels.

Periarteritis nodosa. In the nervous system, this disease causes polyneuropathy and mononeuropathies and, less commonly, focal deficits of the central nervous system or epileptic seizures.

Churg–Strauss syndrome. The main clinical manifestations of this disorder, closely related to periarteritis nodosa, are bronchial asthma and eosinophilia; polyneuritis is the main neurological manifestation.

GANS (granulomatous angiitis of the central nervous system) is a vasculitic disorder, restricted to the cerebral vessels, that causes multiple thrombotic strokes.

Temporal arteritis. Intractable *headache* is the main symptom of this disease. The temporal artery is thickened (at least on one side) and, in advanced disease, no longer pulsates. A more extensive discussion of this disease can be found on page 250.

Wegener granulomatosis is a systemic, necrotizing vasculitis that primarily involves the kidneys and the upper airways, but can also cause mononeuritis (of the cranial nerves as well) and focal manifestations in the central nervous system.

6

Diseases of the Brain and Meninges

Systemic lupus erythematosus only rarely presents with neurological deficits, but more than half of all patients develop neurological and/or psychiatric manifestations as the disease progresses. The most common types are headache, neuropsychological deficits and behavioral abnormalities, focal neurological deficits, and spinal cord transection syndromes, followed by neuritis and myopathy.

Sarcoidosis (Boeck disease) is characterized by the formation of multiple granulomas in the lungs and other internal organs. Depending on their location, granulomas in the nervous system can cause chronic meningitis (p. 113), encephalitic manifestations (diabetes insipidus, hemiparesis, ataxia), cranial nerve palsies, or mononeuritis multiplex (p. 179).

Renal Failure and Electrolyte Disturbances

> Electrolyte disturbances can impair the functioning of the **brain** (impairment of consciousness and/or cognition, generalized epileptic seizures) and of the **neuromuscular junction** (overexcitability, e. g., in tetany due to hypocalcemia; underexcitability, e. g., in disorders of potassium metabolism with episodic paralysis, see p. 271). Electrolyte disturbances, particularly those affecting sodium concentration, are often caused by **renal failure**. In renal disease, the pathological retention of substances normally excreted in the urine has further toxic effects.

Acute renal failure causes *uremic encephalopathy*, which is characterized by progressive impairment of concentration and short-term memory, followed by impairment of consciousness and delirium. These abnormalities of mental state are often accompanied by *dysarthria, gait unsteadiness*, and *ataxia. Myoclonus* and *asterixis* (bilateral, irregular back-and-forth movements of the fingers when the arms are extended; sometimes, analogous motor phenomena in other parts of the body as well) are seen in nearly all patients.

Chronic renal failure may lead to the development of *polyneuropathy* and "*restless legs syndrome*" (p. 261). Patients undergoing dialysis may develop the *dialysis disequilibrium syndrome* (nausea, agitation, delirium, convulsions). Those who have been treated with dialysis for a long time are at risk for *dialysis encephalopathy* (dialysis dementia), with dysarthria, ataxia, and convulsions.

Electrolyte disturbances. Disturbances of sodium concentration alter the serum osmolality and are the type of electrolyte disturbance most commonly causing neurological dysfunction. The neurological condition in such cases can be considered a type of metabolic encephalopathy. **Hyponatremia and hypo-osmolality** cause cerebral edema, which presents clinically with headache, nausea, impaired attention and concentration, epileptic seizures, and a progressive decline of consciousness. **Hypernatremia and hyperosmolality** lower the water content of the brain and, therefore, also its volume, and cause cognitive impairment and a progressive decline of consciousness. The generalized hypercoagulable state characterizing these conditions may lead to venous sinus thrombosis. Alternatively, as the brain shrinks from loss of water, bridging veins may be torn, producing a subdural hematoma.

A rapid return of sodium concentration from below normal (hyponatremic) toward normal values is thought to be the cause of **central pontine myelinolysis**, i. e., bilaterally symmetrical demyelination of the white matter of the base of the pons. Clinically, the disorder presents with impairment of consciousness, dysphagia, dysarthria, and spastic quadriparesis, and sometimes oculomotor dysfunction (horizontal gaze paresis). Severe cases can cause the "locked-in syndrome" (p. 77) or decerebrate rigidity.

Disturbances of potassium, calcium, and magnesium balance, as well as hypophosphatemia, can affect muscular function, sometimes dramatically. **Hypokalemia or hyperkalemia** can cause flaccid paralysis of peripheral neurogenic type, as well as disturbances of myocardial excitability. **Hypocalcemia or hypomagnesemia** causes tetany; **hypercalcemia or hypermagnesemia** causes metabolic encephalopathy with slowing, confusion, and impairment of consciousness. **Hypophosphatemia** causes peripheral weakness.

Malignancy

> Malignant neoplasia can impair the functioning of the nervous system by **direct tumor invasion**, **metastasis** (p. 95), or **long-distance humorally mediated effects** (paraneoplastic syndromes).

Paraneoplastic effects can, in principle, occur in any type of malignancy, but are especially common in *small-cell bronchial carcinoma*. Paraneoplastic syndromes often become clinically evident while the primary tumor is still asymptomatic. They can predominantly affect the central nervous system, the spinal nerve roots, the peripheral nerves, or the muscles. They are diagnosed based on their clinical findings, combined with the identification of the responsible tumor; the diagnosis can be confirmed, in many patients, by the demonstration of more or less specific antineuronal antibodies. Nonetheless, paraneoplastic syndromes are still, in general, diagnoses of exclusion. Some of the paraneoplastic syndromes affecting the nervous system are listed in Table 6.**23**, together with the primary tumors that cause them.

Tabelle 6.**23** **Paraneoplastic syndromes affecting the nervous system**

Syndrome/structure affected	Clinical features	Remarks
Paraneoplastic encephalomyelitis	affects the cerebral hemispheres, limbic system, brainstem, cerebellum, and spinal cord; limbic system involvement is prominent; confusion, agitation, hallucinations, anxiety, depression, epileptic seizures, pyramidal tract signs	occurs in small-cell bronchial carcinoma, less commonly in carcinoma of the breast, ovary, uterus, and other organs; there are subtypes that preferentially affect individual nervous structures, e. g., paraneoplastic myelitis, paraneoplastic retinopathy, opsoclonus–myoclonus syndrome, and stiff man syndrome
Paraneoplastic cerebellar degeneration	rapidly progressive cerebellar ataxia (weeks), disabling truncal and appendicular ataxia, dysarthria, nystagmus, and sometimes other neurological deficits	the most common paraneoplastic syndrome; actually a subtype of paraneoplastic encephalomyelitis; seen in small-cell bronchial carcinoma, ovarian carcinoma, Hodgkin lymphoma
Paraneoplastic polyneuropathy	sensory or, less commonly, sensorimotor polyneuropathy or mononeuropathy	mainly in lung carcinoma
Paraneoplastic syndromes of the neuromuscular junction: myasthenia gravis and Lambert–Eaton syndrome	myasthenic syndrome preferentially affecting the extraocular and bulbar musculature in myasthenia gravis and the limb muscles in Lambert–Eaton syndrome	thymoma (myasthenia gravis); mainly small-cell bronchial carcinoma (Lambert–Eaton syndrome)
Dermatomyositis, polymyositis	progressive muscle weakness; in dermatomyositis, skin changes also	tumors of the breast, lung, stomach, ovary, and intestine

Diseases of the Basal Ganglia

Fundamentals

In general, diseases of the basal ganglia are characterized by either too much or too little **movement impulse**, **movement automatism**, and/or **muscle tone** (p. 18). The typical signs and symptoms of these diseases include:

- an abnormality of movement (in all cases of basal ganglionic disease)
- muscular hyper- or hypotonia (in most patients)
- involuntary movements (often)
- neuropsychological deficits (sometimes).

Elevated muscle tone is often combined with paucity of movement, while diminished muscle tone is often combined with an excess of movement. Thus, extrapyramidal syndromes can be broadly classified into:

- hypertonic–hypokinetic syndromes and
- hypotonic–hyperkinetic syndromes.

Diseases Causing Hypertonia and Hypokinesia

In hypertonic–hyperkinetic syndromes, elevated muscle tone is typically manifest as **rigidity**. Paucity of movement, depending on its severity, is termed either **hypokinesia** (= diminished movement) or **akinesia** (= complete lack of movement). A third so-called "cardinal manifestation," **tremor**, is also commonly present. This clinical triad, called the **parkinsonian syndrome** (or **parkinsonism**), is typically found in **idiopathic Parkinson disease**. This disease, however, is only one possible cause of parkinsonism; there are many others besides, some of which have a clearly identifiable cause. Parkinsonism may be due to an underlying illness or condition other than idiopathic Parkinson disease (**symptomatic parkinsonian syndromes**). In addition, a number of systemic neurodegenerative diseases cause parkinsonism. These diseases are marked by a loss of neurons not only in the basal ganglia, but also in other areas of the CNS, and thus are clinically characterized not only by extrapyramidal manifestations, but also by neurological deficits localizable to other regions of the brain.

Idiopathic Parkinson Disease

Epidemiology. Parkinson disease has an overall prevalence of 0.15 % and a mean age of onset of 55 years. Its age-specific prevalence rises with increasing age, to 1 % in persons over 60 and 3 % in persons over 80.

The etiology of idiopathic Parkinson disease is unknown. There are a number of rare conditions similar to idiopathic Parkinson disease that run in families (so-called *hereditary Parkinson disease*; one well-known variety is the Parkinson-dementia complex seen on the island of Guam). Though most cases of idiopathic Parkinson disease are sporadic, rather than familial, certain genetic factors do appear to play a role in its causation (above all the chromosome segments 2q, 6q, 4q, and 4p).

The neuropathological hallmark of idiopathic Parkinson disease is degeneration of the dopaminergic neurons of the substantia nigra and the locus ceruleus. Hyaline inclusion bodies, called Lewy bodies, are found within the degenerated neurons.

The loss of dopaminergic neurons leads to a degeneration of the nigrostriatal dopaminergic pathway and, therefore, to **dopamine deficiency in the striatum**. This, in turn, results in enhanced activity of striatal glutamatergic neurons, which produces the clinical manifestations of the disease.

Clinical manifestations. The clinical picture is typically characterized by:
- *hypokinesia*, i. e., slowing of movement,
- *increased muscle tone*,
- *abnormal body posture* (stooped head and trunk, flexion at the knees),
- *impaired postural reflexes*,
- often *tremor*,
- later, *neuropsychological deficits*, and
- a number of other manifestations, to be described.

The motor signs (both "plus" and "minus") are often only unilateral, or more marked on one side, when the disease first appears.

Hypokinesia manifests itself as *paucity of facial expression* (mask facies), *reduced frequency of blinking*, and *speech disturbances* (slow, monotonous, unmodulated speech, repetitions). There is little spontaneous movement, and the normal accessory movements (e. g., of the arms during walking) are diminished or absent. The patient's handwriting becomes progressively smaller (*micrographia*). Repeated or alternating movements are performed slowly (dysdiadochokinesia). Axial movements, such as turning around in a standing position or turning over in bed, are difficult to perform. Very severe hypokinesia is sometimes called *akinesia*.

The patient's gait is characterized by a mildly stooped posture, with the head jutting forward, and a small-stepped, often shuffling gait, without accessory arm movements (Fig. 6.**33**). To turn around in a standing position, the patient makes numerous, small turning steps.

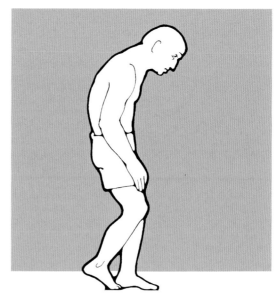

Fig. 6.**33 Typical posture of a patient with Parkinson disease while walking.**

Increased muscle tone is primarily evident as *rigidity* (p. 29, Fig. 3.**22**), felt by the examiner during large-amplitude, passive flexion and extension of the joints. Rigidity is sometimes easier to detect when the patient voluntarily contracts the muscles on the opposite side of the body. Often, during passive movement, the examiner may feel a small, brief, periodically recurring diminution of muscle tone, known as the *cogwheel phenomenon*, which is usually most evident in the radiocarpal joint (Fig. 3.**23**, p. 30). The patient's *postural tone, too*, is elevated; if, for example, the head is lifted off the bed and let go; it may remain suspended in midair for some time (the classic literature spoke of a *"coussin psychique,"* i. e., an imaginary pillow).

Tremor is seen eventually in 3/4 of patients, most often a distal rest tremor at a frequency of 5 Hz. A pronation–supination ("pill-rolling") tremor is highly characteristic. The tremor is present at rest and generally disappears on voluntary movement; it is sometimes increased by mental exertion, concentration, or walking. Some patients have postural and intention tremor in addition to rest tremor (p. 29).

An impairment of postural reflexes, combined with hypokinesia, has the consequence that changes of body posture and orientation in space can no longer be compensated for by reflexive, rapid corrective movements. The most obvious manifestations of this problem are *pro- and retropulsion.* If the patient is pushed while standing still, or stumbles over an obstacle, the movements made to regain balance are too small and too slow, and a fall may result.

Neuropsychological deficits usually appear as the disease progresses. Memory is impaired, cognitive processes are slowed, and there is a tendency toward perseveration: rapid changes in the content of thought are difficult to achieve.

Table 6.**24** **Simplified scale for evaluating the severity of individual signs of Parkinson disease** (Webster, 1968)

1. **Bradykinesia of hands, including handwriting**
   0 = normal
   1 = mild slowing
   2 = moderate slowing, handwriting severely impaired
   3 = severe slowing

2. **Rigidity**
   0 = none
   1 = mild
   2 = moderate
   3 = severe, present despite medication

3. **Posture**
   0 = normal
   1 = mildly stooped
   2 = arm flexion
   3 = severely stooped; arm, hand, and knee flexion

4. **Arm swing**
   0 = good bilaterally
   1 = unilaterally impaired
   2 = unilaterally absent
   3 = bilaterally absent

5. **Gait**
   0 = normal, turns without difficulty
   1 = short steps, slow turn
   2 = markedly shortened steps, both heels slap on floor
   3 = shuffling steps, occasional freezing, very slow turn

6. **Tremor**
   0 = none
   1 = amplitude < 2.5 cm
   2 = amplitude > 10 cm
   3 = amplitude > 10 cm, constant, eating and writing impossible

7. **Facial expression**
   0 = normal
   1 = mild hypomimia
   2 = marked hypomimia, lips open, marked drooling
   3 = masklike facies, mouth open, marked drooling

8. **Seborrhea**
   0 = none
   1 = increased sweating
   2 = oily skin
   3 = marked deposition on face

9. **Speech**
   0 = normal
   1 = reduced modulation, good volume
   2 = monotonous, not modulated, incipient dysarthria, difficulty being understood
   3 = marked difficulty being understood

10. **Independence**
   0 = not impaired
   1 = mildly impaired (dressing)
   2 = needs help in critical situations, all activities markedly slowed
   3 = cannot dress him- or herself, eat or walk unaided

Possible further symptoms and signs include seborrhea, orthostatic hypotension, disturbances of the sense of smell, and constipation.

Classification and quantification. The foregoing clinical manifestations are not all present to equal degrees in every patient. Idiopathic Parkinson disease has the following clinical subtypes:
- the *akinetic-rigid* subtype (without tremor),
- the *tremor-dominant* subtype (with relatively little hypokinesia and rigidity), and
- the *equivalence* or *mixed* subtype (with equally severe tremor, rigidity, and hypokinesia).

The individual clinical manifestations can be *quantified* (e. g., for research purposes, or for long-term patient follow-up) with the aid of the *Webster Rating Scale* (Table 6.**24**) or the very detailed *Unified Parkinson Disease Rating Scale* (UPDRS, not presented here).

Physical findings and other diagnostic tests. The diagnosis is made based on the *typical clinical manifestations* and *characteristic findings* on neurological examination and further diagnostic testing. In addition to hypokinesia, rigidity, tremor, and propulsion and retropulsion, examination generally reveals a weakness of convergence and a persistent glabellar reflex (i. e., lack of habituation of the reflex after repeated glabellar tapping). Ocular pursuit movements are often saccadic. The intrinsic muscle reflexes are normal, however, as are all

modalities of sensory function. CT and MRI of the head reveal no abnormalities; the loss of striatal dopaminergic afferent fibers can be demonstrated with PET or SPECT after the administration of [18]fluorodopa.

Idiopathic Parkinson disease is always a *diagnosis of exclusion*, i. e., all varieties of symptomatic parkinsonism must be ruled out before this diagnosis can be made.

Treatment. Effective therapy alleviates the manifestations of the disease, moving the symptomatic progression curve to the right by some three to five years, but does not affect the disease process as such. The putative early neuroprotective effect of selegiline and similar medications has not yet been confirmed.

Pharmacotherapy replaces the missing dopamine in the striatum. **Dopamine agonists** (e. g., bromocriptine, lisuride, pergolide, ropinirol, or pramipexol) are preferred for initial treatment in younger patients; the effectiveness of these agents, however, matches that of L-DOPA only in the early stages of the disease. The disease manifestations can sometimes be controlled adequately for a few months, and the need for dopaminergic treatment deferred, by using either **amantadine** (thought to enhance dopamine release from nerve terminals) or **selegiline** (an MAO-B inhibitor that slows the degradation of dopamine to homovanillic acid). In older patients, **L-DOPA** is used from the outset. This agent, unlike dopamine itself, crosses the blood–brain barrier; it is converted to dopamine in the central nervous system. It is always given in combination with a decarboxylase inhibitor to prevent its premature degradation in the periphery. A **COMT inhibitor**, such as tolcapone or entacapone, can further increase dopamine bioavailability. Tolcapone, however, is occasionally hepatotoxic and is therefore reserved for otherwise intractable cases.

Neurosurgical treatment consists of the stereotactic implantation of stimulating electrodes into the thalamus, globus pallidus, or subthalamic nucleus for deep brain stimulation. This method has now largely replaced earlier methods involving the creation of permanent lesions.

In addition to medications and surgery, **physical therapy** and **speech therapy** play important roles in patient care, as does adequate psychological support for patients and their families. **Self-help groups** can be very valuable in this regard.

Medication side effects and complications. Prolonged L-DOPA treatment can cause a number of problems:

- **Fluctuations in drug effect** ("on–off" phases, end-of-dose akinesia) can often be improved by the use of sustained-release L-DOPA preparations, division of the daily dose into smaller individual doses at more frequent intervals (perhaps with the use of liquid preparations), and/or the addition of dopamine agonists or COMT inhibitors.
- **Drug-induced dyskinesias**, e. g., peak-dose dyskinesia or hyperkinesia (often manifest as choreiform involuntary movements), are seen in 40% of patients after six months of L-DOPA treatment, in 60% after two years, and in 100% after six years. They are usually more disturbing to patients' families than to the patients themselves.
- **Painful foot dystonia** can be managed with the use of sustained-release preparations in the evening and perhaps by the subcutaneous injection of 2–5 mg of apomorphine, as needed.
- **"Freezing,"** i. e., sudden arrest of movement, is not directly related to the serum concentration of L-DOPA. Various mental techniques can help (carrying a briefcase, etc.).
- **Psychosis** may respond to a reduction of the dose or to the addition of an atypical neuroleptic drug (clozapine, risperidone).
- **Akinetic crisis** is a prolonged phase of extreme rigidity causing complete immobility and accompanied by hyperthermia, hyperhidrosis, other autonomic disturbances, and dysphagia. It is treated with water-soluble L-DOPA and intravenous amantadine.
- **Malignant L-DOPA withdrawal syndrome**, consisting of rigidity, hyperthermia, autonomic disregulation, impairment of consciousness, and elevation of the serum CK, is treated with dopamine agonists and dantrolene.

Prognosis. The tremor-dominant type has a relatively favorable prognosis. L-DOPA treatment can shift the symptomatic progression curve to the right by six to seven years. It is hard to predict which patients will eventually become dependent on nursing care. This tends to occur after about 20 years of illness.

Table 6.25   The differential diagnosis of idiopathic Parkinson disease

Arteriosclerotic parkinsonism
(e. g., in subcortical arteriosclerotic encephalopathy)

Medication-induced parkinsonism
- neuroleptic agents (most common cause)
- reserpine
- flunarizine

Parkinsonism of infectious origin
- postencephalitic parkinsonism (after encephalitis lethargica)
- cerebrospinal syphilis
- AIDS encephalopathy

Normal pressure hydrocephalus

Wilson disease

Repeated blunt trauma to the head (so-called boxer's encephalopathy)

Toxic parkinsonism
- carbon monoxide poisoning (most common cause)
- manganese poisoning
- MPTP

Parkinsonism in the setting of *other neurodegenerative diseases*

Other causes: brain tumor, subdural hematoma, polycythemia vera

Symptomatic Parkinsonism

There are a number of clinical conditions resembling idiopathic Parkinson disease that have another underlying cause or pathophysiological mechanism. The clue to such a condition may be a history of a **precipitating event** (e. g., intoxication, medication use, trauma, or infection) or a **structural abnormality of the basal ganglia** or other brain areas (e. g., multiple arteriosclerotic changes, hydrocephalus) revealed by CT or MRI. A further characteristic of symptomatic parkinsonism is its *relative resistance to treatment with L-DOPA*, in contrast to idiopathic Parkinson disease, which usually responds very well to L-DOPA, at least at first. Moreover, some forms of symptomatic parkinsonism present symmetrically, while idiopathic Parkinson disease often presents asymmetrically. The most important differential diagnoses of idiopathic Parkinson disease are listed in Table 6.**25**.

Degenerative Systemic Diseases Causing Hypertonia and Hypokinesia

The diseases discussed in this section are other, rarer causes of the parkinsonian syndrome.

Progressive Supranuclear Palsy

This disease is also known as Steele–Richardson–Olszewski syndrome.

The underlying neuropathological lesion consists of cellular degeneration in the substantia nigra, globus pallidus, subthalamic nucleus, periaqueductal area of the midbrain, and other brain nuclei.

Clinical manifestations include:

- paucity of movement,
- gait disturbance early in the course of the disease,
- predominantly axial rigidity,
- often, a permanently extended cervical spine (head turned upward),
- frequent falls,
- tendency to fall backward,
- progressive dementia,
- an impairment of vertical gaze movements (particularly downward), with nystagmus.

Course. This disease presents between ages 50 and 70, mainly in men. It progresses rapidly and causes death within a few years.

Multiple System Atrophies (MSA)

This term subsumes a variety of rare diseases that have also been described individually: *olivo-ponto-cerebellar atrophy* (OPCA), *striatonigral degeneration* (SND), *Shy–Drager syndrome* (SDS), and mixed forms of these.

The neuropathological lesion consists of cellular degeneration and gliosis in the substantia nigra, striatum, pons, inferior olive, and cerebellum.

The main clinical manifestations are present to varying extents in the different forms of MSA, each of which has its own characteristic initial presentation:

- bradykinesia, akinesia, rigidity, and rest tremor (seen early in the course of OPCA and SND),
- autonomic dysfunction, including orthostatic hypotension, incontinence, and impotence in men (seen early in the course of SDS),
- ataxia and other cerebellar signs (prominent in OPCA),
- pyramidal tract signs.

The diagnosis is made from the clinical manifestations. Other findings that are compatible with the diagnosis of MSA may include partial brain atrophy, as revealed by MRI, or a reduction of glucose metabolism or of the concentration of dopamine receptors in the striatum, as revealed by PET or SPECT.

Treatment of MSA is generally not very effective, though dopamine agonists tend to be more effective than L-DOPA. The disease usually leads to severe disability within a few years of onset.

Corticobasal Degeneration

Neuropathological lesion of this disease consists of cellular degeneration and gliosis in the substantia nigra and in the precentral and postcentral gyri. The cerebral peduncles are correspondingly diminished in size.

Clinical manifestations, which are asymmetrically distributed, include:

- impaired fine motor control of an arm (early in the course of the disease),
- progressive rigidity and akinesia,
- weakness,
- central sensory disturbances,
- (sometimes) apraxia,
- (sometimes) dystonia.

Treatment with L-DOPA is generally not very effective and patients usually become severely disabled within a few years of the onset of the disease.

Lewy Body Disease

This disease is described below on p. 139.

Diseases Causing Hyperkinesia

These diseases, unlike Parkinson disease, cause "too much" movement, often in combination with diminished muscle tone. The different clinical varieties of hyperkinesia include **chorea, athetosis, ballism and dystonia**, and mixed forms. Each of these disturbances of movement may be due to many different causes. The hyperkinetic extrapyramidal diseases are a heterogeneous group with regard to both phenomenology and etiology.

Table 6.**26** provides an overview of the extrapyramidal diseases that manifest themselves as hyperkinetic syndromes. The more important members of this group are described in greater detail in this section.

Table 6.**26** The diagnostic evaluation of hyperkinetic extrapyramidal syndromes

Syndrome	Features	Etiology	Remarks
Chorea			
Chorea minor	sudden, usually rapid, distal, brief, irregular involuntary movements; hypotonia	autoimmune; streptococcal infection	often a sequela of streptococcal pharyngitis, most commonly in girls aged 6–13 years
Chorea mollis		autoimmune; streptococcal infection	hypotonia is prominent
Chorea gravidarum		3rd–5th month of pregnancy	usually during first pregnancy, often with prior history of chorea minor
Chorea due to antiovulatory agents			rare, reversible with discontinuation of the drug

Continued →

Table 6.**26**   **The diagnostic evaluation of hyperkinetic extrapyramidal syndromes** (Continued)

Syndrome	Features	Etiology	Remarks
Huntington disease		autosomal dominant inheritance	onset usually at age 30 to 50; associated with progressive dementia
Benign familial chorea		autosomal dominant inheritance	onset in childhood, no further progression, no dementia
Choreoacanthocytosis		autosomal recessive	mainly orofacial, tongue-biting, elevated CPK, hyporeflexia, acanthocytosis
Postapoplectic chorea		vascular (prior stroke)	sudden hemichorea and hemiparesis, often combined with hemiballism
Senile chorea		vascular and degenerative	occasional presenile onset, often more severe on one side, occasionally with dementia
Athetosis			
Status marmoratus	Slow, exaggerated movements against resistance of antagonist muscles, predominantly distal, appear uncomfortable and cramped	perinatal asphyxia	soon after birth, increasingly severe athetotic hyperkinesia, often cognitive impairment, sometimes also spasticity
Status dysmyelinisatus		kernicterus of the newborn	present at birth, often with other signs of perinatal brain damage; further progression
Pantothene kinase-associated neurodegeneration (formerly called Hallervorden–Spatz disease)	joint hyperflexion/hyperextension	autosomal recessive disorder of pigment metabolism	choreoathetotic movements beginning at age 5–15 years, rigidity, dementia, and retinitis pigmentosa in one-third of cases; progressive, death by age 30
Hemiathetosis		focal lesion of pallidum and striatum	unilateral, may come about some time after the causative lesion
Ballism/Hemiballism	unilateral, lightning-like, high-amplitude flinging movements of multiple limb segments	ischemic or neoplastic lesion of the subthalamic nucleus	sudden onset, usually with hemiparesis as well
Dystonic syndromes			
Torsion dystonia	slow, tonic contractions of muscles or muscle groups, of shorter or longer duration, usually against the resistance of antagonist muscles	familial syndromes	often in families of Jewish ancestry, onset in the 1st–2nd decade of life with focal dystonia, later rotating movements of head, trunk, and limbs, as well as athetotic movements of the fingers
		symptomatic types	e. g., in Wilson disease, Huntington disease, pantetheine kinase-associated neurodegeneration
Spasmodic torticollis	slow contraction of cervical and nuchal musculature against antagonist resistance, with turning movements of the head	idiopathic, occasionally after cervical spine trauma and various other causes	one-third spontaneous recovery, one-third no change, one-third progression to torsion dystonia
Localized dystonia	see text, p. 134		e. g., writer's cramp, faciobuccolingual dystonia, oromandibular dystonia

Diseases Causing Chorea

The neuropathological basis of chorea consists of degeneration of small neurons, mainly in the putamen and caudate nucleus. This lesion is particularly evident in hereditary chorea (see below).

Clinical manifestations. Chorea consists of *irregular, sudden, involuntary movements* that are usually more pronounced at the *distal* end of the limbs. In some patients, these movements are of low amplitude and look almost normal, resembling nonpathological "fidgetiness"; in others, they are massive and highly disturbing. They can appear on one side ("hemichorea") or both (Fig. 6.**34**). The muscle tone is normal or diminished, there is no weakness or sensory deficit, and pyramidal tract signs are absent. The intrinsic muscle reflexes are normal, except that they may have a second extension phase (*Gordon phenomenon*) if elicited at the same time as an incipient choreiform movement. Choreiform movements, like other types of hyperkinetic movement (see below), are typically enhanced by goal-directed movement, mental stress, or concentration, and subside in sleep and under general anesthesia.

Individual etiologic forms. Chorea has diverse causes and the prognosis depends on the cause.

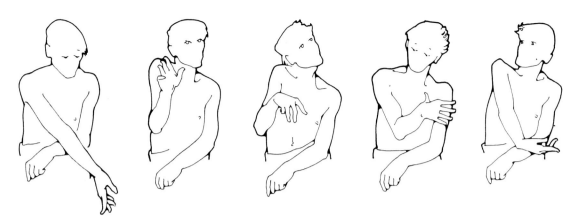

Fig. 6.**34 Senile hemichorea.** Drawings made from a film recording.

Huntington disease (chorea major) is a genetic disorder of autosomal dominant inheritance due to an unstable CAG trinucleotide repeat expansion on chromosome 4. The clinical manifestations generally arise between the ages of 30 and 50 (earlier in patients who inherited the defective gene from their father). Rigidity and pyramidal tract signs are sometimes present at the outset, but, as a rule, *choreiform movements* soon dominate the clinical picture, accompanied by *progressive dementia.* The disease progresses chronically, generally ending in death 10 to 15 years after the onset of symptoms. There is no treatment other than palliative, symptomatic management (see below).

Chorea minor (Sydenham chorea) is the most common etiologic form of chorea. It mainly strikes school-aged girls after an infection with β-hemolytic group A streptococci and is caused by an autoimmune reaction in which antibodies are generated that cross-react with neurons. Within a few days or weeks after an attack of "strep throat," or within a few weeks or months of an attack of rheumatic fever, the patient develops *choreiform motor unrest* (mainly in the face, pharynx, and hands), combined with *irritability* and other *mental abnormalities.* These manifestations resolve spontaneously in a few weeks or months. The usual treatment is with high-dose penicillin for at least 10 days.

Rare types of chorea include *chorea gravidarum* (in pregnant women), *benign familial chorea,* and *postapoplectic hemichorea.*

Treatment. Choreiform movements can be alleviated by *perphenazine, tetrabenazine, tiapride,* and other neuroleptic medications.

Athetosis

The neuropathological basis of athetosis is loss of neurons in the striatum, the globus pallidus, and, less commonly, the thalamus.

Clinical manifestations. Athetosis generally consists of slow, irregular movements mainly affecting the distal ends of the limbs, causing extreme flexion and extension at the joints and correspondingly bizarre postures, particularly of the hands (Fig. 6.**35**). The interphalangeal joints may be hyperextended to the point of subluxation ("*bayonet finger*"). Athetosis is often found in combination with chorea ("choreoathetosis").

Individual forms. *Congenital and perinatally acquired lesions of the basal ganglia* (status marmoratus, status dysmyelinisatus, severe neonatal jaundice = kernicterus) cause bilateral athetosis (*athétose double*), sometimes in conjunction with other signs of brain damage. Choreoathetosis and dystonia are prominent manifestations of iron deposition in the basal ganglia in *pantetheine kinase-associated neurodegeneration. Focal lesions,* too, e. g., an infarct, can produce hemiathetosis.

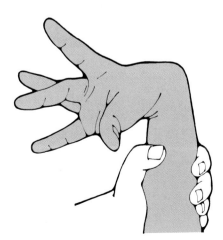

Fig. 6.**35 Hand posture in athetosis.**

Ballism

The neuropathological substrate of ballism is a lesion of the contralateral *subthalamic nucleus* (corpus Luysii) and/or its fiber connections to the thalamus.

Etiology. Ballism is usually due to a focal ischemic process, less commonly to a space-occupying lesion. It may also be the result of severe neonatal jaundice or of a hereditary degenerative disease; it is bilateral in such patients.

Clinical manifestations. Rapid, lightning-like, large-amplitude, unbraked flinging movements of the limbs are seen on one side of the body (*hemiballism*) or both. Unlike chorea, these movements occur mainly at the *proximal* joints. The limbs may be hurled into stationary objects (walls, etc.), causing injury.

Treatment. *Haloperidol* and *chlorpromazine* can alleviate ballistic movements. Stereotactic neurosurgical procedures are rarely indicated.

Dystonic Syndromes

Pathology. There are no characteristic **neuropathological abnormalities** in dystonia. To date, only a few of its etiologic forms have a known pathophysiological basis (e. g., L-DOPA-sensitive dystonia).

Clinical manifestations. Dystonia consists of *slow, long-lasting contractions of individual muscles or muscle groups.* The trunk, head, and limbs assume uncomfortable or even painful positions and maintain them for long periods of time. The various clinical types of dystonia are classified as either *focal*, i. e., affecting individual (small) muscle groups, or *generalized.*

Types of Generalized Dystonia

Torsion dystonias are characterized by slow, forceful, mainly *rotatory movements of the trunk and head*, usually accompanied by athetotic finger movements. Muscle tone is diminished at the onset of the disease. In some cases, hyperkinesia gradually ceases and gives way to hypertonia with a rigidly maintained dystonic posture (*myostatic form*). The various types of *primary torsion dystonia* are mostly of autosomal dominant inheritance, with low penetrance, and have been localized to genes on various chromosomes. The early-onset form is particularly common among Jews of Ashkenazi (Eastern European) ancestry and is due to a genetic defect at the 9p34 locus.

L-DOPA-sensitive dystonia (Segawa disease) is an autosomal recessive disorder due to a genetic defect on chromosome 14q. It usually presents in young girls as a disturbance of gait with dystonic postures or movements of the legs that vary greatly in severity over the course of the day. It is liable to misdiagnosis as a psychogenic disorder. It characteristically responds to low doses of L-DOPA (250 mg, or a little more, daily). A therapeutic test of L-DOPA is worth trying in any young patient with dystonia, including sporadic forms.

Focal Dystonia

Focal dystonia is much more common than generalized dystonia. The abnormal movements are restricted to individual parts of the body or muscle groups. The main types of focal dystonia are the following:

Spasmodic torticollis. In this disorder, slow contraction of individual muscles of the neck and shoulder girdle produce *tonic rotation of the head* to a certain position. It is usually the contralateral sternocleidomastoid muscle that is most prominently affected. Only one-third of all patients with "wry neck" due to spasmodic torticollis undergo a spontaneous remission; a further third later develop other dystonic manifestations. The etiology usually cannot be determined and is presumably multifactorial.

Blepharospasm consists of bilateral tonic contraction of the orbicularis oculi muscle, often with *very prolonged, involuntary eye closure*, during which the patient cannot voluntarily open his or her eyes. It tends to affect older patients, mainly women. Eye closure may be forceful, with visible contraction of the orbicularis oculi muscle, or weak, with a relatively normal external appearance. Cases of the latter type are alternatively designated *lid-opening apraxia*. Misdiagnosis as a psychogenic disturbance is, unfortunately, common.

Dystonia affecting multiple muscles of the head is a subcategory of focal dystonia. The various types of dystonia coming under this heading are not rare when taken together; they include *facio-buccolingual dystonia*, *oromandibular dystonia*, and *Breughel* or *Meige syndrome*. There may also be a relatively *isolated dystonia of the mouth, pharynx, and tongue*, particularly in patients who have been treated with neuroleptics. An acute form can appear as a complication of antiemetic agents such as metoclopramide.

Isolated dystonia has been described for practically every muscle group in the body. Dystonia of this type may be idiopathic or may arise in connection with *nonphysiological (occupational) overuse* of the muscle group in question. Well-known examples include *writer's cramp*, hand dystonia in musicians, and *foot dystonia* in certain other occupations. *Spastic dysphonia* is a focal dystonia of the laryngeal musculature.

Etiology. Precipitating factors for dystonia can be identified in some patients (symptomatic types of dystonia), but the etiology of dystonia usually remains undetermined.

Treatment. Generalized dystonia can be treated with *baclofen, carbamazepine*, or *trihexyphenidyl*, as monotherapy or in combination, but the effect of treatment is usually disappointing. A trial of L-DOPA can be rewarding in some patients (see above). Focal dystonia can be successfully treated with *injections of botulinus toxin A*. Stereotactic neurosurgical procedures for dystonia are currently under investigation and seem to hold some degree of promise.

Other Types of Involuntary Movement

Tremor

Types of tremor. The main *phenomenological distinction* is between **rest tremor** and **action tremor**. The latter, in turn, is subdivided into *postural tremor, isometric tremor* (appearing when a muscle is contracted against constant resistance), and *kinetic tremor* (appearing only during movement). Intention tremor is a type of kinetic tremor that worsens as the limb approaches its target. Tremor can also be classified *etiologically* as **parkinsonian tremor** (discussed above), **psychogenic tremor** (generally of highly variable severity, coarse, and demonstrative), **alcoholic tremor** (fine rest and intention tremor, worse after alcohol withdrawal, better after alcohol consumption), or **essential tremor**. The last named is often misdiagnosed as Parkinson disease.

Essential tremor is the most common type of tremor and often runs in families. It is a predominantly *postural* and sometimes also *kinetic* tremor of the hands; a pure intention tremor is seen in 15% of patients (see p. 29). It may also affect the head in isolation (nodding tremor of the "yes" or "no" type), sometimes including the chin and/or vocal cords. It typically improves after the consumption of a small amount of alcohol and worsens with nervousness or stress. It usually arises between the ages of 35 and 45. Genetic defects causing familial essential tremor have been found on chromosomes 2p22–p25 and 3q. "*Essential tremor plus*" is a combination of this entity with another neurological disorder (e.g., Parkinson disease, dystonia, myoclonus, polyneuropathy, restless legs syndrome).

Further types of tremor that will not be discussed here in any detail include *autonomic (vegetative) tremor, hyperthyroid tremor*, and the tremor of *Wilson disease*.

Treatment. If the tremor is severe enough to interfere with the patient's everyday activities, a *beta-blocker* such as propranolol can be tried; this agent is particularly effective against essential tremor. Primidone, benzodiazepines, and clozapine are further alternatives. *Deep brain stimulation* through an electrode that has been stereotactically implanted in the nucleus ventrointermedius (V.im.) of the thalamus is highly effective but is reserved for severe and medically intractable cases.

Differential diagnosis. Involuntary movements arising from diseases of the basal ganglia must be differentiated from a variety of other movement disorders, which are listed in Table 5.**3** (p. 71).

Cerebellar Diseases

Cerebellar disturbances present clinically with **disequilibrium, truncal,** and/or **appendicular ataxia, impaired coordination,** and **diminished muscle tone** (p. 80). Like disturbances of the cerebral hemispheres, they are usually due either to **vascular processes** (ischemia, hemorrhage) or to **tumors**. Multiple sclerosis is a further, common cause.
In this section, we will also discuss other diseases that may present primarily with cerebellar dysfunction, including infectious, parainfectious, (heredo-)degenerative, toxic, and paraneoplastic conditions, as well as cerebellar involvement in general medical diseases.

The More Common Diseases of the Cerebellum

Acute cerebellar ataxia in childhood arises a few days or weeks after a chickenpox infection, less commonly after another viral illness. The patient is usually a school-aged child. *Unsteady gait, ataxia, tremor,* and *nystagmus* are the characteristic signs; they usually resolve spontaneously and completely within a few weeks.

Acute cerebellitis is similar to the foregoing and affects both children and adults. In older patients, the clinical manifestations may persist.

Atrophie cérébelleuse tardive à prédominance corticale is a historic term encompassing a group of disorders that share the neuropathological finding of extensive loss of Purkinje cells, particularly in the vermian cortex. This is expressed clinically as *unsteady gait, truncal ataxia*, less severe *appendicular ataxia*, and *nystagmus*. The underlying disorder may be a **cerebellar degeneration of genetic or (to date) unexplained etiology** or a **symptomatic involvement** of the cerebellum, e.g., late cerebellar atrophy in chronic alcoholism or subacute paraneoplastic cerebellar cortical atrophy.

Cerebellar heredoataxias are of genetic origin. The enzymatic defects and pathophysiological mechanisms underlying each have not yet been determined, except in a few patients. These disorders are listed together with sporadic and symptomatic forms of cerebellar ataxia in Table 6.**27**.

Spinocerebellar ataxias involve not only the cerebellum, but also the spinal cord (cf. p. 153).

Intermittent cerebellar dysfunction has various causes, among which are *pyruvate dehydrogenase deficiency, Hartnup disease*, and *familial periodic paroxysmal*

Table 6.**27**   **Types of cerebellar ataxia**

Category	Disease	Clinical features	Remarks
Autosomal recessive hereditary ataxias	• Friedreich ataxia	lumbering, broad-based, unsteady gait, progressive from the 1st or 2nd decade onward; later, clumsiness of the hands, explosive speech; typical Friedreich foot (see Fig. 7.**13**); scoliosis, hypotonia	GAA triplet expansion on chromosome 9; impaired synthesis of the protein frataxin
	• Refsum disease (heredopathia atactica polyneuritiformis)	ataxia of gait and limbs beginning in childhood or adolescence, polyneuropathy with areflexia and sensory loss, hearing impairment, retinitis pigmentosa, mental abnormalities	lack of phytanic acid α-dehydrogenase
	• A β-lipoproteinemia (Bassen–Kornzweig syndrome)	progressive ataxia, nystagmus, ophthalmoplegia, polyneuropathy; acanthocytosis, low cholesterol and triglyceride values; vitamin E deficiency	low serum lipoprotein, cholesterol, and triglyceride values
	• Ataxia telangiectasia (Louis–Bar syndrome)	onset in infancy with ataxia and choreoathetosis; frequent lung, ear, nose, and throat infections, slow eye movements; telangiectases in conjunctiva and joint creases	one of the chromosomal fragility syndromes
	• **spinocerebellar ataxia** (different varieties, e. g., deficiencies of hexosaminidase, glutamate dehydrogenase, pyruvate dehydrogenase, ornithine transcarbamylase, or vitamin E	onset usually in the 1st decade, sometimes later, ataxia with variable accompanying deficits, e. g., mental retardation, visual or hearing impairment, polyneuritis, myoclonus, etc.; speech may be loud, deep, and harsh ("lion's voice")	
Autosomal dominant hereditary ataxias	• **cerebellar cortical atrophy** (Holmes type = Harding type III)	onset at age 20 or later, with cerebellar signs	genetically heterogeneous, SCA 5 and SCA 6
	• **olivo-ponto-cerebellar atrophy** (Menzel type = Harding type I)	onset at age 20 or later; cerebellar and noncerebellar signs including optic atrophy, basal ganglionic dysfunction, pyramidal tract signs, muscle atrophy, and sensory deficits, and sometimes dementia	genetically heterogeneous, SCA 1–SCA 4; SCA 3 = Machado–Joseph disease
	• cerebellar atrophy (Harding type II)	onset after age 20 with cerebellar signs and retinal degeneration	corresponds to SCA 7
Sporadic ataxias	• nonhereditary ataxias "atrophie cérébelleuse tardive à prédominance corticale"	onset in late adulthood with slowly progressive gait and truncal ataxia, later arm ataxia ; rarely, nystagmus, muscle hypotonia, and pyramidal tract signs	symmetrical degeneration of Purkinje cells, predominantly in the vermis
Symptomatic ataxias	tumor, infarct, hemorrhage, multiple sclerosis, infection, birth defect, chronic alcoholism, other toxic causes, vitamin E deficiency, hypothyroidism, malabsorption syndrome, sprue, ataxia in gluten hypersensitivity, paraneoplastic, physical	clinical features depend on cause	often with accompanying involvement of other systems and organs

SCA = spinocerebellar ataxia

ataxia. The last named is a genetic disease, due to a defect on chromosome 19p, which responds to treatment with acetazolamide. Intermittent ataxia is also seen in many cases of *multiple sclerosis.*

Cerebellar dysfunction in other diseases is usually manifest as ataxia. *Intoxication* with diphenylhydantoin, lithium, organic mercury, piperazine, 5-fluorouracil, or DDT is a common cause. Others include *infectious diseases,* such as mononucleosis, macroglobulinemia, myxedema, vitamin B deficiency, heatstroke, cerebellar tumors, and cranial polyneuritis (p. 175). There is also a form of gluten-induced ataxia, which may or may not be accompanied by gastrointestinal symptoms. Finally, cerebellar dysfunction may be the presenting manifestation of Creutzfeldt–Jakob disease.

The **differential diagnosis** must include all noncerebellar processes that can cause ataxia: (contralateral) frontal lobe lesions, motor pareses, and disorders affecting the afferent sensory pathways (e. g., polyneuropathy and posterior column disorders). Prolonged confinement to bed by illness ("bed ataxia") and psychogenic mechanisms are further possible causes.

Treatment is possible only when a treatable underlying illness has been identified.

Dementing Diseases

The Dementia Syndrome

> Unlike the terms "mental retardation" and "oligophrenia," both of which refer to congenital disturbances, "dementia" refers to an **acquired degeneration of intellectual and cognitive abilities**, which persists for at least several months or takes a chronically worsening course, leading to major impairment in the patient's everyday life. The clinical picture is dominated by **personality changes** as well as **neuropsychological** and accompanying **neurological** (particularly motor) **deficits**. **Reactive changes**, including insomnia, agitation, and depression, are common.

Causes. Unlike the various types of neuropsychological disturbance that are due to localized brain lesions, dementia is a global syndrome caused by a **diffuse loss of functional brain tissue**. Neuroimaging usually discloses *extensive brain atrophy* or *multifocal lesions in the brain.* The loss of functional tissue is often due to primary (degenerative) brain atrophy, which predominantly affects the cerebral cortex, progresses chronically, and causes irreversible cognitive impairment; in such cases, dementia is the direct consequence and most obvious expression of the causative pathological process (**dementing diseases** in the narrow sense of the term: *Alzheimer disease, Lewy body disease, focal cortical atrophies*). In principle, however, any disease that damages the structure or function of the brain can produce the dementia syndrome (**symptomatic dementia**, usually accompanied by other manifestations of the underlying disease). It is important to realize that nearly 10% of all cases of dementia are due to diseases that can be reversed, or at least kept from progressing further, by appropriate treatment. Early diagnosis and treatment of such patients is crucial for the prevention of worsening dementia. Table 6.**28** contains an overview of the causes of dementia, with an indication of which among these conditions are irreversible, and which are at least partially treatable.

! *All patients with dementia deserve a thorough diagnostic evaluation, because a treatable cause may be discovered.*

Epidemiology. One percent of persons aged 60 to 64, and more than 30% of persons over age 85, suffer from dementia. The most common cause is **Alzheimer disease**, which accounts for 40 to 50% of all patients. The second most common cause, and the most common cause of symptomatic dementia, is **vascular** (i. e., **multi-infarct**) **dementia** (15%); the third most common cause is alcoholism.

General clinical features of the dementia syndrome include neuropsychological deficits, personality changes, and behavioral abnormalities. In particular, the following are seen:
- impairment of short-term and long-term memory,
  - for new content (faulty generation of engrams)
  - and/or for old content (faulty recall);
- *impairment of thinking,* particularly with respect to
  - judgment,
  - problem solving,
  - and symbol comprehension;
- impairment of visuospatial and spatial-constructive functions, aphasia, apraxia;
- impairment of attention;
- reduced drive, initiative, and motivation;
- impaired concentration;
- mild fatigability;
- affect lability and impaired affect control;
- impairment of emotionality and social behavior;
- in some patients, confusion and impairment of consciousness.

General procedure for the diagnostic evaluation of dementia. The diagnosis of the dementia syndrome is based on *thorough history-taking from the patient and from the members of his or her family; a comprehensive general medical and neurological examination;* and *neuropsychological testing.* (The MiniMental Status Test described on p. 39 can be used for screening, but is nonspecific and thus of limited diagnostic value.) *Neuroimaging* (usually MRI) should be performed in every case as part of the search for the underlying etiology, which may also require some or all of the following, depending on the specific clinical situation: *laboratory tests* (complete blood count, electrolytes, hepatic and renal function tests, thyroid hormones, vitamin B_{12}, folic acid, TPHA test, HIV serology, CSF examination, etc.), *EEG, PET,* and *SPECT.*

Differential diagnosis at the syndrome level. It may be hard to differentiate the dementia syndrome from certain other psychopathological states, particularly the following:
- nonpathological diminution of cognitive ability in old age;

Table 6.**28**   **Causes of dementia** (based on the classifications of Whitehouse and of Cummings and Benson)

Degenerative diseases of the nervous system with dementia as their principal manifestation: — Alzheimer disease[1] — Pick disease — frontal lobe degeneration — Lewy body disease	**Epilepsy:** — progressive myoclonus epilepsy[1] — frequent seizures, status epilepticus[2] — diseases causing both dementia and epilepsy[1]
Other degenerative diseases causing dementia: — Parkinson disease[1] — progressive supranuclear palsy[1] — pantetheine kinase-associated neurodegeneration (formerly Hallervorden–Spatz disease) — hereditary ataxias — progressive myoclonus epilepsy[1]	**Demyelinating diseases:** — multiple sclerosis[1] **Systemic diseases, endocrine disorders, and deficiency states:** — hypothyroidism, Hashimoto thyroiditis[2] — hypopituitarism[2] — hepatic encephalopathy[1] — uremic encephalopathy[2] — hypoxic brain injury — hypoglycemia[1]
Cerebrovascular diseases: — multi-infarct syndrome[1] — "strategic" infarcts[1] — Binswanger disease (subcortical arteriosclerotic encephalopathy)[1]	— electrolyte disorders[1] — hypercalcemia, hyperparathyroidism[2] — vasculitis, connective tissue disease[2] — vitamin B_{12} deficiency[2] — pellagra[2] — Wernicke encephalopathy[1] — jejuno-ileal bypass[2]

Infectious diseases:
— HIV, AIDS–dementia complex[1]
— other viral encephalitides and postviral encephalopathies[1]
— prion diseases
  ⊜ kuru
  ⊜ Creutzfeldt–Jakob disease
  ⊜ Gerstmann–Sträussler–Scheinker syndrome
  ⊜ familial fatal insomnia
  ⊜ familial progressive subcortical gliosis
— syphilis (progressive paralysis)[2]
— brain abscesses[2]
— Whipple disease[2]
	Toxic conditions:
	— alcoholism[2]
	— heavy metal poisoning[2]
	— carbon monoxide poisoning
	— organic solvent poisoning[1]
	— medication toxicity[2]
	
	Mental illnesses:
	— depression[2]
	— schizophrenia[2]
	— hysteria[2]

Metabolic disorders affecting the brain: — Wilson disease[2] — disorders of lipid, protein, urea. and carbohydrate metabolism[1] — leukodystrophies	**Hydrocephalus:** — obstructive hydrocephalus[2] — malresorptive hydrocephalus[2]
Neoplasia: — primary brain tumors, metastases[1] — paraneoplastic encephalopathies[1]	**Trauma:** — open trauma with destruction of brain tissue — closed trauma with brain contusions[1] and/or subcortical shear injuries[1]

[1]   preventable, (rarely) curable, or treatable to some extent
[2]   usually curable or, at least, largely treatable

- depression with severely reduced drive (so-called depressive pseudodementia);
- an isolated neuropsychological disturbance (especially aphasia, apraxia, and/or agnosia);
- congenital mental retardation (oligophrenia);
- cognitive impairment by medications or drugs of abuse;
- status epilepticus with partial complex seizures or absences;
- cognitive impairment due to endogenous psychosis.

General aspects of treatment. If the dementia syndrome is found to be due to a treatable condition, **causative treatment** can be instituted, resulting in cure or, at least, the prevention of further progression of dementia. In all other cases, however, dementia responds poorly to treatment, if at all. The current medications for Alzheimer disease provide only modest clinical benefit, often at the cost of side effects. **Various symptoms accompanying dementia can be treated individually**, with major benefit to the patient and his or her family, in-

cluding depression, delusions, insomnia, and agitation. *Training of the remaining cognitive abilities* is also advisable in order to keep the patient functionally independent for as long as possible. In advanced stages, patients often require home nursing visits, or care in a suitable day clinic; removal from the home to a permanent care facility should be deferred for as long as this is practically achievable. *The patient's family* is thus the most important component of treatment. Family members should receive early and thorough information about the patient's disease and, where appropriate, counseling in the ways they can help care for the patient.

The common degenerative diseases of the brain whose major clinical manifestation is dementia are described in greater detail in the next section, and vascular dementia in the section immediately following.

Degenerative Brain Diseases Causing Dementia as Their Most Prominent Manifestation

Alzheimer Disease (Senile Dementia of Alzheimer Type, SDAT)

Alzheimer disease is the paradigmatic example of **cortical** (as opposed to **subcortical**) dementia. In cortical dementia, dementia itself is the main clinical manifestation; subcortical dementia is usually seen as an accompaniment to a motor disturbance.

The neuropathological lesion in Alzheimer disease consists of neuronal loss in the cerebral cortex, particularly in the basal temporal lobe (hippocampus) and the temporoparietal region. Histological examination reveals a paucity of cells and an accumulation of neuritic ("senile") plaques and neurofibrillary tangles. Amyloid angiopathy is often present as well.

Pathogenesis. *Genetic factors* play a role, but not the only role. Familial cases are associated with a defect in chromosome 21q, which contains the amyloid precursor gene. Persons with trisomy 21, i. e., Down syndrome, generally become demented by age 30. In other patients, there is a defect in the apolipoprotein E gene on chromosome 19q. The regularly demonstrable loss of neurons in the nucleus basalis of Meynert, which sends a diffuse cholinergic projection to the frontal cortex, and the finding of a diminished amount of acetylcholine in the brain of persons with Alzheimer disease both imply that the cholinergic system plays a role in pathogenesis. These observations provide the motivation for cholinergic treatment (as described below).

Clinical manifestations. The nonspecific *early manifestations* can include depression, insomnia, agitation, anxiety, and excitability. Within a year, forgetfulness, fatigability, poor concentration, and a lack of initiative appear and slowly worsen, often accompanied by *focal neuropsychological deficits* such as aphasia, apraxia, and disturbances of temporal and spatial orientation. Thereafter, the patient's capacity for abstract thought deteriorates, complex situations can no longer be grasped, and confusion, lack of interest, and the progressive loss of language ultimately lead to the *loss of functional independence and the need for nursing care.*

Diagnosis. *Early recognition and interpretation of the psychopathological deficits* described above is crucial for the diagnosis of the disease, which is often further supported by the typical *neuroimaging findings* (cortical atrophy, wide ventricles; see Fig. 6.**36**). Neuroimaging is also mandatory because it can rule out some of the other causes of the dementia syndrome. Further studies (*hematological, biochemical, and serological blood tests, CSF examination, EEG*) may be indicated, depending on the specific differential diagnostic considerations in the individual patient.

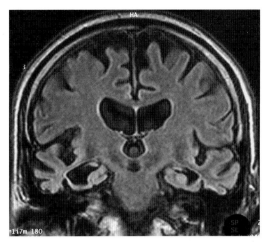

Fig. 6.36 Brain atrophy in dementia. High-grade, symmetrical, mainly frontal atrophy of the cerebral hemispheres in a 64-year-old man. Note the marked atrophy of the temporal lobes as well. The lateral ventricles, including the inferior horns, are markedly dilated, as is the third ventricle. Both external hydrocephalus and internal "hydrocephalus ex vacuo" are present.

Course. Alzheimer disease always progresses. The average life expectancy from the time of diagnosis is eight to nine years.

Treatment. *Cholinomimetic agents* (donezepil or rivastigmine) improve neuropsychological deficits symptomatically but do not halt the progression of dementia. A possible beneficial effect of nonsteroidal anti-inflammatory drugs, including aspirin, is currently being studied. No clear benefit has been shown for high-dose vitamin E, *Ginkgo biloba* preparations, calcium antagonists, or nootropic agents such as piracetam. The most important aspect of treatment in all patients is the management of the accompanying symptoms: *depression* (preferably with selective serotonin reuptake inhibitors), *psychosis* (preferably with clozapine or olanzapine), *insomnia, agitation, and aggressiveness* (preferably with mild neuroleptic agents such as pipamperone, melperone, and clomethiazole). Patients with advanced Alzheimer disease, and their families, can benefit from referral to special outpatient and day care facilities.

Dementia with Lewy Bodies

The hallmark of this common dementing disease is the presence of *Lewy bodies* in the neurons of the cerebral cortex and brainstem. Clinically, *progressive dementia* in these patients is accompanied by certain other characteristic findings: there are highly variable deficits of attention and concentration, as well as frequent, objective *visual hallucinations* and *parkinsonian manifestations* (particularly in patients with early disease onset). Patients often suffer from repeated falls, syncope, brief episodes of unconsciousness, and hallucinatory experiences.

Focal Cortical Atrophies

The dementing diseases belonging to this category, all of them much rarer than Alzheimer disease, are characterized by **localized atrophy of particular areas of the brain**. Histopathological examination reveals gliosis and spongiform changes. The commonest of these conditions is **Pick disease**, classified by some authors as a type of *frontal lobe degeneration.* Patients often manifest frontal personality changes and abnormal social behavior (p. 77) Many cases are familial and of autosomal dominant inheritance. In **primary progressive aphasia**, the language disturbance may precede the development of generalized dementia by several years. In **posterior cortical atrophy**, dementia may be accompanied by the specific neuropsychological deficits of Gerstmann syndrome (p. 78).

Vascular Dementia

SAE-Associated Dementia and Multi-infarct Dementia

Etiology. Vascular dementia, the second most common etiologic category of dementia, is caused either by multiple subcortical lacunar infarcts due to *cerebral microangiopathy* (subcortical arteriosclerotic encephalopathy, SAE: more common type) or by multiple cortical and subcortical infarcts due to *macroangiopathy* or *recurrent embolic stroke* (multi-infarct dementia: less common type). The two types often appear together. The sites and extent of the infarcts determine the severity and progression of the dementia syndrome.

Clinical manifestations. Vascular dementia often strikes patients with preexisting arterial hypertension and/or other vascular risk factors. There may be a history of transient neurological deficits in the past. *Dementia* can arise suddenly or progress in spurts. There may be accompanying *neuropsychological deficits*, such as aphasia, as well as marked *incontinence of affect*: involuntary laughing and crying are common. The *neurological findings* include enhanced perioral reflexes, signs of pseudobulbar palsy (e. g., dysarthria and dysphagia), a tripping, small-stepped gait (old person's gait, "marche à petits pas"), and, sometimes, pyramidal and extrapyramidal signs.

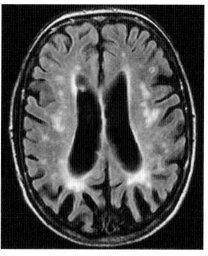

Fig. 6.**37 Vascular encephalopathy as seen by MRI.** There are multiple focal signal abnormalities in the deep white matter, the subcortical region, and the cerebral cortex. The ventricles and subarachnoid space are dilated ("hydrocephalus ex vacuo").

The *psychopathological abnormalities* in patients with predominantly subcortical lesions include apathy, depression, and slowness. Patients can recall old information more easily than they can store new information.

Diagnostic evaluation. Neuroimaging reveals brain atrophy and evidence of multiple focal lesions (usually in the subcortical white matter; see Fig. 6.**37**).

Course. Vascular dementia is, in principle, a progressive illness, but the speed of progression is variable, as it depends on the type and extent of the underlying arteriopathy.

Treatment. The intermediate goal of treatment is *vascular risk reduction* (treatment of arterial hypertension, cardiac arrhythmias, and diabetes mellitus, if present; inhibition of platelet aggregation with aspirin and/ or other drugs). Generally speaking, the treatment is the same as that discussed above for the prevention of ischemic stroke (p. 105).

7 Diseases of the Spinal Cord

Anatomical Fundamentals

The spinal cord is the component of the central nervous system that connects the brain to the peripheral nerves. It contains:

- in the **white matter**, fiber pathways leading from the brain to the periphery and vice versa;
- in the **gray matter**, an intrinsic neuronal system consisting of:

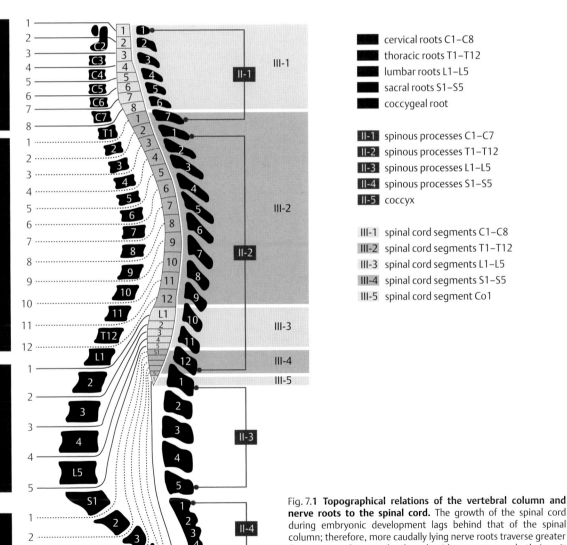

cervical roots C1–C8
thoracic roots T1–T12
lumbar roots L1–L5
sacral roots S1–S5
coccygeal root

II-1 spinous processes C1–C7
II-2 spinous processes T1–T12
II-3 spinous processes L1–L5
II-4 spinous processes S1–S5
II-5 coccyx

III-1 spinal cord segments C1–C8
III-2 spinal cord segments T1–T12
III-3 spinal cord segments L1–L5
III-4 spinal cord segments S1–S5
III-5 spinal cord segment Co1

Fig. 7.1 Topographical relations of the vertebral column and nerve roots to the spinal cord. The growth of the spinal cord during embryonic development lags behind that of the spinal column; therefore, more caudally lying nerve roots traverse greater distances in the spinal subarachnoid space to reach their exit foramina. In the conventional numbering system, the *cervical spinal nerves* exit the spinal canal *above* the correspondingly numbered vertebra, while *all spinal nerves from T1 downward* exit *below* the correspondingly numbered vertebra.

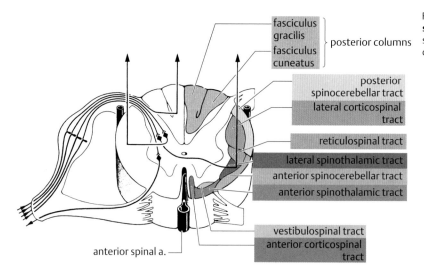

Fig. 7.2 Important fiber tracts of the spinal cord (cross-sectional view). Descending tracts are shown in red, ascending tracts in gray.

Labels in figure: fasciculus gracilis, fasciculus cuneatus } posterior columns; posterior spinocerebellar tract; lateral corticospinal tract; reticulospinal tract; lateral spinothalamic tract; anterior spinocerebellar tract; anterior spinothalamic tract; vestibulospinal tract; anterior corticospinal tract; anterior spinal a.

- *interneurons,* i.e., relay neurons for the conducting pathways and reflex loops;
- *motor neurons* in the anterior horns, whose efferent axons travel in the peripheral nerves;
- *somatosensory neurons* in the dorsal horns (although many sensory neurons are located outside the spinal cord, in the spinal ganglia);
- *nociceptive sensory neurons* in the dorsal horns that receive and transmit impulses mainly from pain and temperature fibers; and
- *autonomic neurons* in the lateral horns.

The topographic relations of the spinal cord, vertebral column, and nerve roots are shown in Fig. 7.1, and the major ascending and descending pathways of the spinal cord are shown in Fig. 7.2. The blood supply of the spinal cord is described below (p. 148).

The Main Spinal Cord Syndromes and Their Anatomical Localization

Diseases of the spinal cord, like those of the brain, can be of **traumatic, vascular, neoplastic, paraneoplastic, infectious, inflammatory, metabolic, endocrine, toxic,** or **hereditary degenerative origin.** The clinical manifestations of spinal cord lesions depend on their **level and extent** and are largely independent of etiology. Thus, the first step in the diagnostic evaluation of spinal cord diseases, as of brain diseases, is *topographical localization,* i.e., the deduction of the level of the lesion from the patient's constellation of neurological deficits. The next step is the *determination of the etiology,* usually based on further criteria (accompanying nonneurological manifestations, temporal course, results of ancillary tests).

Spinal cord transection syndrome is the pattern of neurological deficits resulting from damage of the entire cross-section of the spinal cord at some level. Most acutely arising cases of the complete spinal cord transection syndrome are of either **traumatic** or **ischemic** origin; rare cases are due to inflammation or infection (transverse myelitis) or nontraumatic compression (e. g., by a hematoma or tumor). The clinical features of the spinal cord transection syndrome are:

- dysfunction of all of the ascending sensory pathways up to the level of the lesion, and of the posterior horns and posterior roots at the level of the lesion: there is a **sensory level** below which all modalities of sensation are impaired or, in a complete transection, absent;
- bilateral pyramidal tract dysfunction: **spastic paraparesis or paraplegia,** or, with cervical lesions, **spastic quadriparesis or quadriplegia** (immediately after a trauma, in the phase of "spinal shock" and diaschisis, there is usually flaccid weakness, which subsequently becomes spastic);
- bladder dysfunction;
- dysfunction of the motor neurons of the anterior horn at the level of the lesion: possibly, **flaccid paresis** in the myotome(s) supplied by the cord at the level of the lesion, corresponding **loss of reflexes,** and, later muscle atrophy.

Spinal cord hemisection syndrome (Brown–Séquard syndrome, e. g., caused by a compressing tumor). An anatomical or functional disconnection of one half of the spinal cord exactly to the midline is a rare event. The associated symptoms and signs are described in Table 7.1. Incomplete unilateral lesions are, understandably, more common and present with a subset of these manifestations.

Table 7.**1** **Brown–Séquard syndrome**

Involved structure	Ipsilateral deficits	Contralateral deficits
Pyramidal tract	paresis	
Lateral spinothalamic tract		diminution or loss of pain and temperature sensation (dissociated sensory deficit)
Anterior spinothalamic tract		mildly diminished sense of touch
Vasomotor fibers of the lateral columns	initially, warmth and redness of the skin; sometimes absence of sweating	
"Overload" of the contralateral spinothalamic tract with tactile stimuli?	transient cutaneous hyperesthesia	
Posterior columns	loss of proprioception and vibration sense	
Anterior horns and anterior roots	segmental muscular atrophy and flaccid weakness	
Entering posterior roots	segmental anesthesia and analgesia	

Central cord syndrome is the classic presentation of *syringomyelia* (see below), but can also be due to an intramedullary hemorrhage or tumor. Its clinical features are:
- *pyramidal tract dysfunction*: **spasticity** of the limbs below the level of the lesion; cervical lesions tend to affect the upper limbs more than the lower limbs;
- *interruption of the pain and temperature fibers of the anterior spinal commissure*: bilateral impairment of pain and temperature sensation in the dermatome(s) at the level(s) of the lesion, with preservation of touch (**segmentally restricted dissociated sensory deficit**); in analogous fashion, concomitant involvement of the posterior horn(s), if present, causes segmental impairment of touch sensation, either uni- or bilaterally, depending on whether one posterior horn is affected, or both;
- *dysfunction of the lateral horn/intermediolateral tract*: **autonomic and trophic disturbances** (disturbances of sweating, nail growth, and bone metabolism; hyperkeratosis and edema; all disturbances more pronounced in the upper limbs);
- *possible concomitant involvement of the spinothalamic tracts*: bilateral deficit of pain and temperature sensation below the level of the lesion, with impaired touch sensation;
- *possible concomitant involvement of the motor neurons of the anterior horns* at the level of the lesion: segmentally distributed flaccid weakness, loss of reflexes, and muscle atrophy;
- *sparing of the posterior horns and spinocerebellar tracts*: touch, vibration sense, and proprioception usually remain intact;
- bladder dysfunction.

Bilateral lesion of the anterolateral region of the spinal cord (e. g., ischemia in the territory of the anterior spinal a.) produces the following symptoms and signs:
- *pyramidal tract dysfunction*: depending on the level of the lesion, **quadriparesis (quadriplegia)** or **paraparesis (paraplegia)**, with enhanced intrinsic muscle reflexes and pyramidal tract signs;

- *involvement of the spinothalamic tracts and the pain and temperature fibers crossing in the anterior spinal commissure*: **dissociated sensory deficit** in the entire region of the body **below the level of the lesion**; less commonly, the spinothalamic tracts are spared and there is a **segmentally restricted dissociated sensory deficit**;
- *intact posterior columns*: no impairment of touch or proprioception;
- bladder dysfunction.

Isolated or combined long tract processes (of various causes) present with:
- for example, pure spastic paraparesis (*isolated lesion of the pyramidal tracts*, e. g., in spastic spinal paralysis);
- impaired touch and position sense (*posterior column lesion*);
- ataxia (*lesion of the spinocerebellar tracts and/or posterior columns*);
- combinations of the above (e. g., pyramidal tract and posterior column dysfunction in funicular myelosis, dysfunction of both of these and the spinocerebellar tracts in Friedreich ataxia).

Anterior horn lesions (e. g., spinal muscle atrophy, acute poliomyelitis) cause the following manifestations:
- flaccid weakness of various muscles, muscle atrophy (and fasciculations in chronic processes),
- diminution or loss or reflexes,
- no sensory impairment.

Combined anterior horn and long tract lesions, e. g., in amyotrophic lateral sclerosis (*simultaneous involvement of the anterior horn ganglion cells and of the pyramidal and corticobulbar tracts* due to upper motor neuron degeneration; brisk reflexes).

Conus medullaris syndrome (Fig. 7.3). The conus medullaris is the lower end of the spinal cord and lies in the spinal canal at the L1 level. An isolated conus lesion typically produces:

7

Diseases of the Spinal Cord

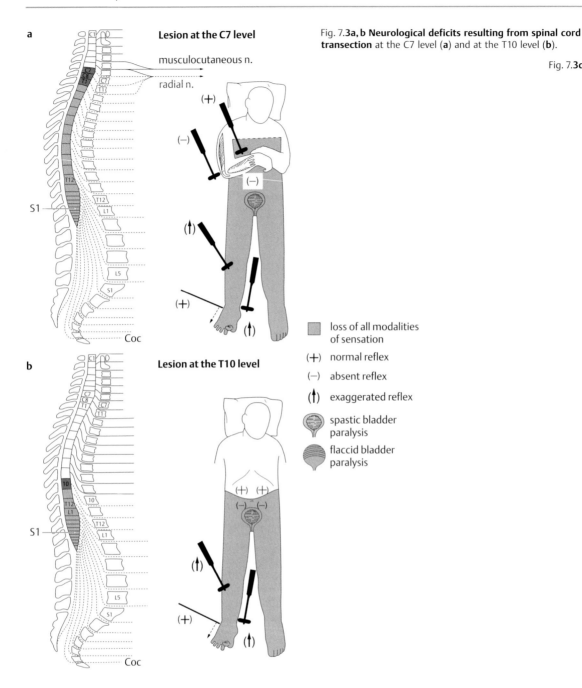

Lesion at the C7 level

musculocutaneous n.

radial n.

Lesion at the T10 level

Fig. 7.**3a, b Neurological deficits resulting from spinal cord transection** at the C7 level (**a**) and at the T10 level (**b**).

Fig. 7.**3c,d** ▷

loss of all modalities of sensation

(+)   normal reflex

(−)   absent reflex

(↕)   exaggerated reflex

spastic bladder paralysis

flaccid bladder paralysis

- bladder dysfunction,
- dysfunctional defecation with sphincter weakness,
- impairment of sexual function,
- possibly a dissociated sensory deficit or complete loss of sensation in the cutaneous distribution of the sacral and coccygeal spinal cord segments (saddle anesthesia);
- usually, preserved motor function and absence of pyramidal tract signs.

Cauda equina syndrome (Fig. 7.3) results from compression of the nerve roots coursing through the spinal canal below the conus medullaris, i. e., below the L1/2 level. Unlike conus medullaris syndrome, it involves a variably severe impairment of sensory and motor function in the lower limbs. Its clinical manifestations are:

- flaccid weakness and areflexia of the lower limbs, without pyramidal tract signs;
- impairment of all sensory modalities in multiple lumbar and/or sacral dermatomes, usually most pronounced in the "saddle" area;
- impaired urination, defecation, and sexual function, with sphincter weakness.

Fig. 7.**3c** Epiconus syndrome and cauda equina syndrome, **d** Conus medullaris syndrome.

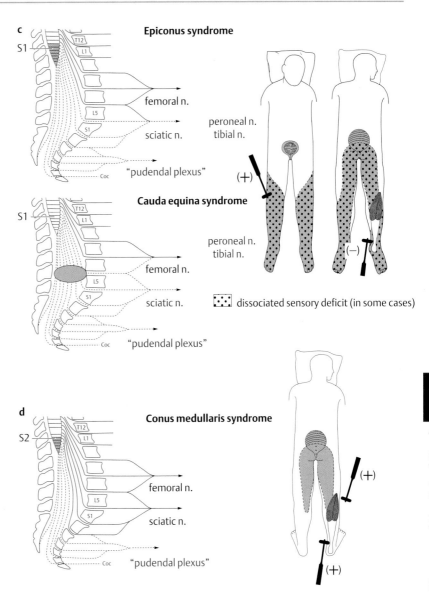

Epiconus syndrome

Cauda equina syndrome

dissociated sensory deficit (in some cases)

Conus medullaris syndrome

Spinal Cord Trauma

Traumatic spinal cord lesions are usually due to **fractures and dislocations of the spine** causing displacement of fragments of bone and/or intervertebral disk. The spinal cord can also be compressed by a **traumatic hemorrhage** in the spinal canal or sustain **direct traumatic compression** in the absence of a fracture. The clinical signs of spinal cord trauma depend on the level and severity of the lesion, as shown schematically in Fig. 7.**3**.

Like traumatic brain injury, spinal cord trauma can be classified by severity:

Spinal concussion. Immediately after blunt trauma to the trunk, a more or less complete spinal cord transec-

tion syndrome arises, usually at a cervical or thoracic level. The neurological deficits regress completely within minutes.

Spinal contusion. The traumatic event has caused *extensive structural damage and compression of the spinal cord*, usually with hemorrhage. There is a **partial or complete spinal cord transection syndrome** (depending on the extent of the lesion), including bladder dysfunction (p. 142) and an initially flaccid paraparesis (paraplegia) or quadriparesis (quadriplegia) (phase of spinal shock, diaschisis). The transection syndrome usually improves no more than partially, if at all.

If a spinal cord contusion is very extensive, the associated cord edema and/or hemorrhage may secondarily lead to compression of the affected segments of the cord within the spinal canal (see **spinal cord compression**, discussed in the next section). As long as this compression is not severe enough to choke off the cord's blood supply and cause infarction, the neural tissue may be able to recover its function again once the traumatic edema has subsided and any hemorrhage has been resorbed.

Practical steps to be taken in acute spinal cord trauma are the following:
- a gentle, nontraumatic neurological examination to determine the level of the lesion;
- directed neuroimaging, usually with plain films followed by MRI, to identify fractures and dislocations of the vertebral column and assess damage of the intraspinal structures, including the spinal cord;

- by means of the foregoing, objective correlation of the anatomic findings with the clinically determined level, extent, and type of spinal cord injury;
- catheterization of the bladder;
- prophylaxis against decubitus ulcers from the beginning, with frequent repositioning of the patient;
- surgical treatment of bony or other injuries, where indicated;
- transfer to a specialized institution for the rehabilitation of patients with spinal cord injuries.

The intravenous administration of high-dose corticosteroids in acute spinal cord injury may have a modest neuroprotective effect, but it is currently unclear whether the benefit of this treatment outweighs the risk of additional complications.

Spinal Cord Compression

Spinal cord compression may develop **acutely** or by **slow progression**. Acute spinal cord compression is usually due to **trauma** (see above) or **hemorrhage** (e.g., epidural hematoma). Slowly progressive compression is usually due to a **tumor**, less commonly an abscess or granuloma. Other causes include **deformities of the spine** (kyphoscoliosis, ankylosing spondylitis), **degenerative narrowing** of the spinal canal (especially in the cervical region, see below), and **massive intervertebral disk herniation**.

Clinical manifestations that are typical of *slowly progressive* spinal cord compression include:
- increasing stiffness or fatigability of the lower limbs,
- more or less rapidly progressive gait impairment,
- bladder dysfunction,
- impaired sensation in one or both lower limbs,
- bandlike paresthesiae around the chest or abdomen,
- back pain.

Diagnostic evaluation. *Neuroimaging* usually provides definitive evidence of spinal cord compression; MRI is generally superior to CT for this purpose.

General aspects of treatment. The treatment is determined by the nature of the compressive lesion and is generally analogous to the treatment of corresponding lesions affecting the brain.

Spinal Cord Tumors

Tumors in the spinal canal can arise from the spinal cord tissue itself (**intrinsic spinal cord tumors**), from the spinal meninges (**meningioma**), or from the Schwann cells of the nerve roots (**neurinoma**). Tumors (particularly **metastases**) can also project into the spinal canal from the vertebral and paravertebral regions. Intrinsic spinal cord tumors are **intramedullary**; leptomeningeal tumors are usually **extramedullary**, though still intradural. Tumors growing into the spinal canal from without are both extramedullary and extradural. Some highly invasive tumors arising in an extramedullary location can infiltrate the substance of the spinal cord, thereby becoming partly intramedullary.

In this section, we will briefly describe the more common varieties of spinal cord tumor.

Extramedullary Tumors

Metastases usually arise from the vertebral bodies and grow into the spinal canal. Their initial symptom is usually *pain*, which may be restricted to the site of the tumor, or else radiate in a radicular distribution. *Paraparesis* can arise quite rapidly thereafter, followed by *bladder dysfunction*. Clinical examination reveals the corresponding *neurological deficits* (pyramidal tract signs, possible sensory level, radicular segmental deficits) and, often, *focal tenderness of one or more spinous processes to percussion*. Neuroimaging studies are essential for the definitive diagnosis (Fig. 7.**4**). The most common primary tumors are carcinomas of the lung and breast, followed by carcinoma of the prostate gland.

Meningiomas arise from the spinal dura mater and account for one-third of all intraspinal masses. They are usually found in the thoracic and lumbar regions. They produce very slowly progressive *gait impairment* and *spastic paraparesis*, often over the course of several years, and have a characteristic appearance in imaging studies (Fig. 7.**5**).

Neurinomas (also called schwannomas) are nearly as common as meningiomas and, like them, are usually found in the thoracic and abdominal regions. They arise from the Schwann cells of the spinal nerve root sheaths. They nearly always present with *radicular pain and radicular deficits*. A neurinoma arising from a nerve root and straddling an intervertebral foramen, so that it has

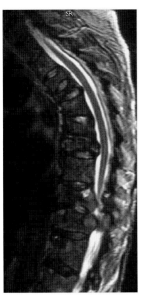

Fig. 7.**4 Metastatic carcinoma of the breast.** The MR image reveals destruction of several thoracic vertebral bodies and spinal cord compression by tumor projecting into the vertebral canal at a mid-thoracic level.

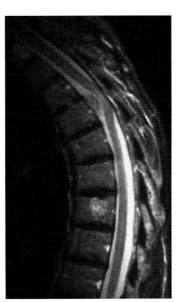

Fig. 7.**5 Extramedullary meningioma** at T4, based on the ventral dura mater. Spinal cord compression is clearly visible. (T2-weighted MR image.)

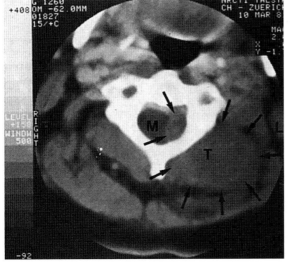

Fig. 7.**6 Neurinoma at C4,** as seen by CT. The arrows indicate the intra and extraspinal portions of the tumor. The intraspinal portion compresses the spinal cord (c). (Image courtesy of the Neuroradiological CT Institute, PD Dr. H. Spiess, Zurich.)

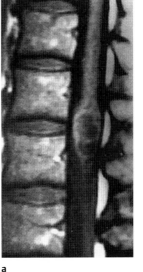

a   b

Fig. 7.**7 Intramedullary ependymoma** in the conus medullaris, as seen in T1-weighted (**a**) and T2-weighted (**b**) MR images. The spinal cord is expanded, especially dorsally.

both intra- and extraspinal portions, is called a *dumbbell* or *hourglass* tumor (Fig. 7.**6**).

Meningeal carcinomatosis and leukemic meningitis can cause clinically evident spinal cord compression, in addition to *pain* (the most common symptom) and *polyradicular neurological deficits.*

Intramedullary tumors are less common. Their manner of presentation depends on their location. The two most common types are astrocytoma and ependymoma; im-

aging studies are essential for definitive diagnosis (Fig. 7.**7**).

Tumors are only one possible cause of slowly compressive spinal cord compression. Another very common cause is discussed in the next section.

Myelopathy Due to Cervical Spondylosis

Cervical myelopathy is often due to degenerative narrowing of the spinal canal with resulting spinal cord compression. Patients with inflammatory diseases of the spine, such as rheumatoid arthritis, are at elevated risk. The initial presentation is often with (*poly-*)*radicular deficits* due to narrowing of the intervertebral foramina; as the spinal canal itself becomes increasingly stenotic, clinically evident *spinal cord compression* develops. Patients typically complain at first of paresthesiae in the fingers and impairment of the sense of touch (examination reveals astereognosis). The intrinsic muscles of the hands may become atrophic. Ultimately—or, rarely, as the sole manifestation—involvement of the *long white matter tracts* produces spastic paraparesis, enhanced reflexes, and pyramidal tract signs. *Neuroimaging* is essential for the establishment of the diagnosis; *MRI* is best (Fig. 7.**8**). Neurosurgical *decompression* of the spinal canal, possibly with spinal stabilization (fusion) at the same procedure, generally arrests the progression of the neurological deficits.

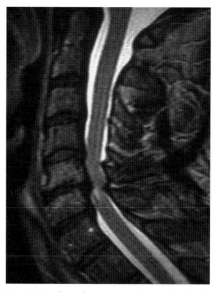

Fig. 7.**8 Myelopathy in cervical spondylosis.** The T2-weighted MR image reveals narrowing of the spinal canal at C5/C6 and C6/C7 both anteriorly and posteriorly because of degenerative spondylotic changes. A signal abnormality in the spinal cord below C6/C7 indicates a lesion induced by compression.

Circulatory Disorders of the Spinal Cord

Vascular lesions of the spinal cord, as of the brain, are of two main types: **hemorrhage** and **ischemia**. The latter is due to blockage of either the arterial blood supply (e. g., because of thrombosis or embolism) or the venous outflow.

Blood Supply of the Spinal Cord

The spinal cord receives arterial blood from three vessels: the unpaired **anterior spinal a.**, which runs down the anterior median fissure of the cord and supplies the anterior two-thirds of its cross-sectional area, and the paired **posterolateral spinal aa.** Each of these spinal arteries is made up of a series of individual segments that are linked with one another along the longitudinal axis and receive arterial blood from various sources (Fig. 7.9). At cervical levels, the anterior spinal a. receives blood mainly from the *vertebral a.* and the *costocervical and thyrocervical trunks*; further down the spinal cord, it is supplied by *segmental arteries* arising from the aorta (spinal branches and radicular arteries, each of which has an anterior and a posterior branch). In the embryo, there is a radicular artery for each spinal segment; postnatally, only six to eight such arteries are still present. The largest of these, called the *great radicular a.* or the *artery of Adamkiewicz*, usually enters the spinal canal between T10 and L2, more commonly on the left side. The anatomy of the spinal vessels is shown in Fig. 7.**9** and the intramedullary blood supply of a cross-section of the cord in Fig. 7.**10**. Venous blood flows out of the spinal cord through radicular veins and into the vena cava.

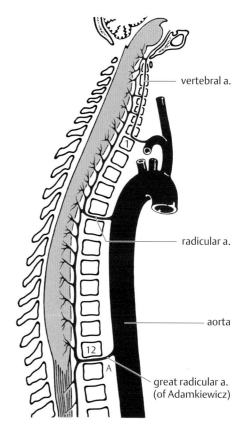

vertebral a.

radicular a.

aorta

great radicular a.
(of Adamkiewicz)

Fig. 7.**9 Blood supply of the spinal cord** (diagram, longitudinal view).

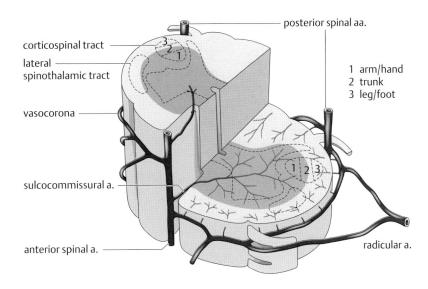

Fig. 7.**10 Blood supply of the spinal cord** (diagram, cross-sectional view). Occlusion of the anterior spinal a. produces infarction in the area shaded in gray.

posterior spinal aa.

corticospinal tract

lateral spinothalamic tract

1 arm/hand
2 trunk
3 leg/foot

vasocorona

sulcocommissural a.

anterior spinal a.

radicular a.

Arterial Hypoperfusion

Global (arterial) myelomalacia. Infarction of the entire cross-section of the spinal cord at a particular level may be due to the occlusion of a local spinal artery or of a radicular artery, or to extraspinal vascular pathology, such as an aortic aneurysm. The clinical presentation is usually an acute spinal cord transection syndrome (complete or partial, see p. 142), though, in some patients, symptoms develop subacutely over the course of a few days, or stepwise. Affected patients usually remain paraplegic, particularly if the ischemic lesion is very extensive.

Anterior spinal artery syndrome. Thrombotic or embolic occlusion of the anterior spinal a. damages the anterolateral aspect of the spinal cord over one or more segments. The characteristic clinical manifestations are described above on p. 143. An occlusion at a distal location along the course of the anterior spinal a., e. g., in a *sulcocommissural artery* (cf. Fig. 7.**10**), may cause a partial Brown–Séquard syndrome (Table 7.1), with preservation of the sense of touch.

Central cord infarction. Infarction of the spinal cord, whether it involves the entire cross-section of the cord or only a part of it, is usually not restricted to a single cord segment in the vertical dimension, but rather tends to involve multiple segments. As part of this process, necrosis affects the motor neurons of the anterior horn, causing flaccid paresis and areflexia at the level of the lesion, in addition to the spastic paresis below the level of the lesion due to involvement of the corticospinal tracts. In a few weeks' time, the flaccid muscles become atrophic. The clinical picture is, therefore, that of a *"peripheral" paralysis at the level of the transection* and also a short distance below it.

Intermittent spinal ischemia is very rare and causes a type of spinal intermittent claudication with fluctuating spastic paraparesis.

Chronically progressive vascular myelopathy can cause slowly progressive spastic paraparesis, as well as muscle atrophy owing to involvement of the anterior horns.

Impaired Venous Drainage

Spinal cord ischemia due to impaired venous drainage is a rare cause of infarction. It is usually due to a *spinal arteriovenous fistula* or *arteriovenous malformation*.

Spinal Arteriovenous Malformations and Fistulae

Arteriovenous malformations are usually found in the thoracolumbar region, while fistulae are usually found at lower lumbar levels (Fig. 4.**10**, p. 51). Both types of vascular anomaly are more common in men. They tend to present between the ages of 10 and 40, often with *(bandlike) pain* as the initial symptom. *Neurological deficits* referable to the spinal cord are often only intermittent at first and are (partially) reversible at this stage; later, they take a chronic, progressive course and become permanent. A dural arteriovenous fistula, for example, can cause chronically progressive spastic paraparesis. These vascular anomalies also occasionally present with spinal subarachnoid hemorrhage. *MRI* is the most important diagnostic study for the establishment of the diagnosis. *Spinal angiography* can provide useful additional anatomical detail.

Hemorrhage in or Adjacent to the Spinal Cord

The function of the spinal cord can be affected by an *intramedullary*, *subdural*, or *epidural hemorrhage*. These types of hemorrhage can arise spontaneously in anti-coagulated patients, or they can be caused by ruptured vascular malformations or trauma. They usually produce *intense pain* and more or less pronounced *neurological deficits*, depending on their site and extent. Hemorrhage in or adjacent to the spinal cord requires immediate diagnostic evaluation and, in some patients, emergency neurosurgical decompression.

Infectious and Inflammatory Diseases of the Spinal Cord

The spinal cord and spinal nerve roots, like the brain, can be infected by bacteria, viruses, and other pathogenic organisms. Combined infection of the brain and spinal cord is common: simultaneous manifestations of encephalitis, meningitis, myelitis, and radiculitis (cf. pp. 116 ff.) can be caused by spirochetes (borrelia, leptospira, treponemes; cf. pp. 209 ff.) and by many viruses. Acute anterior poliomyelitis, on the other hand, affects only the motor neurons of the anterior horns of the spinal cord.

Any infectious or inflammatory disease of the spinal cord, whatever its etiology, is called **myelitis**. The causes of myelitis include direct infection, secondary autoimmune processes in the wake of an infectious disease, and chronic autoimmune inflammatory disease of the central nervous system, such as multiple sclerosis.

The main causes of **acute myelitis** include *viruses* (measles, mumps, varicella-zoster, herpes simplex,

HIV), as well as rickettsiae and leptospira. Postvaccinal and postinfectious myelitis have also been described, as has myelitis in the setting of granulomatous disease. The clinical manifestations range from *progressive spastic paraparesis* to *partial spinal cord transection syndrome*. Myelitis can be visualized by MRI (Fig. 7.11).

Transverse myelitis affects the entire cross-section of the spinal cord, producing a **complete spinal cord transection syndrome**. It has a variety of causes. Often, the neurological manifestations are preceded by *nonspecific flulike symptoms* one to three weeks before onset. The spinal cord deficits usually arise acutely or subacutely and become maximally severe within a few days. *Fever, back pain,* and *myalgia* accompany the acute phase. The *cerebrospinal fluid* displays inflammatory changes (lymphocytic pleocytosis, elevated IgG and total protein concentrations). A *neuroimaging study* (usually MRI) must be performed to rule out a mass or ischemic event. The responsible organism is treated specifically if it can be identified; otherwise, only symptomatic treatment can be given. The spinal cord transection syndrome persists, or resolves less than completely, in two-thirds of all patients.

Acute Anterior Poliomyelitis

Etiology and epidemiology. This disease, caused by a **poliovirus**, almost exclusively affects the *motor neurons of the anterior horn of the spinal cord*. Its incidence in countries with a well-developed public health system has been reduced nearly to zero by prophylactic vaccination. The disease is transmitted by the fecal–oral route under conditions of poor sanitation.

Clinical manifestations. After an incubation period ranging from three to 20 days, **nonspecific prodromal manifestations** arise, consisting of fever, flulike symptoms, and, in some patients, meningeal signs. The prodrome may resolve without further consequence or be followed, within a few days, by a **paralytic phase** (likewise accompanied by fever). Over the course of a few hours or days, *flaccid paralysis* arises in various different muscles or muscle groups; it is asymmetrical, often mainly proximal, and of variable extent and severity. There is *no sensory deficit*, but the affected muscles may be painful and tender.

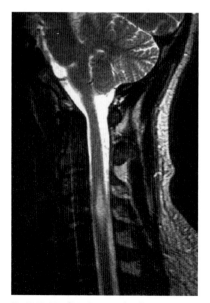

Fig. 7.**11** **Myelitis** (T2-weighted MR image). A spindle-shaped signal anomaly extends from C3 to C5 and expands the spinal cord (which is wider here than the normal cervical enlargement).

Diagnostic evaluation. The diagnosis is based on the typical course and physical findings, combined with an *inflammatory CSF pleocytosis*: at first, there are several hundred cells per microliter, often mainly polymorphonuclear granulocytes. Later, there is a transition to a predominantly lymphocytic picture. The responsible organism (poliovirus) can be identified in the patient's stool.

Treatment. There is no specific etiologic treatment; the most important aspect of treatment is the management of respiratory insufficiency (if present).

Prognosis. Brain stem involvement and respiratory paralysis confer a worse prognosis; in the remainder of patients, paralysis may regress partially or completely in a few weeks or months. There is usually some degree of residual weakness.

Postpolio syndrome. This term refers to two different syndromes. Some authors use it for a *symptom complex seen a few years after the acute illness* in polio patients with residual weakness, characterized by fatigability, respiratory difficulties, pain, and abnormal temperature regulation (with negative polio titers). Others use it for a syndrome with *progressive worsening of residual weakness* occurring decades after the acute illness. Before this problem can be ascribed to the earlier polio infection, other possible causes of weakness must be ruled out, e. g., compression of the spinal cord or spinal nerve roots because of secondary degenerative disease of the spine.

Spinal Abscesses

Spinal abscesses are most often *epidural*, less often subdural, and only rarely intramedullary. The most common pathogen is *Staphylococcus aureus*, which reaches the spinal canal from a site of primary infection outside it by way of the bloodstream (hematogenous spread). The typical clinical features are *general signs of infection* (fever, elevated erythrocyte sedimentation rate, leukocytosis, chills in some cases), *pain*, and *neurological deficits* referable to the spinal nerve roots or spinal cord, depending on the specific anatomic situation. Spinal abscesses usually require prompt surgical treatment, followed by weeks of high-dose antibiotics.

Syringomyelia and Syringobulbia

Syringomyelia, a condition coming under the general heading of **spinal dysraphism**, is sometimes seen in combination with other congenital defects such as the Arnold–Chiari syndrome or spina bifida. It has several different causes; it can be classified into **primary** syringomyelia and **symptomatic** forms due to (for example) hemorrhage, infection, or a tumor.

Syringomyelia is defined by the **pathological finding** of a tubelike or cleftlike **cavity (syrinx) within the spinal cord**, often lined by ependyma, and usually extending over several spinal segments. The cavity may reach all the way up to the medulla, or even the midbrain (*syringobulbia*, *syringomesencephaly*). Mere widening of the central canal of the spinal cord is called *hydromyelia*.

Clinical manifestations of syringomyelia depend on the location of the syrinx within the spinal cord and on its vertical extent; they usually arise in the patient's second or third decade. The typical signs and symptoms are summarized in Table 7.**2**.

Diagnostic evaluation. Syringomyelia can be diagnosed from its typical symptoms and physical findings; the characteristic picture is of a *dissociated sensory deficit* combined with *trophic disturbances*. The diagnosis must then be confirmed with neuroimaging, specifically MRI (Fig. 7.**12**).

Clinical course. Syringomyelia is usually slowly progressive.

Treatment. Neurosurgical methods are occasionally successful. The options include the *Puusepp operation* (opening the posterior aspect of a large syrinx into the subarachnoid space), drainage of the syrinx with a shunt, or operation of an accompanying Arnold–Chiari malformation at the craniocervical junction.

7

Diseases of the Spinal Cord

Table 7.**2** **Common symptoms and signs of syringomyelia**

Symptoms/signs	Localizing significance	Remarks
Spastic paraparesis/ aspastic quadriparesis	pressure of syrinx cavity on the pyramidal tracts	may be unilateral or asymmetric
Muscle atrophy	loss of anterior horn ganglion cells	segmental, usually unilateral
Sensory level	pressure of syrinx cavity on all ascending sensory pathways	differential diagnosis: extramedullary lesion compressing the spinal cord
Uni- or bilateral dissociated sensory deficit below a given level	uni- or bilateral involvement of the ascending spinothalamic tract	highly characteristic
Segmental loss of all modalities of sensation	syrinx involving posterior root entry zone	usually unilateral or asymmetrical; predisposes to burns and other types of mutilating injury
Pain	involvement of entering sensory fibers or ascending spinal cord pathways	
Segmental dissociated sensory deficit	syrinx involving the anterior spinal commissure, thereby interrupting the decussating fibers of the spinothalamic tract	segmental, bilateral, less commonly unilateral
Autonomic disturbances	involvement of the intermediolateral tract in the upper thoracic spinal cord, or of the lateral horns	impaired sweating, succulent edema, osteolytic bone lesions, arthropathy
Trophic disturbances	as above	severe spondylosis, mutilation of the fingers
Kyphoscoliosis	secondary to weakness of the paravertebral muscles	usually later in the course of the disease; rarely congenital
Associated anomalies	part of a disorder of prenatal development	basal impression, Arnold–Chiari malformation, spina bifida, hydrocephalus

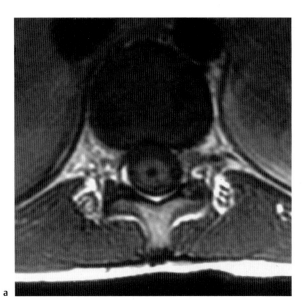
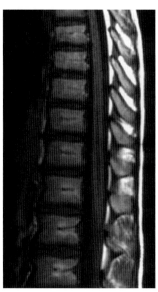

a   b

Fig. 7.**12 Thoracic syringomyelia** (MRI). **a** The axial image reveals the expanded central canal as a cavity (syrinx) in the middle of the spinal cord. **b** The sagittal image shows the syrinx extending from T4 to the lower border of T8.

Diseases Mainly Affecting the Long Tracts of the Spinal Cord

The diseases described up to this point affect both the gray and the white matter of the spinal cord. Other diseases of the spinal cord remain confined to the white matter, primarily involving one or more of its long tracts. The origin of these diseases is **genetic** in many patients (e. g., the spinocerebellar ataxias) but can also be **metabolic** (e. g., vitamin B$_{12}$ deficiency), **endocrine, paraneoplastic,** or **infectious.**

Hereditary Diseases of the Long Tracts of the Spinal Cord

Some of the spinocerebellar ataxias have already been described above in Chapter 6 (p. 136); there are a number of other diseases that mainly affect the *long tracts* of the spinal cord. Their pathophysiology is well understood in only a few patients, not (yet) understood in others.

Friedreich Ataxia

This *autosomal recessive* hereditary disease is due to a defect on chromosome 9. Its major **pathological findings** include cell loss in the dentate nucleus and combined **degeneration of the spinocerebellar tracts, pyramidal tracts, and posterior columns.**

Clinical manifestations. The disease usually becomes manifest in the second decade, initially through *signs of posterior column degeneration* and then through *spasticity* and *cerebellar signs.* Typical findings include:
- progressive *(spinal) ataxia* with *disequilibrium,* particularly when walking with the eyes closed;

- diminution or *loss of intrinsic muscle reflexes;*
- *impaired proprioception;*
- in advanced stages of the disease, *cerebellar dysarthria.*

Diagnostic evaluation. The diagnosis is based on the typical symptoms and signs. Physical examination characteristically reveals the following:
- a typical *deformity of the foot* due to the pathological abnormality of muscle tone (Fig. 7.**13**),
- *intracardiac conduction abnormalities,*
- often *kyphoscoliosis,*
- sometimes optic nerve atrophy, nystagmus, pyramidal tract signs, and distal muscle atrophy,
- psychopathological changes tending toward *dementia.*

Course. Friedreich ataxia is chronically progressive and causes invalidism within a few years of onset. It sometimes takes a protracted course.

Treatment. No effective treatment is known.

Familial Spastic Spinal Paralysis

This *genetically heterogeneous syndrome* can be inherited in X-linked, autosomal dominant, or (most commonly) autosomal recessive fashion. Its pathophysiological hallmark is *degeneration of the pyramidal tracts,* more severe at caudal levels, due to diffuse loss of neurons in the primary motor cortex. This condition is thus caused by **isolated disease of the first (upper) motor neuron,** as opposed to the spinal muscular atrophies, which involve isolated disease of the second (lower) motor neuron (as will be described further below). Clinically, spastic spinal paralysis is characterized by *spastic paraparesis, usually beginning in childhood and then progressing slowly over many years,* with exaggerated reflexes, pyramidal tract signs, and increasing gait impairment ("scissors gait" due to adductor spasticity).

Nongenetic Diseases of the Long Tracts of the Spinal Cord

Funicular myelosis is caused by **vitamin B$_{12}$ deficiency.** The latter, in turn, may be due either to inadequate dietary intake or to impaired resorption, owing to a lack of sufficient *gastric intrinsic factor* (e. g., in atrophic gastritis, or after gastrectomy). The pathological findings include **demyelination of the posterior columns, posterior roots,** and **pyramidal tracts;** in later stages of the disease, other tracts of the spinal cord, and the cerebral white matter, can be affected as well. There is often, but by no means always, an accompanying hyperchromic, megaloblastic *anemia* with macrocytosis, and the patient's skin is pale yellow. Neurological examination reveals an *ataxic gait, impaired proprioception,* and, rarely, other sensory deficits. These abnormalities may arise subacutely (over a few weeks) or acutely (over a

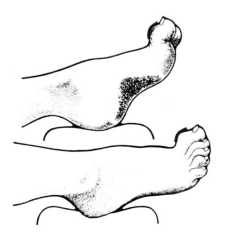

Fig. 7.**13 The typical foot deformity in Friedreich ataxia** ("Friedreich foot").

7

Diseases of the Spinal Cord

few days). The *intrinsic muscle reflexes are diminished* because of posterior root involvement, *pyramidal tract signs* are common, and *mental abnormalities* may be seen, ranging to dementia. The diagnosis rests on the demonstration of vitamin B_{12} deficiency. Vitamin B_{12} must be given as rapidly as possible, preferably by the intramuscular route.

Long tracts of the spinal cord can also be involved in *paraneoplastic syndromes, tabes dorsalis* due to neurosyphilis (pp. 116 f.), *adrenoleukodystrophy* (p. 122), and a number of *congenital metabolic diseases.*

Diseases of the Anterior Horns

Isolated diseases of the anterior horn cells are mostly of **genetic (spinal muscular atrophies)** or infectious origin (acute anterior poliomyelitis, p. 150). **Amyotrophic lateral sclerosis,** in which there is simultaneous degeneration of the anterior horn cells and the corticospinal and/or corticobulbar tracts, is usually **sporadic.**

The typical clinical features of diseases involving chronic loss of anterior horn cells are summarized in Table 7.**3**. Some of these diseases are described in further detail in this section.

Spinal Muscular Atrophies

These diseases are due to a genetic defect on chromosome 5 that causes **isolated degeneration of the second (lower) motor neurons,** i.e., the motor neurons of the anterior horn cells and the cranial nerve nuclei. The result is the typical clinical syndrome of anterior horn degeneration described above (flaccid weakness, muscle atrophy, loss of reflexes, fasciculations). The main clinical types of spinal muscular atrophy are classified according to their *age of onset* and the *pattern of motor deficits* that they cause:

- In the early infantile type (**Werdnig–Hoffmann**), *neonates and infants* suffer from rapidly progressive muscle weakness, beginning in the *muscles of the pelvic girdle*. The affected children can survive for no more than a few years.

Table 7.**3** **Diseases with chronic involvement of the anterior horn ganglion cells***

Disease	Affected structures	Symptoms and signs	Remarks	Etiology
Infantile spinal muscular atrophy (Werdnig–Hoffmann)	anterior horn ganglion cells of the spinal cord (and bulbar motor neurons)	muscle atrophy and weakness, hypotonia, fasciculations of the tongue	affects infants and small children; rapidly fatal	autosomal recessive inheritance (?); gene on chromosome 5
Pseudomyopathic spinal muscular atrophy (Kugelberg–Welander)	anterior horn ganglion cells of the spinal cord	muscle atrophy and fasciculations, progressive gait disturbance, no bulbar involvement	children and adolescents, usually begins in the lower limbs, slowly progressive	irregular dominance; gene on chromosome 5
Adult spinal muscular atrophy (Aran–Duchenne)	anterior horn ganglion cells of the spinal cord	muscle atrophy, weakness, and fasciculations	younger adults; begins distally (hands)	usually isolated, of unknown etiology; occasionally due to syphilis
Proximal spinal muscular atrophy of the shoulder girdle (Vulpian–Bernhardt)	anterior horn ganglion cells of the spinal cord	muscle atrophy, weakness, and fasciculations in the shoulder girdle region	adults; slowly progressive	unknown; occasionally due to syphilis
Amyotrophic lateral sclerosis (sometimes including true bulbar palsy)	anterior horn ganglion cells of the spinal cord, perhaps also motor cranial nerve nuclei, pyramidal tracts, and corticobulbar tracts	muscle atrophy and weakness, fasciculations, bulbar palsy with dysarthria and dysphagia, spasticity, pyramidal tract signs	adults, rapidly progressive and lethal; juvenile (familial) cases are less common and have a relatively benign course	usually sporadic, rarely familial

* A number of rarer neurological diseases affect the anterior horn ganglion cells as one component of a wider disease process; these include Creutzfeldt–Jakob disease, orthostatic hypotension, diabetic amyotrophy (?), metacarcinomatous myelopathy, organic mercury poisoning, and others.

- Pseudomyopathic spinal muscular atrophy (**Kugel-berg–Welander**) becomes symptomatic *between the 2nd and 10th years of life*. The *pelvic girdle* is most severely affected at first, as in the early infantile type, but the weakness and atrophy progress more slowly, and the overall prognosis is much more favorable. The first signs of disease are progressive quadriceps weakness, disappearance of the patellar tendon reflex, and, sometimes, pseudohypertrophy of the calves.
- Types that become symptomatic *from the third decade onward* tend to be *generalized*, though the initial presentation tends to be either *mainly distal* (**Aran–Duchenne**) or *mainly proximal* (**Vulpian–Bernhardt**). The Aran–Duchenne type often presents with atrophy of the intrinsic muscles of the hand, the Vulpian–Bernhardt type with scapulohumeral atrophy. The latter is now considered a subtype of familial amyotrophic lateral sclerosis (see below); it affects not only the muscles of the limbs, but also those of the trunk and respiratory apparatus (Fig. 7.**14**).

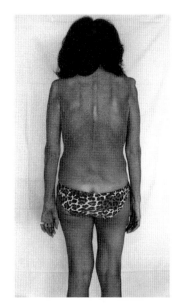

Fig. 7.**14 Spinal muscular atrophy** in a 46-year-old woman. There is marked atrophy of the muscles of the shoulder girdles, arms, and hands, as well as of the paravertebral musculature.

Amyotrophic Lateral Sclerosis (ALS)

This disease, also known as motor neuron disease (MND), is characterized by **combined degeneration of the first and second motor neurons**. Its clinical features are thus a combination of flaccid paresis, muscular atrophy, and spasticity.

Epidemiology. Three-quarters of patients are men, most of them between the ages of 40 and 65. More than 95% of cases are *sporadic*; the rare *familial* cases are thought to be due to a defect of the Cu/Zn superoxide dismutase gene.

Neuropathological hallmark of this disease is *loss of anterior horn cells*, combined with *degeneration of the pyramidal and corticobulbar tracts* and of the *Betz pyramidal cells* of the precentral gyri.

Characteristic clinical manifestations are:
- *weakness and atrophy* of the muscle groups of the limbs and trunk (including the respiratory apparatus) and/or the bulbar muscles (tongue, throat), progressing slowly over months,
- *fasciculations*,
- *exaggerated reflexes*,
- (in some patients) pyramidal tract signs,
- intact sensation,
- often *muscle cramps* and *pain*.

Course. At first, there is circumscribed, asymmetrical, *predominantly distal muscle atrophy*, which is usually most obvious in the intrinsic muscles of the hands. There may be accompanying pain or fasciculations, which are often evident only on prolonged observation. As the disease progresses, muscle atrophy spreads proximally. Spasticity gradually appears as well; it is usually only mild at first and may indeed remain so over the ensuing course of the disease. The *intrinsic muscle reflexes* are usually *brisk*, more than one would expect in view of the concomitant atrophy and weakness, but py-

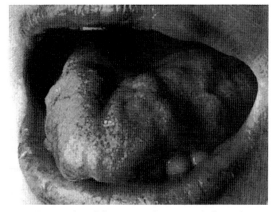

Fig. 7.**15 Atrophy of the tongue** due to true bulbar palsy in a 65-year-old woman with amyotrophic lateral sclerosis.

ramidal tract signs are not necessarily demonstrable. The *bulbar muscles are also involved* in about 20% of patients, as manifested by atrophy, weakness, and fasciculations of the tongue (Fig. 7.**15**), dysarthria, and dysphagia (*true bulbar palsy*). Involvement of the corticobulbar tracts is indicated by *exaggerated nasopalpebral, perioral* and *masseteric reflexes*, and by involuntary laughter and crying, which are often present.

Treatment. *Riluzole* marginally slows the progression of the disease. There is no other specific treatment.

Prognosis. ALS takes a chronically progressive course. Death usually ensues within one or two years, although a minority of patients survives longer.

8 Multiple Sclerosis and Other Myelinopathies

Fundamentals

The common feature of all diseases affecting myelin is a **pathological abnormality** or **total destruction of myelin sheaths**, primarily in the central nervous system. Deficient myelin formation is caused by **congenital enzyme defects** in a small subgroup of these diseases (the leukodystrophies, p. 121), but, in most of them, myelin is lost later in life, for reasons that are currently not well understood. **Immunological (autoimmune) processes** and **metabolic disturbances** appear to play important roles. The most common demyelinating disease is **multiple sclerosis**.

Myelin

Most axons are surrounded by a myelin sheath. The myelin sheaths of the central nervous system are composed of the cell membrane of *oligodendroglia*, which is wrapped around the axon to form a multilaminar structure, as seen in the illustration on p. 2.

The myelin sheath enables the axon to conduct impulses more rapidly (see p. 4); thus, loss of myelin lowers conduction velocity, producing clinical manifestations of neuronal dysfunction. The myelination of the central nervous system reaches its final extent in the first few years of postnatal life. Each layer of a myelin sheath is 7.5 microns thick and is composed of two lipoid and two proteinaceous monomolecular layers. In the genetic myelinopathies, the *primary development of myelin is deficient*; in the metabolic and autoimmune demyelinating diseases, *originally intact myelin is attacked and destroyed*. The most common demyelinating disease, multiple sclerosis, is described in further detail below.

Multiple Sclerosis

Multiple sclerosis (MS) is a **chronic** disease of the central nervous system. It usually presents with **episodic neurological deficits**, which, later on in the course of the disease, tend not to reverse fully, leaving increasingly severe residual deficits whose summation causes **progressively severe disability**. The clinical manifestations are very diverse because **widely separated areas of the CNS are affected** and **the temporal course of the disease is variable**.

"Disseminated encephalomyelitis" is a synonym for multiple sclerosis. In French, the disease is called "sclérose en plaques," as it was named by Charcot; related terms are used in the other Romance languages.

Epidemiology. The incidence in temperate zones is four to six new cases per 100 000 persons per year and the prevalence is greater than 100 per 100 000. MS is particularly common in northern Europe, Switzerland, Russia, the northern U.S.A., southern Canada, New Zealand, and southwest Australia. Women are affected about four times as commonly as men. The initial attack usually oc-

curs in the second or third decade, only rarely in a child or older adult.

After ischemic stroke, multiple sclerosis ranks second among all neurological diseases as a cause of chronic disability.

Pathological anatomy. There are *disseminated foci of demyelination in the central nervous system* (brain and spinal cord), sometimes with destruction of axons as well. Local, reactive gliosis is found at the sites of older foci. Thus, "sclerosis" develops at "multiple" locations, giving the disease its English name.

Pathogenesis. The pathogenetic mechanisms underlying MS are still poorly understood. The most promising hypothesis at present is that an *infection* of neurons and glia occurs in childhood, after which the genome of the pathogenic organism remains in the nervous system. The pathogenic genome is then reactivated on multiple occasions through influences of various kinds; this reactivation, in turn, impairs the functioning of the oligodendroglia, producing episodes of demyelination. According to this hypothesis, CNS demyelination and the generation of antibodies against myelin are merely secondary consequences of the disease process, rather than the cause of MS. An effect of the primary infection outside the central nervous system might explain the lymphocyte abnormalities that are also observed in MS.

Another hypothesis is that an infection induces a *(cell-mediated) autoimmune reaction against normal or virally infected components of the nervous system.*

In any case, multiple sclerosis clearly involves a reactive process that can be set in motion by more than one precipitating factor. This explains why foci can arise in such diverse locations in the central nervous system and why the temporal course of the disease is so variable.

Many different exogenous factors have been proposed as putative causes of MS, but no clear causal relationship has yet been demonstrated for any of them.

Course. The temporal course of multiple sclerosis (Fig. 8.**1**) can be characterized:
- by the episodic appearance of new neurological deficits (**relapsing type**), which can then:
  - remit completely or almost completely,
  - leave residual deficits of greater or lesser severity, or
  - (rarely) fail to regress at all;
- by episodic worsening at first, followed by steady progression (**secondary progressive type**);
- by steady progression from the beginning (**primary progressive type**), as is most commonly seen in older patients with paraparesis; or
- by steady progression with interspersed episodes of acute worsening (**progressive relapsing type**).

Clinical manifestations and neurological findings. The general clinical features of MS are summarized in Table 8.**1**. The neurological deficits present in each individual patient depend on the number and location of the demyelinating foci. The following are among the more characteristic disease manifestations and physical findings:

Retrobulbar neuritis is usually unilateral. Over the course of a few days, the patient develops an *impairment of color vision*, followed by a *marked impairment of visual acuity* (finger counting is barely possible). *Orbital pain* is often present and the patient may see *flashes of light on movement of the globe.* These problems begin to improve in one or two weeks and usually resolve completely. The temporal side of the optic disc becomes pale three or four weeks after the onset of symptoms. Retrobulbar neuritis rarely affects both eyes, either at the same time or in rapid succession. Recurrences are rare. If retrobulbar neuritis is an isolated event in a patient otherwise free of neurological disease, the probability that other clinical signs of multiple sclerosis will appear in the future is roughly 50%. This probability is greater if pathological changes are seen in the CSF (see below) or on an MRI scan (cf. Fig. 8.**3**, p. 159).

Disturbances of ocular motility. *Diplopia*, particularly due to *abducens palsy*, is a common early symptom but nearly always resolves spontaneously. Later, typical findings are *nystagmus* (often dissociated) and *internu-*

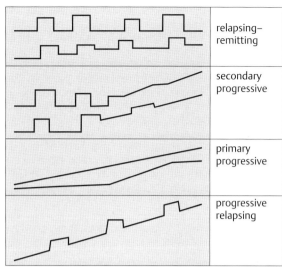

Fig. 8.**1 The temporal course of multiple sclerosis:** four major types.

Table 8.**1   Clinical features of multiple sclerosis**

Symptoms and signs	Remarks
Repeated attacks	– separated in time after each attack – either complete recovery or residual deficit
Diverse sites in CNS affected	– multiple, distinct sites may be involved in a single attack – different sites are usually involved in different attacks – rarely, successive attacks may have similar clinical manifestations (particularly when the lesions are in the spinal cord)
Progressive neurological impairment	– cumulative progression, with worse residual deficits after each attack – steady progression independent of attacks (particularly in late-onset disease)

clear ophthalmoplegia (p. 188), often without any subjective correlate. Internuclear ophthalmoplegia in a young patient is relatively specific for multiple sclerosis.

Lhermitte sign (positive neck-flexion sign). Active or passive forward flexion of the neck induces an "electric" paresthesia running down the spine and/or into the limbs.

❗ Retrobulbar neuritis, disturbances of ocular motility, sensory deficits, and Lhermitte sign are common early findings in multiple sclerosis.

Pyramidal tract signs and exaggerated intrinsic muscle reflexes may be present early in the course of the disease. *The abdominal cutaneous reflexes are absent.* Later on, in almost all patients, *spastic paraparesis* or *quadriparesis* develops.

Cerebellar signs are practically always present in advanced MS, including *impaired coordination, ataxia,* and, frequently, a very characteristic *intention tremor* (Fig. 3.**20** [p. 28], Fig. 8.**2**).

Gait impairment often becomes severe early in the course of the disease. Typically, the combination of *spastic paraparesis* and *ataxia* results in a spastic–ataxic, uneven, uncoordinated, and stiff gait (p. 14, Fig. 3.**2**).

Sensory deficits are found early in the course of the disease in about half of all patients. *Vibration sense in the lower limbs is nearly always impaired. Pain* is not uncommon; sometimes there is even a *dissociated sensory deficit.*

Bladder dysfunction is present in about three-quarters of all patients (generally in association with spasticity); disturbances of defecation are much rarer. Bladder dysfunction is sometimes an early manifestation of the disease. *Urge incontinence* is highly characteristic, i. e., a sudden, almost uncontrollable need to urinate, perhaps leading to "accidents" and bedwetting. Patients often do not mention bladder dysfunction until they are directly asked about it.

Ictal phenomena of various types are not uncommon. It is still debated whether MS causes epileptic seizures. About 1.5 % of persons with MS suffer from *trigeminal neuralgia,* which may alternate from one side to the other. *Acute dizzy spells* can occur, as can *paroxysmal dystonia, dysarthria,* or *ataxia.* The characteristic so-called *tonic brainstem seizures* consist of paroxysmal, often painful, tonic stiffness of the muscles on one side of the body. The lower limb is hyperextended, the upper limb flexed (Wernicke–Mann posture). The patient remains fully conscious. Tonic brainstem seizures are often provoked by a change of position; they last less than one minute and are followed by a refractory period of a half hour or more in which no further seizures can occur. Tonic brainstem seizures and most other MS-associated ictal phenomena respond to treatment with carbamazepine or other antiepileptic drugs.

Mental disturbances are not severe early in the course of the disease. Later on, however, many patients develop *psycho-organic changes* and *psychoreactive and depressive disturbances.* Psychosis is very rare.

The typical clinical findings in multiple sclerosis are shown schematically in Fig. 8.**2**.

Diagnostic evaluation. The typical **physical findings** (see above) reveal the involvement of multiple areas of the nervous system by lesions separated in space and time. The following ancillary tests are also useful:
- **Neuroimaging studies,** particularly *MRI,* typically reveal *abnormal white matter signal* in the periventricular regions and the corpus callosum. Active MS plaques take up contrast medium (Fig. 8.**3**).
- **Cerebrospinal fluid** examination reveals a mild *elevation of the total protein concentration,* mild *lymphocytic and plasma cell pleocytosis,* and, in 90 % of patients, *oligoclonal banding* (demonstrable by isoelectric focusing, Fig. 8.**4**).
- **Electrophysiological testing:** delayed latency of the visual evoked potentials is typical.

Treatment. *Individual acute episodes (relapses)* are treated with high-dose steroids, e. g., methylprednisolone 500 mg i. v. per day for five days, followed by oral prednisone, initially 100 mg per day and then in tapering doses, for two weeks. Patients with frequent re-

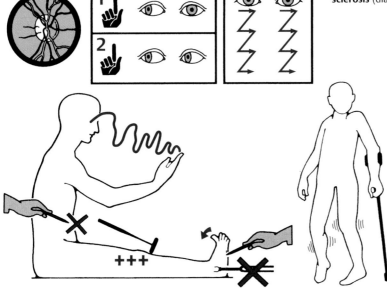

Fig. 8.**2 Common physical findings in multiple sclerosis** (diagram).

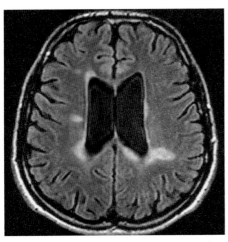
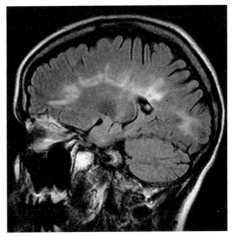

a

b

Fig. 8.**3 MRI of the brain in multiple sclerosis. a** Asymmetrically scattered foci of abnormal signal, affecting only the white matter, are seen in the periventricular regions and at the anterior and post-erior ends of the lateral ventricles. There is mild internal hydro-cephalus. **b** There are typical signal abnormalities in the corpus cal-losum, extending into the white matter of the hemispheres.

lapses are treated over the long term with the **immune modulator** β-**interferon**, at a dose of (for example) 8 × 10^6 IU s.c. q.i.d. for three or four days every week. This lowers the number of relapses per year by about 30%. **Copolymer-1**, a synthetic mixture of amino acids, has a comparable effect when injected subcutaneously every day. β-Interferon is also thought to be an effective treat-ment for the secondary progressive forms of MS. In general, these drugs can slow the progression of the dis-ease, but they cannot stop it. Thus, **general treatment measures** remain very important: patient education, symptomatic treatments (antispasmodic drugs, treat-ment of bladder infections, etc.), psychological and re-habilitative treatment (especially physical therapy).

Differential diagnosis. Generally speaking, when a patient presents with an isolated neurological deficit that would be typical of MS, the differential diagnosis must include all other conditions that could produce that deficit. Even recurrent and relapsing neurological deficits referable to more than one part of the nervous system (the typical clinical picture of MS) do not by themselves establish the diagnosis. The most important elements of the differential diagnosis are listed in Table 8.**2**.

Prognosis. Patient survival 10 years after the onset of MS is nearly the same as that of a normal control popu-lation, and the total life span is reduced by no more than a few years. Advanced age at the onset of disease confers a worse prognosis, but only the disease takes a primary or secondary progressive course. Further unfavorable prognostic factors include cerebellar and brainstem signs, rapid initial progression, and a brief interval be-

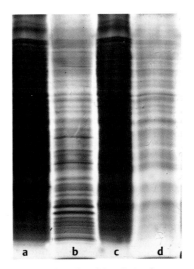

a   b   c   d

Fig. 8.**4 Oligoclonal bands in the serum (a) and CSF (b) of a patient with multiple sclerosis;** compare with the serum (**c**) and CSF (**d**) of a normal control subject.

tween the onset of disease and the first relapse. The patient's condition five years after onset is closely corre-lated with their condition 10 and 15 years after onset, particularly with respect to cerebellar and pyramidal tract signs. About one-third of patients have no major disability 10 years after onset and a few percent still have none 25 years later.

! *Multiple sclerosis sometimes takes a "benign" course.*

Table 8.**2** **Differential diagnosis of multiple sclerosis**

Clinical manifestation	Possible alternative diagnoses	Useful criteria for differential diagnosis
Lhermitte sign	status post traumatic brain injury, status post radiotherapy; pathological process in the thoracic spinal cord, the dorsal cervical spinal cord, or the junction of the spinal cord and medulla; vitamin B_{12} deficiency	accompanying history and physical findings
Intermittent visual loss	amaurosis fugax in carotid stenosis; amblyopic attacks in papilledema	age of the patient, signs of intracranial hypertension, duration of episodes, cervical bruits
Optic disc pallor	optic nerve compression by a mass	slowly progressive visual impairment; mass on CT
Paresis of extraocular muscles	diabetic mononeuritis; compression of one or more cranial nerves by a mass, e. g., at the skull base or in the region of the cavernous sinus	diabetes, pain; tumor or aneurysm on CT or MRI
Nystagmus	disease affecting the cerebellum	other cerebellar signs
Progressive spastic paraparesis	<ul><li>spinal cord compression</li><li>arteriovenous fistula</li><li>spastic spinal paralysis</li><li>parasagittal mass</li></ul>	<ul><li>slow progression, sensory level</li><li>relapsing course</li><li>no relapses or remissions; purely motor deficit</li><li>possibly, headache</li></ul>
Intermittent paraparesis	<ul><li>vascular spinal cord lesion (e. g., arteriovenous malformation)</li><li>benign spinal cord tumor (e. g., lipomatosis after prolonged steroid treatment)</li></ul>	<ul><li>very rapid or sudden worsening</li><li>look for a sensory level; is it constant or variable?</li></ul>
Symptoms and signs arising from multiple foci in the CNS, all at once or with relapses and recurrences	multiple vascular lesions in the CNS	simultaneous involvement of other organs (e. g., coronary artery disease, occlusive peripheral vascular disease) vascular risk factors

Other Demyelinating Diseases of Unknown Pathogenesis

In addition to the genetic, immune-mediated, and metabolic myelinopathies, there are a number of other demyelinating diseases whose causes remain unknown. These diseases are briefly listed and characterized in Table 8.**3**.

Table 8.**3** **Rarer demyelinating diseases**

Disease	Clinical manifestations	Special features
Concentric sclerosis (Baló sclerosis, periaxial encephalitis)	onset at any age, slow progression, associated with dementia	concentric bands of demyelination
Acute disseminated encephalomyelitis (ADEM)	acute multiple sclerosis; simultaneous appearance of symptomatic foci in the brain and spinal cord; acute onset, with fever; peripheral nervous system also involved	MRI shows foci that arose simultaneously; histopathological examination shows axonal injury as well; dramatic course; responds to cortisone and immunosuppressive drugs
Neuromyelitis optica (Devic disease)	simultaneous appearance of symptomatic foci in the optic nerve and spinal cord; mainly affects young women	elevated CSF protein; no oligoclonal bands in CSF; inflammatory axonal damage
Subacute myelo-optic neuropathy (SMON)	ascending paresthesiae and weakness of the lower limbs, appearing days or weeks after a gastrointestinal illness; the optic nerve is also involved in one-third of patients	most common in Japan; many patients have a prior history of oxyquinoline use

9 Epilepsy and Its Differential Diagnosis

Types of Epilepsy

An epileptic seizure is produced by a **temporally limited, synchronous electrical discharge of neurons in the brain**. It presents as a variable combination of motor, somatosensory, special sensory, autonomic, and/or behavioral disturbances, which arises suddenly and may last for a few seconds or a few minutes. On rare occasions, seizure activity persists for more than 20 minutes and may go on for hours, or even longer, without interruption (status epilepticus). The epileptic event may affect a circumscribed area of the brain (partial or **focal seizures**), or both cerebral hemispheres at the same time (**generalized seizures**). An impairment of consciousness is found in generalized seizures and in so-called complex focal seizures. In their differential diagnosis, epileptic seizures must be carefully distinguished from other sudden events involving neurological deficits and disturbances of consciousness.

Epidemiology. It has been calculated that 0.5 % of all individuals suffer from epileptic seizures. The child of a parent with idiopathic epilepsy has a 4 % likelihood of suffering from it.

Pathophysiology. Epileptic seizures are due to dysfunction of neurons in the brain, which expresses itself electrophysiologically as an abnormality of the fluctuations of electrical potential that are seen in an electroencephalogram (EEG, p. 54). (If the surface EEG is normal, such abnormalities can be revealed by recording with depth electrodes.) The underlying cause is an *imbalance of excitatory and inhibitory potentials*, with predominance of excitatory neurotransmitters such as glutamate and aspartate, or diminished activity of inhibitory neurotransmitters such as GABA. The synchronous discharge of neurons in a particular area of the brain is accompanied by a local increase in blood flow.

Etiology. Epileptic seizures can be produced by structural lesions in the brain (so-called epileptic foci: scar, tumor, congenital malformation), by metabolic disturbances (e. g., hypoglycemia), or by toxic influences (e. g., alcohol). These are all types of **symptomatic epilepsy**. In contrast, the **idiopathic epilepsies** involve a genetic predisposition to epileptic seizures, in the absence of a structural lesion. The **cryptogenic epilepsies** are presumed to be of symptomatic origin, although their cause cannot (yet) be demonstrated. Molecular genetic techniques have made it possible to trace certain forms of focal epilepsy back to abnormalities of specific gene loci.

Not uncommonly, more than one etiologic factor is at work: thus, diseases of the brain are more likely to produce epileptic seizures in persons with an inherited predisposition to seizures than in other, normal individuals.

General characteristics of epileptic disorders are the following:
- Epileptic seizures are *events of sudden onset*, which occur with *variable frequency* (generally in the range of a few seizures per year to several per day).
- They often present with *motor phenomena* (in particular, repetitive, clonic twitching or changes of muscle tone) and sometimes with *somatosensory*, *special sensory*, and/or *autonomic manifestations*.
- Depending on their type, they may involve an *impairment or loss of consciousness*, or consciousness may be preserved during the seizure.
- The seizure may be preceded by premonitory symptoms of various kinds (*auras*, e. g., nausea, ascending warmth, or a feeling or unreality).
- In some patients, seizures occur in response to specific *provocative* and *precipitating factors* (sleep deprivation, alcohol withdrawal, medications, strobe lighting, hyperventilation, fever).

Classification of the Epilepsies

Epilepsy can be **classified** according to a number of criteria, including:
- **Etiology**, e. g.:
  - "genuine/idiopathic," genetic,
  - symptomatic,
  - cryptogenic.
- **Age of onset**, e. g.:
  - epilepsy of childhood or adolescence,
  - epilepsy of adulthood,
  - late epilepsy (age 30 and up; always suspect a primary organic disease).
- Setting in which seizures are most frequent, e. g.:
  - sleep epilepsy,
  - epilepsy on awakening.
- EEG correlate and corresponding topographical localization, e. g.:
  - generalized epilepsy,
  - focal (partial) epilepsy.
- finally, the clinical manifestations of each seizure.

Clinical classification of seizures. The nomenclature for the different clinical types of epileptic seizure proposed by the International League Against Epilepsy is reproduced in Table 9.**1**, with the addition of a few further designations that are currently in general use.

Table 9.**1**   **Classification of epileptic seizures** as proposed by the International League Against Epilepsy

1.   Partial (focal, localized) seizures
1.1   *Simple partial seizures (without alteration of consciousness)*
1.1.1   with motor signs
        focal motor without Jacksonian march
        focal motor with Jacksonian march
        versive
        postural
        phonatory (vocalization without interruption of speech)
1.1.2   with somatosensory or special sensory symptoms
        (elementary hallucinations)
        somatosensory
        visual
        auditory
        olfactory
        gustatory
        vertiginous
1.1.3   with autonomic symptoms or signs
        epigastric sensations, diarrhea
        pallor
        sweating
        blushing
        gooseflesh
        pupillary dilatation
1.1.4   with mental symptoms and/or disturbances of higher
        cerebral function (almost always involving alteration of
        consciousness, i. e., more common in complex partial
        epilepsy)
        dysphasia
        dysmnesia (e. g., déjà vu)
        cognitive (twilight states, altered sense of time)
        affective (anxiety, agitation)
        illusions (e. g., dysmorphopsia)
        structured hallucinations
1.2   *Complex partial seizures (with disturbance of consciousness,*
        sometimes beginning with simple manifestations only)
1.2.1   simple partial onset, followed by disturbance of conscious-
        ness with simple partial features, followed by disturbance
        of consciousness with automatisms
1.2.2   with disturbance of consciousness at onset
        with isolated disturbance of consciousness
        with automatisms
1.3   *Partial seizures with secondary generalization to a tonic–*
        clonic (GTC) seizure (synonymous terms: GTC seizures with
        partial or focal onset; secondarily generalized partial
        seizures)
1.3.1   simple partial seizures with secondary generalization
1.3.2   complex partial seizures with secondary generalization
1.3.3   simple partial seizures that develop into complex partial
        seizures and then become secondarily generalized

2.   **Generalized seizures**
2.1   *Absence seizures*
        with isolated disturbance of consciousness
        with automatisms
        with mild clonic component
        with atonic component
        with tonic component
        with autonomic component
2.2   *Atypical absences*
        altered muscle tone may be more prominent; seizures
        may begin and end gradually, rather than abruptly
2.3   *Myoclonic seizures*
        single
        multiple
2.4   *Clonic seizures*
2.5   *Tonic seizures*
2.6   *Tonic–clonic seizures*
2.7   *Atonic seizures*

3.   **Unclassifiable seizures**

Practical Clinical Management of a Suspected Epileptic Seizure

History and physical examination. A *precise history* is of the essence for the diagnosis of epilepsy and its differentiation from other, nonepileptic disorders (see below). A description of the seizures should also be obtained from *someone other than the patient*, if possible, because patients usually suffer amnesia for the seizures. The questions to be asked are summarized in Table 9.**2**. When performing the physical examination, the examiner should pay special attention to: (1) any physical evidence that a seizure has occurred; and (2) any signs of a neurological or general medical disease that might have caused the seizure (Table 9.**3**).

General diagnostic aspects. If the clinical findings suggest that an epileptic seizure has occurred, a series of laboratory studies and ancillary tests should be performed. These are indicated as part of the initial evaluation of every case of suspected epilepsy and mainly serve to detect, or exclude, any possible symptomatic cause of the seizure (Table 9.**4**).

General therapeutic aspects. If the diagnosis of pilepsy can be made securely based on the clinical findings and further testing, an appropriate course of therapy must be decided upon. Any underlying cause of symptomatic epilepsy should be treated (**causal treatment**); moreover, the predisposition to seizures can be treated **symptomatically** with one or a combination of medications (**antiepileptic drugs**, AEDs). Not every epileptic seizure implies a need for treatment. In many patients of a first seizure, it may be best to wait and see whether the event will repeat itself, as long as this presents no special danger and the patient agrees. The decision whether to treat with medications must always be taken on an individual basis, with due consideration of the patient's personality, life situation, occupation, and so forth. The following situations, however, are generally held to indicate treatment:

- two or more epileptic seizures within six months;
- seizures in the setting of a known disease of the brain (encephalitis, cerebral hemorrhage, tumor, etc.);
- epilepsy-typical potentials on EEG;
- initial status epilepticus.

Some general guidelines for the treatment of epilepsy are summarized in Table 9.**5**. Table 9.**6** provides an overview of the major antiepileptic drugs that are currently available and the indications for each.

Table 9.**2** Questions for history-taking in the aftermath of a suspected epileptic seizure

1. About the current seizure:
- Premonitory signs?
- Amnesia?
- Loss of consciousness?
- Manner of waking up?
- Postictal fatigue?
- Injuries?
- Tongue biting?
- Urinary or fecal incontinence?
- Provocative factor?

2. Past history:
- Family history of epilepsy?
- Past events possibly causing brain damage?
  - Perinatal injury (left handedness, strabismus, psychomotor retardation)?
  - Meningitis, encephalitis?
  - Head trauma?
- Prior episodes of loss of consciousness or related disturbances?
  - Febrile seizure(s) in childhood?
  - Unconsciousness?
  - Bedwetting (possibly due to nocturnal grand mal seizures)?
  - Twilight states? (ask specifically about partial complex seizures and déjà vu)
- If epileptic seizures have occurred in the past:
  - When was the first one?
  - When was the most recent previous one?
  - Frequency?
  - Characteristics of each seizure?
  - EEG obtained? If so, with what result?
  - Antiepileptic medications taken, if any:
    Which medications?
    Dosage?
    Taken regularly as directed?
    With what effect on seizures?
    Any side effects?

Table 9.**4** Ancillary tests that may be useful in the aftermath of a suspected epileptic seizure

1. Evidence that a seizure has occurred
- laboratory tests: elevation of CK; elevation of serum prolactin level (a few minutes after the seizure)

2. Clues implicating an underlying disease as the cause of the seizure
- *EEG:* if a routine EEG is normal, EEG with special provocative maneuvers may be indicated (e. g., sleep deprivation, hyperventilation)
- *brain imaging* (MRI is more sensitive than CT) to detect, or rule out, a structural lesion of the brain
- *lumbar puncture* if meningitis and/or encephalitis is suspected
- *further laboratory testing* (routine laboratory parameters and additional, specific ones depending on the clinical situation)

Table 9.**3** Important points for physical examination in the aftermath of a suspected epileptic seizure

1. Evidence that a seizure has occurred
- tongue bite
- urinary or fecal incontinence
- conjunctival hemorrhage
- external injuries
- bone fracture
- shoulder dislocation

2. Clues implicating an underlying disease as the cause of the seizure
- neurological deficits evident on physical examination, and/or signs of intracranial hypertension (esp. papilledema); both are indications of an underlying organic disease of the brain
- abnormal mental status; may indicate an intoxication, or an adverse effect of a medication or illicit drug
- general medical conditions (evidence of metabolic or endocrine disturbances, evidence of heart disease that may be causally related to a possible episode of cerebral ischemia)

Table 9.**5** General principles of the treatment of epilepsy

- thorough patient education
- avoidance of precipitating factors (regular sleep habits, no excessive alcohol consumption, avoidance of strobe lights)
- treatment of the underlying illness, if any (e. g., resection of a meningioma)
- if pharmacotherapy is indicated: choice of a suitable medication for the particular seizure type (cf. Table 9.**6**)
- gradual increase of the dose till seizure control is achieved, or intolerable adverse effects arise. Beware of treatment failure through underdosing: the adverse effect threshold varies greatly from patient to patient and must be crossed, or nearly so, before a medication can be declared ineffective
- meticulous follow-up for possible adverse effects, with especially close observation in the initial phase of treatment
- checking for compliance, e. g., with serum levels, if medications appear to be ineffective
- if therapy with the first agent tried is truly ineffective despite maximal dosing and adequate compliance, change to another agent of first choice, in gradual and overlapping fashion
- combination therapy only if monotherapy fails
- determination of serum levels when:
  - poor compliance is suspected
  - drug toxicity is suspected
  - drug interactions are suspected, particularly those involving enzyme induction
  - an already high dose is to be raised even further
  - medicolegal questions arise, particularly with respect to driving
- guidelines for the cessation of pharmacotherapy: the patient should be free of seizures for at least 2 years; the EEG should be free of potentials typical for epilepsy; traditionally, the medication is slowly tapered off over several months (though the need for this has not been fully demonstrated); the patient and family must be explicitly told that seizures may recur during or after the tapering phase

Epilepsy and Its Differential Diagnosis

9

Table 9.**6**   **Antiepileptic drugs of choice depending on the type of seizure** (after Donati, in Hess). Drugs of second and third choice are listed in alphabetical order

	Partial seizures with or without generalization	Absences	Primary generalized tonic–clonic seizures	Myoclonic seizures	West syndrome (salaam seizures)	Lennox–Gastaut syndrome (myoclonic–astatic seizures)	Rolandic epilepsy (benign epilepsy of childhood and adolescence, with central spikes on EEG)
1st choice	carbamazepine valproate	valproate ethosuximide	valproate	valproate	valproate vigabatrin	valproate	carbamazepine sulthiame (not available in USA)
2nd choice	gabapentin lamotrigine oxcarbazepine phenytoin tiagabine topiramate levetiracetam	lamotrigine	lamotrigine	clonazepam ethosuximide lamotrigine	ACTH	ACTH clobazam felbamate	valproate
3rd choice	vigabatrin clonazepam phenobarbital primidone	clonazepam	phenobarbital primidone	primidone	clonazepam	carbamazepine phenytoin	phenytoin

Generalized Seizures

> Generalized seizures involve both cerebral hemispheres, either from the outset of seizure activity, or when an initially focal seizure becomes secondarily generalized (see below). They typically involve an obvious **impairment of consciousness. Abnormalities of muscle tone** are always present and there are often **involuntary**, **repetitive motor phenomena** involving both sides of the body (clonic or myoclonic activity; see also Table 9.**1**).

The more common types of generalized seizure are described in this section.

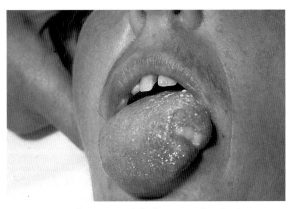

Fig. 9.**1 Tongue bite incurred during a grand mal seizure.**

Tonic–Clonic Seizures (Grand Mal Epilepsy)

Pathogenesis and etiology. A grand mal seizure may be **idiopathic**; in such patients, it is usually primarily generalized ("centrencephalic"). It may also be due to a circumscribed brain lesion (**secondary generalization**). The cause can sometimes be inferred from the findings of the clinical history, imaging studies, and EEG, though it often remains obscure.

Clinical manifestations. Grand mal seizures are the most common and most impressive type of epileptic seizure and also the most familiar to nonprofessionals. Such seizures are sometimes heralded by an *aura* (see above) and a loud cry or shout. Next, the patient *acutely loses consciousness* and *falls to the ground*, and the muscles are *tonically contracted*: the limbs are extended, and the trunk and neck are hyperextended. About 10 seconds later, there follows a *rhythmic, clonic, generalized twitching of all muscles of the body*, accompanied by cyanosis of the face, frothing at the mouth, and possibly by a tongue bite and urinary or fecal incontinence. The twitching persists for a minute or a little longer and is followed by a period of initially deep unconsciousness. Within a few minutes, a gradual transition begins to a phase of confusion and somnolence (*postictal twilight state*) and then to the return of normal consciousness.

The entire seizure typically lasts about 10 minutes. The patient may remember the aura but is otherwise entirely amnestic for the seizure event. Afterward, the patient is tired and may complain of myalgia. A tongue bite (Fig. 9.**1**), urinary or fecal incontinence, and fall-related injuries may be evident. Shoulder dislocation and vertebral or other fractures are rare.

Diagnostic evaluation. Even in the interictal period, the electroencephalogram may reveal the typical picture of synchronous, generalized spikes and waves in all electrodes (Fig. 9.**2**).

Treatment . The medication of first choice for the treatment of grand mal epilepsy is **valproate** (Table 9.**6**).

Absences (Petit Mal)

Absences are very brief seizures involving a momentary diminution of consciousness, rather than a complete loss of consciousness. They most commonly occur in children and adolescents.

Etiology. Like other types of childhood epilepsy, absences are **idiopathic**.

Clinical manifestations. Motor phenomena are not always seen; if present, they are only mild (blinking, automatisms, loss of muscle tone, brief clonus). In the simplest type of absence epilepsy, **petit mal epilepsy of school-aged children**, the seizures often seem to be no more than brief periods of "*absent-mindedness*": the child stares fixedly with eyes turned upward, blinks, and may make movements of the tongue or mouth, or pick at his or her clothes. These types of movements are called *petit mal automatisms*. The entire event lasts no more than a few seconds. Absences usually occur multiple times per day. The examining physician may be able to provoke an absence by having the patient hyperventilate.

Diagnostic evaluation. The **electroencephalogram** reveals a pathognomonic pattern of bursts of synchronous, generalized spike-and-wave activity at a frequency of about 3 Hz. These can be provoked by hyperventilation (Fig. 9.**3**).

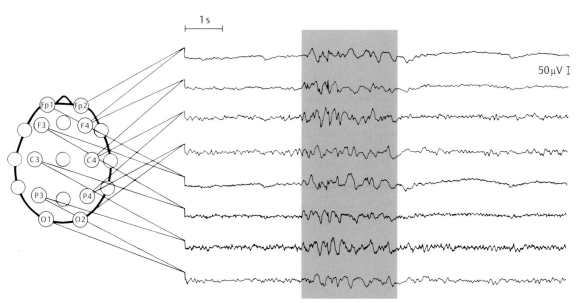

Fig. 9.**2 Interictal EEG in a patient with grand mal seizures**, showing a synchronous paroxysm of generalized, partly atypical spikes and waves.

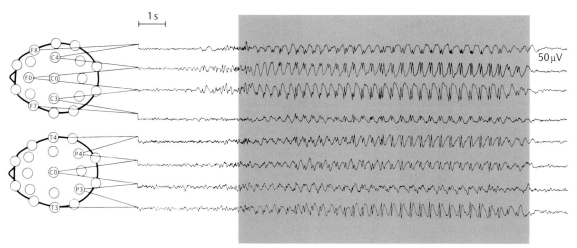

Fig. 9.**3 EEG in a patient with absence seizures,** showing generalized spikes and waves at 3–4 Hz, induced by hyperventilation.

Table 9.**7**   **Epilepsy syndromes mainly or exclusively affecting children**

Syndrome	Age group	Features	Remarks
West syndrome (propulsive petit mal, infantile spasms, salaam spasms)	1st year of life	Rocking and nodding movements, twitching of the trunk, forward thrusting of the arms; seizures are very frequent	Often seen in brain-damaged, retarded children. Typical EEG finding: hypsarrhythmia
Febrile seizures	0–5 years	Generalized seizures in febrile children	Later development of true epilepsy is not uncommon
Myoclonic–astatic petit mal (Lennox–Gastaut syndrome)	0–8 years	Variable loss of muscle tone (ranging from nodding to collapse and falling), very brief unconsciousness; frequent seizures	More common in boys; seizures of this type often occur in association with tonic seizures
Typical absences	1–13 years	Very brief period of unconsciousness, rare falls, occasional minor motor phenomena (picking at clothes), vacant stare; many times a day, precipitated by hyperventilation	Sometimes found in association with grand mal seizures (mixed epilepsy); EEG typically shows 3 Hz spike-wave pattern (Fig. 9.**3**)
Myoclonic seizures (impulsive petit mal)	2nd decade and onward into adulthood	Irregular rocking twitches, more frequent on awakening, no loss of consciousness	Later often combined with grand mal seizures
Benign focal epilepsy of childhood and adolescence	1st and 2nd decades	Focal twitching, usually during sleep; patient is conscious during seizures that occur when he/she is awake; one-third also have generalized seizures	Multiple subtypes; typical EEG pattern with biphasic centro-temporal spikes; good prognosis for spontaneous recovery

Treatment. The medications of first choice for the treatment of absences are **valproate** and **ethosuximide**.

Prognosis. About one in four affected children become free of seizures during puberty; in the remainder, seizures persist. One half of these patients with persistent absence seizures will go on to develop grand mal seizures as well.

Atypical Absences and Other Types of Epilepsy In Childhood

The other types of childhood epilepsy are summarized in Table 9.**7**.

Partial (Focal) Seizures

> Focal seizures are always due to a **circumscribed lesion in the brain**. The specific manifestations of the seizure correspond to the site of the lesion. Unlike generalized seizures, which always involve an impairment of consciousness, focal seizures may occur with the patient remaining fully conscious (**simple partial seizures**). They can, however, involve an impairment of consciousness, in which case they are called **complex partial seizures**. The excitation arising in the epileptic focus may spread to the entire brain and thereby provoke a **secondarily generalized grand mal seizure**. In such patients, the initial focal phase may be very brief and is not always clinically recognizable.

Figure 9.**4** schematically represents the clinical manifestations that can be expected in focal seizures arising from various brain areas. The major types of focal seizure will be described in detail in the remainder of this section.

Simple Partial Seizures

Simple partial seizures can be purely motor, mixed sensory and motor, or purely sensory (either somatosensory or special sensory). They are, by definition, not accompanied by an impairment of consciousness, though they may undergo secondary generalization.

Individual types of simple partial seizure. A simple partial seizure may involve **focal motor twitching** on one side of the body, or sensory disturbances that suddenly arise in a circumscribed area of the body. Focal twitching confined to a very small area (e.g., a hand) and lasting for a very long time (hours or more) is called **epilepsia partialis continua** (of Kozhevnikov).

In a **Jacksonian seizure**, the motor (or sensory) phenomena rapidly spread to the entire ipsilateral half of the body ("*Jacksonian march*"). If the seizure focus lies in the precentral or the supplementary motor area, the seizure will be of **adversive** type: the patient's head and eyes turn tonically to the opposite side, while the contralateral arm is abducted and elevated. If the seizure focus lies in the visual or auditory cortex or the neighboring association areas, the seizure may consist of, or begin with, auditory or visual sensations, or even scenic images.

Diagnostic evaluation. The focal nature of the seizure, or its focal origin (in the case of secondarily generalized seizures), is demonstrated not only by the clinical manifestations, but also by the **electroencephalogram**, which displays localized epileptic activity over the seizure focus (Fig. 9.**5**).

Treatment. The medications of first choice for the treatment of focal seizures are **carbamazepine** and **oxcarbazepine**.

Fig. 9.**4 Localization of focal epileptic seizures.** The type of attack depends on the site of the focal lesion (adapted from Foerster).

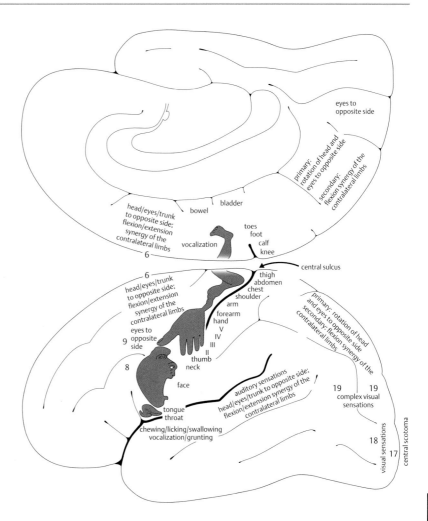

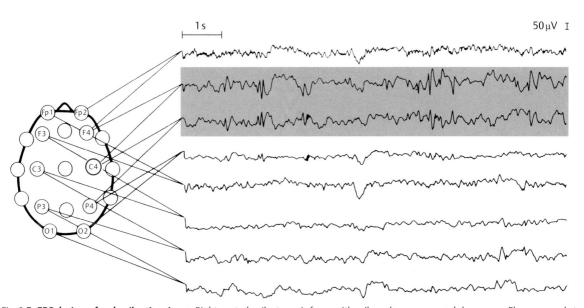

Fig. 9.**5 EEG during a focal epileptic seizure.** Right central epileptogenic focus with spikes, sharp waves, and slow waves. Phase reversal at electrode C4.

Table 9.**8**   Clinical manifestations of partial complex seizures (temporal lobe epilepsy)

Category	Manifestations	Remarks
Sensory disturbances	Dizziness, dysmorphopsia (macropsia, micropsia, everything seems to be far away), gustatory sensations, unpleasant olfactory sensations	Uncinate fits
Autonomic phenomena	Shortness of breath, palpitations, nausea, salivation, dry mouth, hunger, urge to urinate, abdominal sensations	Often, ascending sensation from stomach to throat
Behavioral and psychomotor manifestations	Traumatic experience, feeling of unreality, feeling of unfamiliarity (jamais vu), forced thoughts, déjà vu, déjà vécu, unfounded anxiety or rage, hallucinations, twilight states	
Twilight states	Automatic, semiorganized, but inappropriate behavior, e. g., picking at clothes, senseless moving around of objects, etc. (twilight attacks); long-lasting, semiorganized complex behaviors that may even involve travel over a long distance (twilight state, fugue épileptique)	Amnesia for these states
Temporal syncope	Collapse, usually immediately following one of the above phenomena, typically with only brief unconsciousness	No sudden falling
Psychomotor status epilepticus	Very long persistence of the above phenomena, or repeated occurrence with less than full recovery in between	Rare

Complex Partial Seizures

This type of seizure was previously known as *psychomotor epilepsy* or, alternatively, *temporal lobe epilepsy.* It is due to a lesion in the limbic system, usually in the temporal lobe, but sometimes in the frontal lobe.

Etiology . The most common cause of complex partial seizures is a **perinatal lesion** of hypoxic origin (mesial temporal sclerosis or hippocampal sclerosis). Other causes include **congenital developmental anomalies** (e. g., disorders of neuroblast migration), trauma, and brain tumors.

Clinical manifestations. Complex partial seizures have *sensory*, *behavioral*, *psychomotor*, and *autonomic manifestations*, which are described in further detail in Table 9.**8**.

Which of these manifestations will be present in the individual patient depends on the precise location of the epileptic focus. The manifestations may vary to a mild extent from seizure to seizure, though an unvarying, stereotypical course is more common.

In addition to the manifestations mentioned above, many patients report experiencing *déjà vu* and related phenomena, i. e., the strong, but nonetheless inaccurate, feeling of having already seen or experienced what one is seeing or experiencing at the moment. Patients whose seizure focus lies in the uncinate gyrus also have *olfactory hallucinations*, or, as they are called, *uncinate fits*. These are often produced by a mass in the temporal lobe.

Illustrative case description: The patient's seizures begin suddenly, with a peculiar feeling of distance from his surroundings. Everything seems to be far away, unreal, and like a dream. At the same time, he notices a strange sensation in the pit of his stomach, ascending to his neck. He may also have palpitations or shortness of breath. On some occasions, his consciousness is more

severely affected: he stares blankly ahead, makes chewing and swallowing movements, produces gagging noises, and fails to respond to questions. He picks at his clothes, makes purposeless hand movements, and sometimes falls over. Rarely, when he is in this "twilight state," he carries out complex activities, perhaps even a "*fugue épileptique.*" The entire episode usually lasts one or a few minutes, but may last much longer.

Diagnostic evaluation. Complex partial seizure activity can generally be diagnosed from its typical clinical picture. The **EEG** reveals temporal slow waves or spikes. In the interictal period, however, it is usually normal.

Treatment. The medications of choice for complex partial seizures, as for simple partial seizures, are **carbamazepine** and **oxcarbazepine**. Alternatively, valproate can be used.

Status Epilepticus

Status epilepticus refers to a prolonged, uninterrupted epileptic seizure, or multiple seizures occurring in rapid succession without recovery in between.

> ! *Generalized (grand mal) status epilepticus, in which the patient does not regain consciousness between seizures, is a life-threatening emergency because of the danger of respiratory complications and ensuing cerebral ischemia.*

In **absence status** the patient is not unconscious, but rather confused or mildly dazed, with inappropriate behavior. The EEG is diagnostic.

Complex partial status epilepticus can be mistaken for an acute psychotic episode.

Treatment. Grand mal status epilepticus should be treated with a bolus dose of a **benzodiazepine**, e. g., diazepam 10–20 mg i. v., followed by **intravenous phenytoin** (by slow push or drip) or **valproate** (IV push followed by drip). If seizure activity does not stop within 40 minutes, the patient must be *intubated and ventilated* and put in artificial coma with a barbiturate such as *thiopental* or *propofol*.

Petit mal status epilepticus and psychomotor status epilepticus respond to *clonazepam* 2–4 mg i. v.

Episodic Neurological Disturbances of Nonepileptic Origin

Because the clinical presentations of epileptic seizures are so highly varied, their differential diagnosis necessarily includes a wide variety of conditions. Any episodic loss of consciousness, impaired motor function, or fall might be due either to an epileptic seizure or to a nonepileptic event of another etiology, as will be discussed in this section.

Episodic neurological disturbances of nonepileptic origin can be classified into four major types, as follows:
- transient loss of consciousness and falling;
- falling without loss of consciousness;
- loss of consciousness without falling; and
- episodic movement disorders without loss of consciousness.

Episodic Disturbances with Transient Loss of Consciousness and Falling

Table 9.9 provides a quick overview of nonepileptic disturbances of this type (and, for completeness, also includes some that are of epileptic origin). Only the more important ones are described in greater detail in this section.

Table 9.**9** **Clinical features of various conditions causing brief loss of consciousness and falls**

	"Falling sicknesses"	Found in:	Precipitating factors	Prodromal phenomena
Syncopal attacks	*orthostatic hypotension (vasomotor collapse)*			yawning, tinnitus, feeling of heat, epigastric pressure
	chronic sympathetic autonomic failure	Shy–Drager, tabes dorsalis		
	medications	diuretics, antihypertensives, β-blockers/L-Dopa	prolongued standing; rapidly standing up from a lying position	
	adolescents	possibly due to anemia		
	reflex circulatory syncope (vagal inhibition)			
	vagovasal syncope	hyperventilation / heat, fright, etc.	intense emotion / pain	
	swallowing syncope	glossopharyngeal neuralgia	paroxysms	
	carotid sinus syndrome	elderly men	carotid pressure	
	pressor syncope (inadequate venous return)			
	coughing/laughing syncope	persons with emphysema	coughing fit / laughing fit	
	micturition syncope	men, alcohol	urination while standing	
	"extension syncope"/squatting	children, possibly on purpose	hyperextension / squatting and pressing!	
	primary cardiovascular syncope			
	cervicobrachial stenosis	subclavian steal syndrome / aortic arch syndrome / e. g., subaortic stenosis	physical / exertion / (arm)	
	cardiac anomalies/heart failure			
	"sinoatrial syncope"	cardiac arrhythmias	sometimes induced by intense emotion	fright, anxiety
	Adams–Stokes attack	grade III A–V block	independent of position	often without warning
	respiratory affect seizure			
	cyanotic affect seizure	infants / school-aged children	anger/spite / fright / pain	
	"white" affect seizure			

Continued →

Epilepsy and Its Differential Diagnosis

9

Table 9.**9**   **Clinical features of various conditions causing brief loss of consciousness and falls** (Continued)

	"Falling sicknesses"	Found in:	Precipitating factors	Prodromal phenomena
falling attacks	true reflex "vestibular" syncope (Tumarkin syndrome)	Ménière disease paroxysmal positioning vertigo	head movements (sometimes)	dizziness (sometimes) vertigo
	intermittent vertebrobasilar ischemia	elderly patients vascular risk factors	head turning (sometimes)	nausea, dizziness visual disturbances, etc.
	cryptogenic falling attacks in women	middle-aged women	only while walking	no prodromal phenomena
	cataplectic falling	isolated, or in the setting of narcolepsy	intense emotion laughing fright	without warning
epilepsy	"temporal lobe syncope"	psychomotor epilepsy	intense emotion (sometimes)	psychomotor aura possible
	grand mal seizure	possibly several times/day any age	sleep deprivation alcohol	aura possible
	drop attacks (myoclonic–astatic)	Lennox–Gastaut syndrome (children)		
psychogenic	hysterical falling (with impairment of consciousness)	neurotic disorders psychological gain		
	simulated falling attacks/seizures {	may occur in patients who also have true epileptic seizures malingering ("compensation neurosis")	attacks occur only before an "audience"	

Syncope

Syncope is a *very brief loss of consciousness* during which the affected individual falls to the ground. It is due to a very brief loss of function of the brainstem reticular formation, which, in turn, is usually caused by temporary ischemia and tissue hypoxia. Syncope can be of **vasomotor** or **cardiogenic** origin.

Reflex circulatory syncope, the commonest kind of syncope, can be precipitated by intense emotion (e. g., the sight of blood, anticipatory anxiety), heat, prolonged standing, or physical pain. The affected person becomes dizzy, sees black spots before his or her eyes, turns pale, breaks out in a sweat, and then collapses to the ground. Wakefulness and full orientation are regained at once in most patients.

Etiologic subtypes of reflex circulatory syncope include *idiopathic vasomotor collapse in adolescents, pressor syncope* after prolonged coughing, *micturition syncope, swallowing syncope,* and *extension syncope* (mainly seen in younger patients who stand up too quickly from a squatting position). *Orthostatic syncope* is a feature of many neurological diseases (e. g., multisystem atrophy). *Carotid sinus syncope* is rarer than once thought. *Vestibular syncope* occurs, e. g., in acute paroxysmal positioning vertigo.

Cardiogenic syncope is especially common in older patients. Its causes include *cardiac arrhythmias* (third-degree AV block, sick sinus syndrome, tachycardias) and other types of *heart disease* (e. g., valvular aortic stenosis, atrial myxoma, and chronic pulmonary hypertension with cor pulmonale).

"Convulsive syncope": syncopal episodes are sometimes accompanied by brief, clonic muscle twitching. This may make a syncopal episode even harder to distinguish from an epileptic seizure.

Episodic Falling without Loss of Consciousness

Drop Attacks

In a so-called *drop attack*, the patient suddenly falls to the ground without braking the fall. Consciousness is apparently preserved during the event; in some patients, however, the patient may, in fact, lose consciousness without realizing it afterward, and too briefly for others to observe. Some drop attacks are due to *atonic epilepsy*, others to *basilar ischemia*. *Cryptogenic drop attacks* have been described in older women ("climacteric drop syncope"). Finally, drop attacks can be caused by basilar impression and other structural abnormalities of the craniocervical junction.

Table 9.**10** **Distinguishing features of the narcolepsy–cataplexy and sleep apnea syndromes**

Aspect	Narcolepsy–cataplexy	Sleep apnea
History	30–50 % positive family history, onset usually in 2nd or 3rd decade of life	negative family history, onset usually in middle or old age
Daytime sleep	usually in sleep-promoting situations, patient feels rested afterward; there are also hypovigilant twilight states	overwhelming need to sleep; patient does not feel rested afterward
Nighttime sleep	often restless, nightmares, sometimes sleep paralysis, patients sometimes do not feel rested in the morning, no headache	loud snoring, respiratory pauses lasting more than 10 seconds (hallmark), diminished O_2 saturation of the blood, sometimes angina pectoris during sleep, patients usually do not feel rested in the morning, headache
Other features	cataplectic states, e. g., loss of affective tone, hypnagogic hallucinations and automatic behavior, no dementia	no cataplexy, sometimes hypnagogic hallucinations and automatic behavior, perhaps (reversible) dementia
Clinical findings	sometimes short, stocky habitus	usually men, almost always obese, often hypertensive, occasional anomaly of nasopharynx
Ancillary tests: • EEG	often signs of somnolence, short sleep latency, early REM sleep, frequent alternation with nonREM sleep	unremarkable
• Other	HLA-DR2 constellation	no specific HLA type

Cataplexy

Cataplexy, a component of the **narcolepsy–cataplexy syndrome**, may present with the clinical picture of an unexplained, atonic fall. Directed history taking then reveals some or all of the **five cardinal symptoms** of cataplexy:

- *disturbance of wakefulness*, usually with brief and restorative naps during the day (in sleep-promoting situations);
- *falls*, due to sudden loss of muscle tone, precipitated by fright or other emotions (affective loss of muscle tone), and perhaps brief local loss of tone in individual muscle groups;
- *disturbance of nighttime sleep*, with nightmares;
- *sleep paralysis*, i. e., brief inability to move on awakening;
- partial hypovigilance states and hallucinatory experiences, mostly while falling asleep (*hypnagogic hallucinations*).

The diagnosis of this disorder, which tends to occur in families, is made on clinical grounds and confirmed by the following **objective findings:**

- HLA-DR2 constellation and characteristic EEG abnormalities (SOREM = sleep-onset REM = early REM sleep stages);
- frequent somnolence;
- the appearance of REM sleep during the first hour of nighttime sleep, and
- frequent alternation of REM sleep with typical, deep sleep (Fig. 9.**6**).

Important clinical aspects of the differential diagnosis of the narcolepsy–cataplexy syndrome—in particular, its distinction from sleep apnea syndrome—are listed in Table 9.**10**.

Differential diagnosis: sleep apnea syndrome. This syndrome mainly affects middle-aged and elderly men who snore loudly. Typical manifestations, other than *snoring* are *motor unrest during sleep* and *repeated respiratory pauses* due to airway displacement. When one of these pauses occurs, the patient becomes half awake, with a start, before beginning to breathe again. The repeated pauses interfere considerably with sleep. The patient awakens the next day feeling *poorly rested*, often complaining of *headache*; the next day, he or she is tired, falls asleep repeatedly, and may suffer from impaired intellectual performance or even (reversible) dementia. The diagnosis is established by polysomnography. Treatment with *continuous positive-pressure respiration*, through a mask, during nighttime sleep often results in dramatic improvement.

Episodic Loss of Consciousness without Falling

Certain *metabolic disturbances* (e. g., hypoglycemia) and *electrolyte disturbances* (particularly hyponatremia), as well as *endocrine diseases* (hypothyroidism, hypoparathyroidism), can cause episodic loss of consciousness. Unconsciousness can also be the most prominent manifestation of *tetany*, e. g., in hyperventilation; other signs include Chvostek sign, paresthesiae of the fingers and mouth, and tonic muscle contractions, with carpopedal spasm.

Episodic Movement Disorders without Loss of Consciousness

The following nonepileptic movement disorders must be distinguished from focal motor epilepsy:

- **Focal, repetitive twitching** of various types: *hemifacial spasm* is a synchronous involuntary contraction, at irregular intervals, of muscles innervated by the facial nerve on one side of the face. *Tics* and

Normal sleep profile

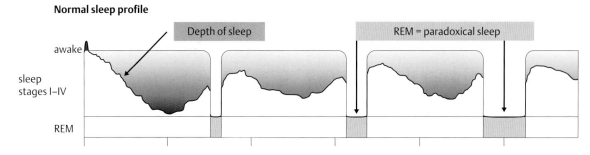

Sleep profile in narcolepsy–cataplexy syndrome

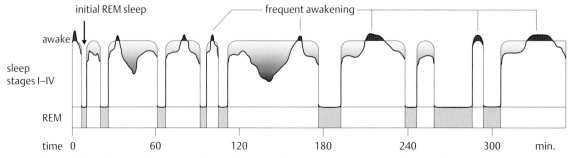

Fig. 9.**6 Sleep profile in the narcolepsy–cataplexy syndrome** (below) compared to a normal sleep profile (above).

blepharospasm are usually bilateral. *Palatal nystagmus* is due to a lesion of the olive or the central tegmental tract. *Myoclonus* and *myorrhythmia* are usually not confined to a particular muscle or muscle group, but tend to migrate from one to another.

- **Episodic, generalized motor processes** include *paroxysmal choreoathetosis*, which may be familial or due to multiple sclerosis, and *tonic brainstem seizures*, which are likewise a feature of MS (p. 158).

10 Polyradiculopathy and Polyneuropathy

Fundamentals

In this chapter, we will describe the characteristic syndromes produced by lesions affecting multiple nerve roots or peripheral nerves simultaneously (**polyradiculopathy** and **polyneuropathy**, respectively). If nerve roots *and* peripheral nerves are affected, the disorder is termed **polyradiculoneuropathy**. These very heterogeneous syndromes can be classified in various ways. Today, they are most commonly classified according to the following criteria:

- **Temporal course:** polyradiculoneuropathy may present acutely with complete or partial remission, or it may take a chronically recurrent or chronically progressive course.
- **Etiology:** polyradiculoneuropathy may be of metabolic, endocrine, toxic, genetic/hereditary, infectious, inflammatory, autoimmune, or paraneoplastic origin.
- **Pathology:** the functioning of the nerve roots and/or peripheral nerves may be impaired either by demyelination or by axonal degeneration. Slowing of nerve conduction early in the course of the illness is a distinguishing feature of demyelinating polyradiculoneuropathy.

The general manifestations of polyradiculopathic and polyneuropathic disorders include:
- paresis,
- diminution or absence of reflexes,
- muscle atrophy,
- sensory deficits and positive sensory phenomena (paresthesia, dysesthesia),
- pain (in some patients),
- predominantly distal symptoms and signs in a symmetrical distribution, or, in other patients, asymmetrical severity,
- usually beginning in the lower limbs,
- with more or less rapid progression,
- with variable involvement of the autonomic nervous system.

The extent, severity, and distribution of these manifestations vary from patient to patient. In addition, predominantly radiculopathic processes are clinically distinguishable from exclusively neuropathic processes. These two types of illness are, therefore, presented separately in the following sections.

Polyradiculitis

This term refers to an **inflammatory process affecting many spinal nerve roots** (most commonly the anterior ones), usually with simultaneous involvement of the proximal segments of the peripheral nerves. Inflammation of the nerve roots or nerves is usually not caused by infection, but rather by immune-mediated processes, e. g., an autoallergic radiculitis or neuritis following a prior, possibly asymptomatic viral or bacterial infection. **Clinical variants** of polyradiculitis are distinguished from one another by the degree of acuity and predominant localization of symptoms and signs. The **acute** form, **Guillain–Barré syndrome**, is the most common; the **chronic** form (**CIDP** = chronic inflammatory demyelinating polyradiculoneuropathy) is rarer, as is **localized polyradiculoneuritis**, which exclusively affect either the cranial nerves or the nerves of the cauda equina. Demyelinating processes are the main pathophysiological mechanism of polyradiculitis. Axonal degeneration is also present, to a varying degree, in CIDP, which explains its protracted course.

Classic Polyradiculitis (Landry–Guillain–Barré–Strohl Syndrome)

Acute polyradiculitis is characterized by **rapidly ascending paresis**, accompanied by at most mild sensory disturbances. In severe cases, the cranial nerves and autonomic system can be involved. Weakness usually improves spontaneously in all involved muscles (those that became weak first recover last). The prognosis is favorable.

Epidemiology. This illness, usually called Guillain–Barré syndrome for short, can appear at any age. Its annual incidence is between 0.5 and 2 cases per 100 000 persons. It tends to appear in the spring or fall.

Etiology and pathogenesis. This syndrome probably has more than one cause. Often, no precipitating factor can be identified. In some patients, the illness is preceded by *Mycoplasma* pneumonia or by infection with varicella-zoster virus, paramyxoviruses (mumps),

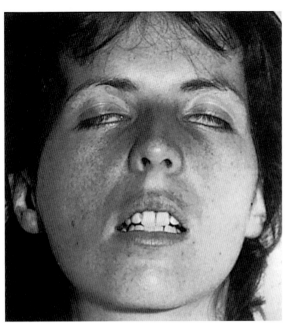
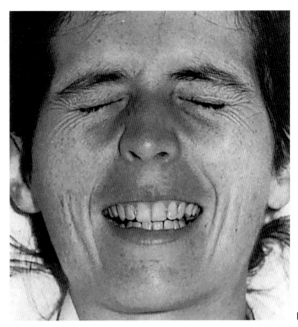

a   b

Fig. 10.**1** **Bilateral peripheral facial nerve palsy in Guillain–Barré polyradiculitis: a** acute phase, **b** after recovery. (From: Mumenthaler, M.: *Didaktischer Atlas der klinischen Neurologie*, 2nd edn, Springer, Heidelberg, 1986.)

HIV, Epstein–Barr virus (infectious mononucleosis), or *Campylobacter jejuni*. The last-named organism often produces axonal lesions and is associated with a particularly severe form of the illness. Immunological processes play an important role in pathogenesis; in particular, there is an elevated concentration of antimyelin antibodies. Finally, anti-GD1a antibodies are found in the rarer forms of the illness that involve axonal degeneration, but not in the more common, demyelinating forms (see above).

Clinical manifestations. The first sign is *weakness of the lower limbs*, beginning distally, occasionally some time after a preceding upper respiratory or gastrointestinal infection. There is no fever. *Weakness ascends within a few hours or days*, so that the patient becomes unable to walk. Distal paresthesiae and sensory disturbances are present in most patients, but are much less disturbing to the patient than the weakness.

Though the weakness ascends rapidly, its ultimate extent is variable. In very severe cases, the upper limbs, diaphragm, and accessory muscles of respiration are affected, as well as the muscles of the head and neck that are supplied by the cranial nerves. Dysphagia and bilateral facial palsy result (Fig. 10.**1**). Respiratory failure often develops rapidly and is a life-threatening condition requiring prompt treatment with intubation and artificial ventilation. In addition, *involvement of the autonomic nervous system* can cause life-threatening abnormalities of blood pressure regulation, cardiac rhythm, central respiratory drive, and, rarely, bladder function.

Diagnostic evaluation. The diagnosis is generally made from the *clinical findings* and confirmed by the charac-

teristic finding of *albumino-cytologic dissociation* in the CSF. This term refers to an elevation of the CSF protein concentration without any accompanying elevation of the cell count; the finding may not be present, however, until two or three weeks after the onset of illness. *Electrophysiological studies* usually reveal focal demyelination with conduction block, or, less commonly, axonal lesions.

Treatment. In severe cases, with profound weakness and rapidly progressive respiratory dysfunction, an intravenous infusion of *immunoglobulins* is indicated (0.4 g/kg body weight for five consecutive days). Another course can be given in four weeks, if necessary. *Plasmapheresis*, too, is effective and is recommended for all patients with rapidly ascending paresis and impending respiratory failure, even if the patient can still walk. Such patients should be hospitalized in an *intensive care unit*, so that their circulatory and respiratory function can be closely monitored and they can be intubated at once, if necessary. In milder cases, *general supportive care* often suffices: routine nursing, prophylaxis against venous thromboses, urinary catheterization if needed, and, later, physical therapy.

Prognosis. The prognosis is generally favorable. Intensive care may be needed in the acute phase, but, once this is past, the weakness usually resolves in all affected muscles (those that became weak first recover last). Recovery may take several months, however, or even up to two years in very severe cases. Most of the deaths caused by Guillain–Barré syndrome are complications of prolonged immobility (pneumonia, pulmonary embolism) or of autonomic dysfunction (respiratory failure, sudden cardiac death).

Chronic Inflammatory Demyelinating (Recurrent) Polyneuropathy (CIDP)

> CIDP, a chronic form of polyradiculitis, has a similar pathophysiological mechanism to Guillain–Barré syndrome, the corresponding acute form. The weakness and autonomic dysfunction are usually less severe, but they last longer. The clinical manifestations fluctuate in severity, often taking a relapsing and remitting or chronically progressive course.

Pathogenesis. The idiopathic form of this condition is presumed to have an immunological basis. Immunoglobulins are found in the CSF and immunoglobulin deposits are seen in biopsy specimens of the sural nerve. There are also forms of CIDP associated with HIV or systemic lupus erythematosus.

Clinical manifestations. CIDP differs from classic, benign Guillain–Barré polyradiculitis in the following ways:
- chronic or relapsing-remitting course (more than four weeks),
- possibly subacute course,
- pain is common,
- asymmetrical distribution of neurological deficits,
- recurrent cranial nerve involvement,
- marked elevation of CSF protein concentration, often combined with an elevated IgG index and pleocytosis,
- central nervous manifestations are more common than in Guillain–Barré syndrome,
- electroneurography reveals evidence of focal demyelination or axonal damage.

Diagnostic evaluation. Electrophysiological studies reveal slowing of nerve conduction, partial conduction blocks, and a delayed F wave.

Treatment. CIDP is treated with corticosteroids or immunosuppressive agents (cyclophosphamide) for a long period. Immunoglobulins and plasmapheresis are also used, sometimes in combination with immune suppression.

! *Although corticosteroids are indicated in the treatment of CIDP, they are only of questionable benefit in Guillain–Barré syndrome.*

Prognosis. The prognosis is unfavorable: 10% of patients die of the disease, 25% remain severely disabled, and 5 to 10% have recurrences.

Multifocal Motor Neuropathy (MMN)

This is a special form of CIDP (see above).

Clinical manifestations. MMN is characterized by asymmetrical, slowly or rapidly progressive weakness with muscle atrophy and, sometimes, fasciculations (which may make MMN difficult to distinguish from ALS). There may also be dysarthria and sensory deficits. Some reflexes are lost.

Diagnostic evaluation. Electrophysiological studies reveal sporadic, circumscribed conduction blocks, and laboratory testing often reveals elevated anti-GM1 titers.

Treatment. MMN is treated like other forms of CIDP.

Cranial Polyradiculitis

Polyradiculitis of the cranial nerves may be a component of ascending polyradiculitis, in which case it generally arises only after the limbs have become paretic. Sometimes, however, it is the first, predominant, or only clinical manifestation of polyradiculitis. The differential diagnosis of such patients must always include borreliosis and chronic meningitis (p. 112).

Miller Fisher Syndrome

Clinical manifestations. This special form of cranial polyradiculitis, which mainly affects younger male patients, is characterized by
- ophthalmoplegia,
- ataxia,
- areflexia,
- (sometimes) pupillary involvement (e. g., Adie pupil),
- (sometimes) facial nerve palsy,
- elevated CSF protein concentration,
- (sometimes) accompanying brainstem signs.

Treatment. Miller Fisher syndrome has a favorable prognosis and generally needs no specific treatment.

Polyradiculitis of the Cauda Equina

This rare type of polyradiculitis, also called Elsberg syndrome, is characterized by isolated involvement of the sacral roots, producing distal weakness and areflexia of the lower limbs and sphincter dysfunction. Many patients are presumably due to borreliosis or a herpes virus infection.

Polyradiculopathy and Polyneuropathy

10

Polyneuropathy

Fundamentals

Polyneuropathy is a condition affecting multiple peripheral nerves, usually simultaneously, though possibly in more or less rapid sequence. The clinical manifestations are usually symmetrically distributed and slowly progressive. The first signs of polyneuropathy are practically always in the lower limbs. Its causes are many.

Etiology. The common causes of polyneuropathy are listed in Table 10.**1**.

Pathogenesis. A variety of harmful influences affect peripheral nerves in different ways and produce correspondingly different histopathological lesions. Initial

Table 10.**1**   **Causes of the more common types of polyneuropathy**

Hereditary polyneuropathy
- hereditary motor and sensory neuropathies
- neuropathy with tendency to pressure palsy
- porphyria
- primary amyloidosis

Polyneuropathy due to a metabolic disorder
- diabetic neuropathy:
  - symmetric, mainly distal type
  - asymmetric, mainly proximal type
  - "mononeuropathy"
  - amyotrophy or myelopathy
- uremia
- cirrhosis
- gout
- hypothyroidism

Polyneuropathy due to improper or inadequate nutrition

Polyneuropathy due to vitamin B$_{12}$ malabsorption

Polyneuropathy due to dysproteinemia or paraproteinemia

Polyneuropathy due to infectious disease
- leprosy
- mumps
- mononucleosis
- typhoid and paratyphoid fever
- typhus
- spotted fever
- HIV infection
- diphtheria
- botulism
- tickborne diseases (borreliosis)

Polyneuropathy due to arterial disease
- polyarteritis nodosa
- other collagenoses
- atherosclerosis

Polyneuropathy due to sprue and other malabsorptive disorders

Polyneuropathy due to exogenous toxic substances
- ethanol
- lead
- arsenic
- thallium
- triaryl phosphate
- solvents (e. g., carbon disulfide)
- drug toxicity (isoniazid, thalidomide, nitrofurantoin)

Polyneuropathy of other causes
- serogenic
- malignant neoplasia
- sarcoidosis

damage of the *neuronal nuclei*, as in diabetes mellitus, leads to secondary, distal, retrograde axonal degeneration. On the other hand, primary damage to *axons* leads to Wallerian degeneration of the distal axon segments, as seen in many toxic polyneuropathies. The *Schwann cells* are another possible "target" of pathogenic influences, e. g., dysproteinemia. Loss of Schwann cells leads to demyelination.

General clinical manifestations. Polyneuropathy is usually characterized by:
- first signs usually appearing distally in the lower limbs,
- paresthesiae in the toes or soles of the feet, mainly at night,
- tingling,
- muffled sensation on the soles, "as if I had socks on,"
- loss of the Achilles' reflexes,
- diminution or loss of vibration sense, beginning distally.
- as the condition progresses, there is paresis of the short toe extensors on the dorsum of the foot, as well as of the interossei (the patient can no longer spread his or her toes),
- later, paresis of the long toe extensors and foot extensors,
- producing bilateral foot drop,
- finally, sensory disturbances and weakness spread to the upper limbs as well.

Diagnostic evaluation. When the *typical clinical findings* reveal the presence of polyneuropathy, a *series of laboratory tests* is performed to determine its etiology (particularly a complete blood count, electrolytes, glucose, CRP, electrophoresis, daily blood sugar profile, glucose tolerance test, HbA$_{1c}$, renal and hepatic function tests, serum vitamin B$_{12}$ and folic acid levels, vasculitis parameters, TSH, and perhaps further endocrine tests and tumor markers). *Electroneurography* reveals a variable degree of impairment of impulse conduction, depending on etiology. If the underlying lesion is primarily axonal, *EMG* reveals evidence of denervation or neurogenically altered potentials. The *CSF protein concentration* is elevated in many types of polyneuropathy (e. g., diabetic polyneuropathy); in rare cases, CSF examination may yield evidence of an infectious process. Sural nerve biopsy is an additional means of distinguishing axonal from demyelinating forms of polyneuropathy, if the findings of ENG and EMG are inconclusive; it may also provide direct evidence of certain etiologies (e. g., vasculitis).

Particular Etiologic Types of Polyneuropathy

The types of polyneuropathy that are clinically most important, either because they are common or for other reasons, are described in the following sections.

Table 10.**2** **Hereditary motor and sensory neuropathies** (after Dyck)

Type of HMSN	Inheritance pattern	Age at onset	Muscle weakness and atrophy	Sensory deficit	Nerve conduction velocity	Other remarks
Type I Charcot–Marie–Tooth disease	autosomal dominant	2nd to 4th decade	mainly distal, beginning in the feet and calves, later in the hands and forearms; pes cavus	none or mild, mainly acral	markedly slowed	peripheral nerves thickened; sural n. biopsy reveals axonal degeneration, de- and remyelination, onion-skin structures
Type II neuronal type of peroneal muscle atrophy	autosomal dominant	2nd to 4th decade	distal atrophy, mainly in the feet and calves; pes cavus	mild, mainly acral	mildly slowed	peripheral nerves not thickened; sural n. biopsy reveals axonal degeneration, no onion-skin structures
Type III Dejerine–Sottas hypertrophic neuropathy	autosomal dominant	1st decade	rapidly progressive weakness in legs and hands	marked, mainly acral	severely slowed	peripheral nerves thickened; sural n. biopsy reveals hypo-, de-, and remyelination, onion-skin structures, only thin myelinated fibers
Type IV hypertrophic neuropathy in Refsum disease	autosomal recessive	1st–3rd decade	mainly distal	marked, mainly distal	markedly slowed	sensorineural hearing loss; occasional retinitis pigmentosa; thickened peripheral nerves; sural n. biopsy reveals axonal degeneration, de- and remyelination, onion-skin structures; phytanic acid accumulation in various tissues
Type V HMSN with spastic paraparesis	autosomal dominant	2nd decade or later	mainly distal muscle atrophy and spastic paraparesis	none or mild	normal or mildly slowed	sural n. biopsy may reveal reduced number of myelinated fibers
Type VI HMSN with optic atrophy	autosomal dominant or recessive	highly variable	mainly distal	none or mild	normal or mildly slowed	visual loss, progressive blindness; thickened nerves in rare cases
Type VII HMSN with retinitis pigmentosa	autosomal recessive	variable	mainly distal	mild	slowed	retinitis pigmentosa

Hereditary Motor and Sensory Neuropathies (HMSN)

The current classification of hereditary polyneuropathies is given in Table 10.**2**.

HMSN Type I (Charcot–Marie–Tooth disease) is the most common hereditary polyneuropathy, with a *prevalence* of two per 100 000 persons. It is *genetically* subdivided into Type Ia, caused by duplication on chromosome 17p11, and Type Ib, caused by a point mutation on chromosome 1q22–23. *Clinically*, its earliest manifestation is pes cavus (Fig. 10.**2a**), later followed by atrophy of the calf muscles, while the thigh muscles retain their normal bulk ("stork legs," "inverted champagne-bottle sign," Fig. 10.**2**). As the disease progresses, predominantly distal muscle atrophy is seen in the upper limbs as well (Fig. 10.**2c**). Distal sensory impairment may not arise until much later and even then is usually only mild. *Electromyography* reveals marked slowing of nerve conduction; *histopathological examination* of a sural nerve specimen reveals axonal degeneration, myelin changes, and onion-skinlike Schwann cells. HMSN Type I progresses very slowly. Patients can often keep working until the normal retirement age or beyond.

Hereditary neuropathy with predisposition to pressure palsies (HNPP) is an autosomal dominant disorder due to a point mutation in chromosome 17p11.2–12. *Clinically*, patients develop recurrent pressure palsies of individual peripheral nerves, even after very light pressure. The *histopathological* substrate of the disorder is an abnormality of the myelin sheaths of peripheral nerves. Microscopy reveals sausagelike, segmental swelling of the sheaths ("*tomaculous neuropathy*").

Diabetic Polyneuropathy

Epidemiology. Diabetic polyneuropathy is the second most common type of polyneuropathy (only the alcohol-induced type is more common). It typically afflicts persons aged 60 to 70 who have suffered from diabetes for five to 10 years or more and 20 to 40% of diabetics have it to some degree. In 10% of patients with diabetic neuropathy, it is only the diagnostic evaluation of neuropathy that brings the underlying diabetes to light.

10

Polyradiculopathy and Polyneuropathy

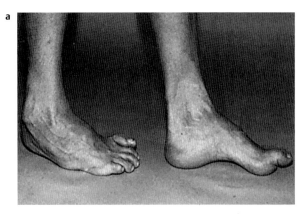

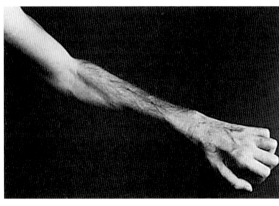

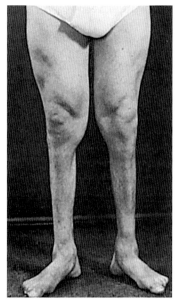

Fig. 10.**2 Hereditary motor and sensory neuropathy (HMSN),** type I (**a** and **b**) and type II (**c**). **a** Pes cavus. **b** Severe calf atrophy with normal muscle bulk in the thighs ("stork legs"). **c** Atrophy of the distal forearm muscles and of the intrinsic muscles of the hand. (From: Meier, C., Tackmann, W.: Die hereditären motorisch-sensiblen Neuropathien. *Fortschr Neurol Psychiat* 50:1982.)

Pathogenesis. Polyneuropathy is caused both by diabetic angiopathy and by the direct effect of elevated blood sugar. *Axonal degeneration* is usually the most prominent histological finding, though segmental demyelination sometimes predominates.

Clinical manifestations. *Irritative sensory symptoms* are most prominent at first, including paresthesia and, often, burning dysesthesia of the feet. Typically, *Achilles reflexes are absent* and there is a *mainly distal impairment of touch and position sense.* It is only later that about half of the affected patients develop *motor deficits.* The condition may present with an asymmetrical neurological deficit, or with isolated disease of an individual nerve, such as cranial nerves I–II, IV, and VI or the femoral n. *Disturbances of autonomic innervation* are also typical: dry, often reddened skin, bladder dysfunction, orthostatic hypotension, tachycardia, diarrhea, and impotence in young male diabetics. The effects of diabetes on the nervous system are listed in Table 10.**3**.

Treatment. *Optimal glycemic control* is of paramount importance. The *pain* of diabetic neuropathy, which is often severe, can be treated with carbamazepine, gabapentin, thioctic acid, clomipramine, or local capsaicin ointment. These drugs can also be combined with neuroleptic agents.

Toxic Polyneuropathies

The numerous substances that can cause a toxic polyneuropathy will not all be listed here. We will merely illustrate the breadth of the clinical spectrum of toxic polyneuropathy by describing two very different, highly characteristic syndromes.

Though **alcoholic polyneuropathy** is very common, its *pathogenesis* is not fully understood. In addition to the direct effects of ethanol and acetaldehyde, alcoholics often suffer from nutritional deficiencies. Further contributing factors include possible defects of the enzymes alcohol dehydrogenase and acetaldehyde dehydrogenase. *Clinically,* intense pain in the lower limbs is often the most prominent symptom. Many patients also suffer from muscle cramps. The intrinsic muscle reflexes are diminished; Achilles reflexes are usually absent. Proprioception is impaired *and* touch and vibration sense are diminished distally. The calves are often tender to deep pressure. The dorsiflexors of the feet are weak. *Motor conduction* in the peroneal n. is slowed. The major finding of *sural nerve biopsy* is axonal degeneration.

Triaryl phosphate poisoning will serve here as an example of an acute toxic neuropathy whose manifestations can persist, either fully or in part. This substance is found in certain mineral oil derivatives used in industry. Their erroneous use as cooking oil leads to a *clinical syndrome* manifested at first by diarrhea and one to five weeks later by fever and other constitutional symptoms.

Tabelle 10.3 **Effects of diabetes mellitus on the nervous system**

Site	Manifestation	Special features
Central nervous system	cerebrovascular accidents spinal cord ischemia	
Peripheral nervous system	polyneuropathy: ● sensorimotor	distal, perhaps painful, symmetric, gradually worsening paresthesiae or burning pain in the feet, absent Achilles reflexes, diminished vibration sense, hypesthesia in a stocking distribution, occasional dorsiflexor weakness, occasional toe ulcers and joint destruction
	● proximal asymmetric	mainly affects lumbar plexus or femoral nerve, unilateral, acute, painful, weakness of hip flexors and quadriceps m., diminished knee-jerk reflexes, positive reverse Lasègue sign, hypesthesia in femoral n. distribution, occasional similar findings in upper limbs, spontaneous improvement possible (as in mononeuropathy, see below)
	mononeuropathy: ● CN III (most common)	painful, affects only extraocular muscles, regresses within a few months
	● other peripheral nerve	e. g., thoracic nerves with abdominal muscle weakness
Autonomic nervous system	bladder dysfunction impotence diarrhea necrobiosis lipoidica osteoarthropathy ulcers	sphincter disturbance, atonic flaccid bladder in younger male patients chiefly at night polycyclic cutaneous atrophy in women particularly in the toes particularly on the soles of the feet

Ten to 38 days after the exposure, flaccid paresis appears in the feet and then, within a few days, in all four limbs. Sensation is also impaired. In many patients, the deficits resolve only in part, or not at all, and spasticity of central origin frequently develops over the ensuing years. *Histopathological examination* reveals axonal lesions both in peripheral nerves and in the central nervous system.

Mononeuropathies and Mononeuritis Multiplex

Mononeuropathy is a neuropathy affecting a single peripheral nerve; *mononeuritis multiplex* is a type of peripheral neuropathy in which single nerves are affected one after the other, in a highly variable temporal sequence. As for their *pathogenesis*, most cases of these two entities are due to a vasculopathy, such as diabetic microangiopathy, polyarteritis nodosa, systemic lupus erythematosus, Sjögren syndrome, Wegener granulomatosis, or atherosclerosis. *Clinically*, they are characterized by asymmetrically distributed weakness, sensory deficits, or autonomic dysfunction in the distribution of a single peripheral nerve, or, in later stages of mononeuritis multiplex, in the distribution of multiple peripheral nerves. Other manifestations of the underlying illness are usually present as well, e. g., constitutional symptoms such as fever, night sweats, and weight loss, an elevated erythrocyte sedimentation rate, and symptoms referable to the internal organs.

Polyradiculopathy and Polyneuropathy

10

11 Diseases of the Cranial Nerves

Fundamentals

The cranial nerves can be affected by disease in isolation, or as a component of a wider disease process. Cranial nerve deficits are caused by **lesions of their nuclei or tracts** in the brainstem, or of the **peripheral course** of the nerves themselves and their branches.

The anatomical relationships of the cranial nerves to the base of the skull are shown in Fig. 3.**3** (p. 17), while their anatomical course and distribution are summarized in Table 3.**3** (p. 17). The causes and clinical manifestations of cranial nerve lesions are discussed in detail in this chapter.

Disturbances of Smell (Olfactory Nerve)

Anatomy. The peripheral olfactory receptors can only be excited by substances dissolved in fluid. The *receptors of the olfactory mucosa* project their axons through the cribriform plate to the *olfactory bulb* (Fig. 3.3, p. 17), which lies on the floor of the anterior cranial fossa, beneath the frontal lobe. After a synapse onto the second neuron of the pathway in the olfactory bulb, olfactory fibers travel onward through the *lateral olfactory striae* to the *amygdala* and other areas of the *temporal lobe*. Olfactory fibers also travel by way of the *medial olfactory striae* to the *subcallosal area* and the limbic system.

Clinical manifestations. Techniques for examining the sense of smell are discussed on p. 16. Only the following types of olfactory disturbances are relevant to neurological diagnosis:

Anosmia. A more or less complete loss of the sense of smell is usually due to *disorders of the nose*, most commonly rhinitis sicca. The most common neurological cause of anosmia is *traumatic brain injury* resulting in a brain contusion and/or traumatic avulsion of the olfactory fibers as they traverse the cribriform plate. The anosmia regresses in one-third of patients, but distortions of olfactory perception, so-called *parosmias*, often persist, sometimes in the form of unpleasant *kakosmia* (see below). Anosmia is the characteristic symptom of an *olfactory groove meningioma* and is often its initial manifestation. Rarer causes of hyposmia include Paget disease, Parkinson disease, prior laryngectomy, and diabetes mellitus. Medications often alter or impair the sense of smell. Anosmia always carries with it an impairment of the **sense of taste** (*ageusia*). The differential perception of gustatory stimuli requires not only an intact sense of taste, but also an intact sense of smell.

Olfactory hallucinations—usually in the form of spontaneous kakosmia—are produced by epileptic discharges from a focus in the anterior, medial portion of the temporal lobe. These hallucinations are sometimes called *uncinate fits*.

Neurological Disturbances of Vision (Optic Nerve)

Visual disturbances can be caused by **lesions of the retina or of its connections** with the visual cortex. Depending on the etiology, the disturbance may consist of an **impairment of visual acuity** (ranging to total blindness) or a visual field defect, and these

problems may appear either suddenly or gradually. In addition, the site of the lesion determines the type of visual field defect that will be present and whether it will affect only one eye or both. A simple clinical rule is that lesions of the retina and optic nerve impair visual acuity, while lesions of the optic chiasm and distal components of the visual pathway (from the optic tract to the visual-cortex) produce visual field defects, usually sparing visual acuity. Retrochiasmatic lesions impair visual acuity only when they are bilateral.

Visual Field Defects

A visual field defect is defined as the absence of some part of the normal visual field. The manual confrontation technique for examining the visual field is shown on p. 19 and the use of special instrumentation for this purpose is presented on p. 65.

The diagnostic assessment of a visual field defect involves, first, **localization** of the underlying lesion to a particular part of the visual pathway on the basis of the characteristics described above; and, second, **determination of the etiology** on the basis of the clinical history, other findings of the neurological examination, and the results of ancillary tests.

Types of visual field defect and their localization. Visual field defects may be either monocular or binocular. **Monocular** visual field defects are caused by unilateral retinal lesions or by partial lesions of the optic n., while **binocular** ones are caused by unilateral lesions of the visual pathway from the optic chiasm onward (cf. Fig. 3.6, p. 19).

The following types of visual field defect are characterized by their **spatial configuration**:

- **Hemianopsia:** the defect occupies one half of the visual field (right or left).
- **Quadrantanopsia:** the defect occupies one quarter of the visual field.
- **Scotoma:** the defect occupies a small spot or patch within the visual field. So-called central scotoma is due to a lesion affecting the macula lutea or its efferent nerve fibers, resulting in an impairment of central vision and thus a reduction of visual acuity.
- **Temporal crescent:** this is a preserved area of vision in the far lateral visual field on the side of a near-hemianopic visual field defect. The cause is a lesion of the contralateral occipital lobe sparing the rostral portion of the visual cortex on either side of the calcarine fissure.

Homonymous and heteronymous visual field defects. If a binocular visual field defect involves a corresponding area of the visual field in both eyes (e. g., the right half of the visual field in both eyes), it is called a **homonymous** visual field defect. For example, a lesion of the *right* optic tract, lateral geniculate body, optic radiation, or visual cortex produces a *left homonymous hemianopsia*, while a lesion of any of these structures on the *left* produces a *right homonymous hemianopsia* (cf. Fig. 3.6, p. 19). A lesion along the course of the optic radiation or in the visual cortex may affect only part of the radiating fibers or cortex, causing a homonymous defect that is less than a complete hemianopsia: thus, depending on the site and extent of the lesion, there may be a *homonymous quadrantanopsia* or *homonymous scotoma.*

In contrast, a *lesion of the optic chiasm* produces a **heteronymous** visual field defect: most such lesions affect the decussating fibers derived from the nasal half of each retina, thereby causing a *bitemporal hemianopsia* or *bitemporal quadrantanopsia.* The visual field defect lies in the temporal half of each visual field, i. e., in the right half of the visual field of the right eye and the left half of the visual field of the left eye.

If a tumor, such as a pituitary adenoma, compresses the optic chiasm from below, there is initially an *upper bitemporal quadrantanopsia*, which is only later followed by bitemporal hemianopsia. If a tumor compresses the optic chiasm from above (e. g., a craniopharyngioma), there is initially a *lower bitemporal quadrantanopsia*, and later bitemporal hemianopsia.

If a tumor compresses the optic chiasm from one side, it will affect not only the decussating medial fibers, but also the uncrossed fibers from the retina on that side. The resulting visual field defect involves the entire visual field on the side of the lesion in addition to temporal hemianopsia on the opposite side.

Etiologic classification of visual field defects. A visual field defect that arises suddenly is generally due to either **ischemia** or **trauma**. The "gestalt" of the visual field defect, too, can provide a clue to its etiology: thus, a temporal crescent is highly characteristic of a **vascular lesion**. A slowly progressive visual field defect suggests the presence of a **brain tumor**. In such patients, the patient may fail to notice the visual field defect, particularly if the tumor lies in the right parietal lobe. There may be **visual hemineglect** accompanying, or instead of, a "true" visual field defect. The patient ignores visual stimuli in the affected hemifield, even though he or she may still be able to see them; and, if the patient truly cannot see stimuli in that hemifield, he or she is nonetheless unaware of the defect. Neuroimaging studies generally reveal the site and nature of the underlying lesion (Fig. 11.1).

Special types of visual field defect. In the **Riddoch phenomenon**, the patient cannot see stationary objects in the affected area of the visual field, though movement can be perceived. In **palinopsia**, the perception outlasts the stimulus: the patient continues to "see" the presented image long after it has been removed. This phenomenon is produced by right temporo-occipital lesions.

Diseases of the Cranial Nerves

11

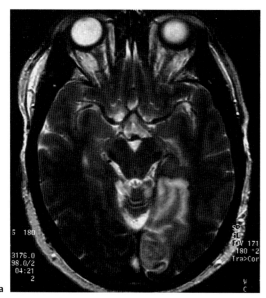
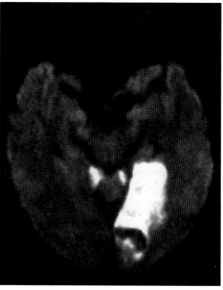

a

b

Fig. 11.1 **Infarct in the territory of the left posterior cerebral a.** in a patient with right homonymous hemianopsia. MR image. **a** The axial T2-weighted image reveals abnormally bright signal in the cerebral cortex and in the underlying white matter, as well as a small hemorrhage within the infarct. **b** The diffusion-weighted MRI reveals diminished diffusion of protons and water molecules in the first few days after the event. Fresh infarcts are very well seen in this type of study. The hemorrhage, too, is visible in this case.

Impairment of Visual Acuity

Sudden unilateral loss of vision, as long as its cause does not lie in the eye itself, is usually due to a **lesion of the optic nerve.** The sudden onset of the defect implies that it has been caused by *ischemia.* A defect of this type may be permanent, e. g., in occlusion of the central retinal a. due to temporal arteritis or embolization from an atheromatous plaque in the carotid a., or it may be temporary, in which case it is called *amaurosis fugax* (transient monocular blindness). Rarely, transient visual loss can be produced by a disturbance of neural function, such as migraine (retinal migraine). **Papilledema,** too, can be accompanied by episodes of sudden visual loss (amblyopic attacks). **Ocular causes** should not be forgotten in the differential diagnosis, e. g., retinal detachment, preretinal hemorrhage, or central vein thrombosis. Correct diagnosis requires a precise clinical history and meticulous examination of the optic disc and fundus.

Sudden bilateral loss of vision may be due to **bilateral retinal ischemia,** e. g., on standing up in a patient with aortic arch syndrome. Certain types of **intoxication** can also rapidly produce bilateral optic nerve lesions, e. g., methanol poisoning, which causes blindness within hours. Yet, bilateral visual loss of more or less sudden onset is much more commonly due to **simultaneous ischemia of both occipital lobes.** Such events are often preceded by hemianopic episodes and loss of color vision as prodromal manifestations. The possible causes include embolization into the territory of the posterior cerebral aa. on both sides simultaneously and compressive occlusion of the posterior cerebral aa. by an intracranial mass. Patients often deny that they cannot see (anosognosia). Despite the severe visual loss, the pupillary light reflex is still present, because the pathway for visual impulses to the lateral geniculate body, where the fibers for the reflex branch off, remains intact. The visual evoked potentials (VEP, p. 56 and Fig. 4.19, p. 59), however, are pathological.

Progressive impairment of visual acuity in one or both eyes. *Unilateral* impairment is due to a process causing more or less rapid, progressive damage to the optic nerve or chiasm. **Retrobulbar neuritis** (inflammation of the optic n. between the retina and the chiasm) and **optic papillitis** (inflammation of the optic n. at the level of the optic disc) cause unilateral visual loss within two days or a little longer. Progressive, unilateral visual loss should also always prompt suspicion of a **mass**: optic glioma, for example, is a primary tumor within the optic n. that is more common in children and an optic sheath meningioma can compress the nerve from outside. Retrobulbar neuritis rarely occurs *bilaterally*, sometimes in combination with myelitis. Further causes of bilateral loss of visual acuity are *Leber hereditary optic atrophy* and *tobacco-alcohol amblyopia*. In the latter condition, the most prominent initial finding is an inability to distinguish the colors red and green. *Vitamin B_{12} deficiency* can cause progressive optic atrophy in combination with polyneuropathy.

Pathological Findings of the Optic Disc

This is an area requiring close collaboration between the neurologist and the ophthalmologist.

Papilledema is usually a reflection of *intracranial hypertension*, but it can also be seen in infectious and inflammatory disorders, such as syphilis. The typical findings include a somewhat enlarged, hyperemic optic disc with blurred margins, enlarged veins, and usually hemorrhages (Fig. 11.2). Inexperienced clinicians often have difficulty distinguishing papilledema from other changes of the optic disc.

Optic nerve atrophy is a *permanent residual finding after lesions of the optic n.* The extent of visual loss, however, need not reflect the degree of visible atrophy. The optic disc is pale all the way to the disc margin, which remains sharp. These findings are typically seen after retrobulbar neuritis, for example (Fig. 3.4, p. 18), but also after optic nerve compression (whether from outside, as by a meningioma, or from inside by an optic glioma). Further causes of optic nerve atrophy include chronic papilledema, syphilis, Leber hereditary optic nerve atrophy (LHON, a mitochondrial disease occurring in men), many types of spinocerebellar degeneration, ischemia, and exogenous intoxication.

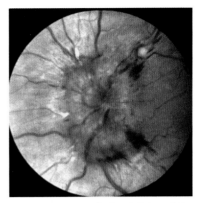

Fig. 11.**2 Acute papilledema** (left eye) in a patient with a brain tumor. The optic disc is swollen, with blurred margins and small, linear hemorrhages.

Disturbances of Ocular and Pupillary Motility

Eye movements enable the fixation of gaze and the visual pursuit of objects that are in motion relative to the observer, whether the object itself of the observer is actually moving. The **anatomical substrate** of eye movements consists of the frontal and posterior eye fields, whose major projections descend to the paramedian pontine reticular formation (PPRF) on both sides of the pons. The PPRF, in turn, controls movements for horizontal gaze, as well as movements for vertical gaze through its interaction with the midbrain reticular formation. Vestibular afferent input and cerebellar connections also play important roles in the control of eye movements. **Lesions of these supranuclear structures**, whatever their etiology, cause horizontal or vertical gaze palsy or internuclear ophthalmoplegia. Clinically, it is important to distinguish **nuclear** from **infranuclear disturbances** of the oculomotor, trochlear, and abducens nerves, all of which can have a variety of causes. In addition, the motor functions of the brainstem, including eye movements, can also be disturbed in myasthenia gravis, muscle diseases, and orbital processes, any of which can cause diplopia. **Pupillary motility** can be altered by many different disease processes. Retinal and optic nerve lesions affect the afferent arm of the pupillary light reflex loop, while oculomotor nerve lesions affect its efferent arm. In the former case, the pupil constricts only upon illumination of the ipsilateral eye; in the latter case, the pupil is dilated and remains so regardless of which eye is illuminated. **Loss of the sympathetic nerve supply** to the eye causes Horner syndrome.

Fundamentals of Eye Movements

The anatomical substrate of eye movements consists of the following structures:

- **cortical areas** in the frontal, occipital, and temporal lobes, in which the impulses for voluntary, conjugate eye movements and ocular pursuit movements are generated;
- a number of important **gaze centers in the brainstem** (particularly the paramedian pontine reticular formation, PPRF, and midbrain nuclei) that relay the cortical impulses onward to the motor nuclei innervating the eye muscles in such a way that coordinated movements of the eyes can occur along the three major axes (horizontal, vertical, and rotatory movements). Special white matter tracts play an important role in this process, particularly the medial longitudinal fasciculus (MLF, Fig. 11.3);
- finally, the **motor nuclei** and **cranial nerves** that innervate the eye muscles (cf. Fig. 3.8a, p. 21);
- the entire process is also affected by cerebellar impulses and by vestibular impulses that enter the central nervous system through the eighth cranial nerve.

Types of eye movement. Eye movements can be divided into the following types:

- **Saccades** are rapid conjugate movements that are executed voluntarily or in reflex fashion in response to stimuli of various kinds. They serve to fix a new object in the center of vision. Small microsaccades have an angular velocity of 20°/s, larger ones up to 700°/s. Saccades are the elementary type of rapid eye movement.
- Once the gaze has been fixated on a given object, **slow pursuit movements** serve to keep it in view if it is moving. The pursuit system is responsible for executing these conjugate eye movements: from the

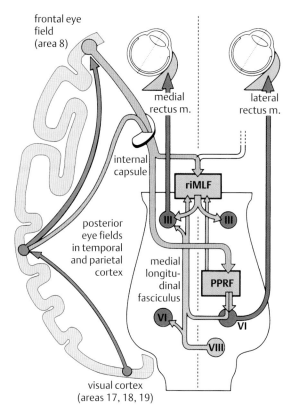

frontal eye field (area 8)

medial rectus m.

lateral rectus m.

internal capsule

riMLF

III III

posterior eye fields in temporal and parietal cortex

medial longitudinal fasciculus

PPRF

VI VI

VIII

visual cortex (areas 17, 18, 19)

Fig. 11.3 Anatomical substrate of conjugate eye movements. The diagram shows the anatomical pathways for a conjugate movement to the right: neural impulses flow from the cortical eye fields of the left hemisphere to the right PPRF and onward to the nucleus of the right abducens n. Impulses in the abducens n. induce contraction of the lateral rectus m. of the right eye. Meanwhile, cortical impulses also travel by way of the medial longitudinal fasciculus to the nucleus of the left oculomotor n., and impulses in this nerve induce contraction of the medial rectus m. of the left eye. Thus, lesions of the hemispheres or of the PPRF result in a palsy of conjugate horizontal gaze (hemispheric lesion: contralateral gaze palsy, PPRF lesion: ipsilateral gaze palsy). On the other hand, lesions of the medial longitudinal fasciculus cause an isolated loss of adduction of one eye during horizontal eye movement (internuclear ophthalmoplegia). Vertical eye movements are generated by the midbrain reticular formation (riMLF, p. 188), which receives input from both the cerebral cortex and the PPRF.

visual cortex in the occipital lobe, impulses travel to the eye fields of the temporal lobe ("medial superior temporal visual area," MST) and the neighboring parietal cortex. These areas are interconnected with the paramedian pontine reticular formation (PPRF) and with the cerebellum. Impulses from the PPRF control the nuclei of the eye muscles either directly or by way of interneurons.

- Disturbances of the pursuit system cause pursuit movements to break up into saccades. If the saccade system is also damaged, gaze palsy can result (see below).
- Convergence movements serve to fix a nearby object in view and involve simultaneous adduction of both eyes.

Oculomotor Disturbances

Nystagmus

In purely descriptive terms, nystagmus is an **involuntary**, **repetitive**, **rhythmic movement of the eyes**. Nystagmus is often, but not always, pathological.

! *Nystagmus is sometimes physiological.*

Examples of physiological nystagmus include optokinetic nystagmus (p. 186) and the type of vestibular nystagmus that is induced by rotation in a swivel chair. End-gaze nystagmus (p. 185) is also physiological, as long as it occurs symmetrically in both directions. Pathological nystagmus, on the other hand, indicates the presence of a lesion in the anatomical structures subserving eye movements. A large number of components in this system can be damaged and nystagmus has a correspondingly wide spectrum of possible causes (see below).

Phenomenological classification of nystagmus. As already discussed to some extent in Chapter 3, nystagmus can be characterized according to various criteria:

- **Jerk vs. pendular nystagmus**: most types of nystagmus are either of the "jerking" type, i.e., with a fast and a slow phase, or pendular (back-and-forth).
- **Direction of beat in relation to the three major axes of eye movement**: one speaks of horizontal, vertical, or rotatory nystagmus.
- **Direction of beat in relation to the midline of the eye**: nystagmus may beat to the left, to the right, upward, downward, or diagonally.
- In saltatory nystagmus, the **direction of beat is defined, by convention, as that of the rapid phase**, even though the slow phase is actually the pathological component and the rapid phase is a physiological correction for it, serving to return the eyes to their original position.
- Nystagmus can be **spontaneous** (p. 185) or else present only in response to **specific precipitating stimuli** (e. g., position, change of position, a rotatory or thermal stimulus to the vestibular system, or a particular direction of gaze → gaze-evoked nystagmus, p. 185).
- The examiner must also determine whether nystagmus is equally severe in both eyes, or whether it is weaker or perhaps nonexistent in one eye. Nystagmus that is unequal in the two eyes is also called **dissociated nystagmus**.

A mainly phenomenologically oriented listing and illustration of the most important types of nystagmus and their causes, is found in Table 11.1 and Fig. 11.4.

There are a few rarer types of nystagmus whose phenomenology is quite complex and not easily described by the criteria listed above. These types of nystagmus are summarized in Table 11.2.

Table 11.**1** **Important physiological and pathological types of nystagmus** (after Henn)

Type of nystagmus	Physiological	Pathological	Remarks
Optokinetic nystagmus	must be symmetrically present	if asymmetric, dissociated, slowed, or absent	can be seen and tested by having the patient fixate on the pattern on a rotating drum
Vestibular nystagmus	must be symmetrically present	if asymmetric, dissociated, or absent	elicited by lavage of the external auditory canal with cold or warm water (always after otoscopy to exclude a tympanic defect); also elicitable by rotating the patient in a swivel chair, if Frenzel goggles are worn to prevent fixation
Spontaneous nystagmus	up to 5°/second is normal in the dark	if present in light	unidirectional: the nystagmus always beats in the same direction, independent of the direction of gaze; can be inhibited by visual fixation; may be due to a central or peripheral vestibular lesion Grade III: present in all directions of gaze Grade II: visible with gaze straight ahead or in the direction of the nystagmus Grade I: visible only with gaze in the direction of nystagmus Head-shaking nystagmus: occurs only after vigorous shaking of the head
Gaze-evolved nystagmus (p. 26)	never	always pathological	beats in the direction of gaze; defined as nystagmus in binocular visual field; lesion always central
End-gaze nystagmus (p. 26)	if symmetric	if asymmetric or dissociated	defined as nystagmus in monocular visual field
Positional nystagmus		always pathological	elicited by rapidly placing the patient supine with the head hanging down 30° and to one side (Hallpike maneuver); latency of one to several seconds, then increasing intensity for a few seconds and equally rapid decline; accompanied by a strong feeling of rotation and dizziness; the nystagmus is mainly rotatory, clockwise when the head hangs down and to the left, counterclockwise when it hangs down and to the right; the response diminishes (habituates) on repeated elicitation
Pendular nystagmus		always pathological, but does not indicate active disease	sinusoidal to-and-fro movement increasing with attention or monocular fixation; usually congenital, rarely acquired
Nystagmus in the vestibulo-ocular suppression test		always pathological	when the patient is passively rotated en bloc while keeping the arms in forward extension and staring at the thumbs, visual fixation normally completely suppresses vestibular nystagmus; if nystagmus does appear, this indicates a lesion of the vestibulocerebellum or of its afferent or efferent connections; the test can be falsely positive with inadequate fixation

Diseases of the Cranial Nerves

11

Topical classification of pathological nystagmus. Often, the type of nystagmus that is present already provides a clue to the site of the lesion:

- **Gaze-paretic nystagmus.** This type of nystagmus may be due to *disease of the eye muscles* themselves, or to a *lesion of the cranial nerves innervating the eye muscles* or of the corresponding *brainstem nuclei*. Gaze-paretic nystagmus is usually slow, coarse, and in the direction of the impairment of gaze.
- **Vestibular nystagmus** is due to a lesion of the *vestibular organ* itself or of the *vestibular n.* or its *nuclei in the brainstem*. It typically appears as a spontaneous nystagmus beating away from the side of the lesion, regardless of the direction of gaze (nystagmus in a fixed direction, cf. Table 11.**1**). Vestibular nystagmus

is typically inhibited by fixation; it is sometimes observable only if fixation is abolished by having the patient wear Frenzel goggles or shake the head rapidly.

- **Gaze-evoked nystagmus** beats in the direction of gaze and indicates a *lesion in the brainstem* or its *afferent or efferent connections with the cerebellum*. If caused by a unilateral cerebellar lesion, it can be highly asymmetrical or even beat only to the side of the lesion. In such patients, gaze-evoked nystagmus can be difficult to distinguish from vestibular nystagmus.
- **Nystagmus due to brainstem lesions.** Vestibular spontaneous nystagmus, gaze-evoked nystagmus, upbeat or downbeat vertical nystagmus and posi-

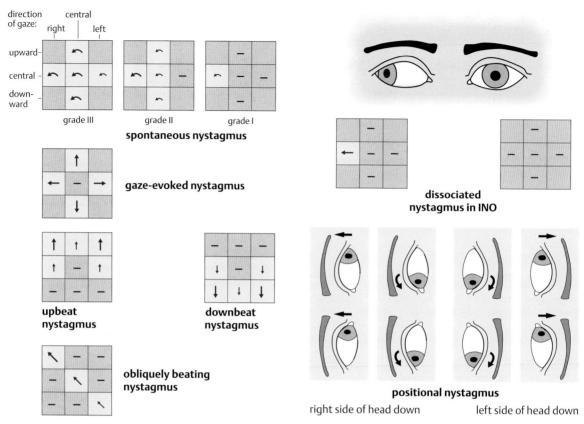

Fig. 11.**4 The most important types of nystagmus.** For each type of nystagmus, the figure shows the intensity and direction of beating, depending on the direction of gaze.

tional and/or positioning nystagmus can all indicate the presence of a brainstem lesion. These types of nystagmus are often rotatory or dissociated (as in internuclear ophthalmoplegia).

- **Positioning nystagmus** is a predominantly rotatory nystagmus lasting several seconds after changes of position of a particular type; it is found in benign paroxysmal positioning vertigo, a disorder of the *peripheral portion of the vestibular system* (p. 202).
- **Congenital pendular nystagmus** is characterized by conjugate, pendular eye movements that increase with attention or monocular fixation. It is normally well compensated. There is *no underlying, pathological structural lesion.*

Physiological nystagmus. The most important example is optokinetic nystagmus. This normal phenomenon serves to stabilize the visual image of a moving object on the retina and thus has the same purpose as the vestibulo-ocular reflex.

Optokinetic nystagmus consists of slow pursuit movements alternating with rapid return movements (saccades). The return movements occur whenever the moving object "threatens" to leave the visual field. If the object is moving very rapidly, optokinetic nystagmus can be voluntarily suppressed. Absent, asymmetrical, or dissociated optokinetic nystagmus is pathological.

Vestibulo-ocular reflex (VOR) is a function of the labyrinth that serves to stabilize gaze fixation on rapid movement of the head: it produces a compensatory eye movement in the direction opposite the head movement. Slower head movements do not need to be compensated for by the vestibular system, as the ocular pursuit system suffices to keep gaze fixated in this case (see above, p. 183). Vestibular nystagmus can be suppressed by fixation on an object moving in tandem with the head (nystagmus or VOR suppression test, see below). An inability to suppress the VOR by fixation is pathological.

Nystagmus suppression test (= VOR suppression test). In this test, the subject stretches both arms forward, holds his or her thumbs up, and fixates gaze on them. When the subject is then rapidly rotated around the long axis of the body, there is normally no nystagmus, because vestibular nystagmus can be suppressed by visual fixation (Fig. 11.**5**). If nystagmus does appear, this indicates a lesion in the cerebellum or its connections with the vestibular apparatus of the brainstem.

Table 11.**2** **Rare types of nystagmus**

Type	Characteristics	Localization	Cause (examples)
Seesaw nystagmus	alternating movement of one eye upward and the other eye downward, with simultaneous rotation; various other kinds of eye movement can resemble this type of nystagmus	oral brainstem and diencephalon	tumor, multiple sclerosis, vascular, syringobulbia
Downbeat nystagmus	vertical nystagmus with downward rapid component	caudal medullary lesion, vitamin B_{12} deficiency	as above; phenytoin intoxication, drugs of abuse
Convergence nystagmus	slow abduction followed by rapid adduction of both eyes	(rostral) midbrain tegmentum	as above
Retractory nystagmus	jerking movements of both eyes back into their sockets, usually accompanied by other oculomotor disturbances	midbrain tegmentum	rare: tumor, multiple sclerosis, vascular
Nystagmus with eyelid response	vertical nystagmus with upward rapid component accompanied by simultaneous rapid raising of upper lid	pons and periaqueductal region	often vascular
Monocular nystagmus	in internuclear ophthalmoplegia; as an ictal phenomenon in epilepsy	medial longitudinal fasciculus	very rarely ictal
Opsoclonus (gaze myoclonus, dancing eyes)	spontaneous, grouped, variably rapid, nonrhythmic conjugate eye movements, irregularly "dancing" back and forth	brainstem and cerebellum	paraneoplastic, neuroblastoma, multiple sclerosis, encephalitis
Ocular bobbing	rapid, nonrhythmic downward beating of the eyes, which stay down for a few seconds, then slowly return to the original position; when it appears unilaterally, the other side is usually blocked by a paresis of the extraocular muscles (usually oculomotor nerve palsy); may also be accompanied by simultaneous palatal nystagmus	pons, compression by cerebellar hemorrhage (lesion of central tegmental tract)	tumor, ischemia, hemorrhage
Gaze dysmetria	overshooting movements when redirecting gaze to a new target, followed by compensatory corrections (ocular apraxia)	cerebellar	e. g., multiple sclerosis
Ocular flutter (ocular myoclonus)	rapid, irregular back-and-forth movements around the point of fixation	as for opsoclonus and gaze dysmetria	

Fig. 11.**5 Nystagmus suppression test.**
The patient extends the arms, fixates gaze on his or her own thumbs, and is then rapidly rotated "en bloc" by the examiner. In a normal individual, gaze fixation on the thumbs prevents the appearance of nystagmus. Failure to suppress nystagmus indicates a central lesion, usually in the cerebellum.

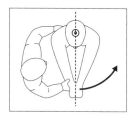
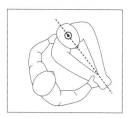
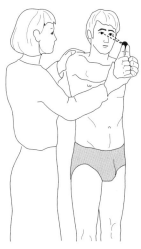
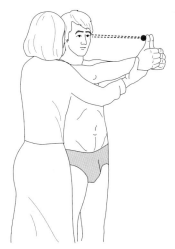

Supranuclear Oculomotor Disturbances

These disturbances are defined as those in which the voluntary movements and involuntary pursuit movements of *both* eyes are simultaneously impaired. The eyes generally remain parallel to each other, but they cannot be moved together in the horizontal or vertical plane. The lesion lies above the level of the cranial nerve nuclei and is thus "supranuclear." In disorders of the brainstem, supranuclear lesions may coexist with nuclear lesions, so that a skew deviation can also be present.

Horizontal Gaze Palsy

A patient with horizontal gaze palsy cannot make a conjugate movement of the eyes to the right, to the left, or (rarely) in either direction. The causative lesion may be at any of several sites in the central nervous system:

- **cortical centers** generating the impulses for horizontal gaze movements, particularly the frontal eye field of the *frontal lobe*;
- the paramedian pontine reticular formation (PPRF), which receives the impulses from the higher cortical centers and relays them to the ipsilateral abducens n. nucleus (innervation of the lateral rectus m.) and simultaneously, by way of interneurons, to the contralateral oculomotor n. nucleus (innervation of the medial rectus m.). This projection lies within the medial longitudinal fasciculus (MLF, Fig. 11.3). The result is an ipsilateral, conjugate, horizontal gaze movement (i.e., to the left on activation of the left PPRF and to the right on activation of the right PPRF);
- a **lesion of the abducens n. nucleus** has the same effect as a PPRF lesion, i.e., a conjugate horizontal gaze palsy to the side of the lesion (see above).

Lesions of the frontal eye field. This field occupies area eight in the middle frontal gyrus. The right eye field generates conjugate gaze movements to the left and the left eye field generates conjugate gaze movements to the right. When the frontal eye field is affected by an acute lesion, the influence of the contralateral field predominates for a few hours (or, rarely, days), so that the eyes (and the head) deviate to the side of the lesion: *déviation conjuguée*, the patient "looks at the lesion." Déviation conjuguée is usually accompanied by contralateral hemiparesis.

Active gaze movements toward the midline rapidly become possible again; so, later, do movements to the opposite side. As contralateral movements begin to re-emerge, they are accompanied by *gaze-paretic nystagmus*, whose rapid component beats away from the side of the lesion.

Lesions of the posterior hemispheric cortex. Horizontal gaze palsy due to an occipital lesion is often accompanied by hemianopsia. The gaze palsy is characterized by saccadization of ocular pursuit movements and optokinetic nystagmus (p. 185) is impaired.

Lesions of the paramedian pontine reticular formation (PPRF) affect the last supranuclear "relay station" for horizontal gaze movements. They usually cause long-lasting or permanent *gaze palsy to the side of the lesion*.

Lesion of the abducens n. nucleus affects not only the neurons whose axons constitute the sixth cranial nerve, but also interneurons that connect the nucleus by way of the adjacent medial longitudinal fasciculus (MLF) to the contralateral oculomotor n. nucleus, which innervates the contralateral medial rectus m. *The clinical picture is initially very similar to that of a PPRF lesion.* PPRF lesions, however, spare the vestibulo-ocular connections in the MLF and do not directly involve the cranial nerve nuclei subserving eye movement; thus, in PPRF lesions, the gaze palsy can be overcome by a vestibular stimulus. In contrast, gaze palsy due to a lesion of the abducens n. nucleus cannot be overcome either voluntarily or through any kind of reflex.

Vertical Gaze Palsy

Impairment of upward or downward conjugate gaze is always due to a **midbrain lesion** involving either the *rostral interstitial nucleus* of the medial longitudinal fasciculus (the Büttner–Ennever nucleus) or its *efferent fibers* (Fig. 11.3). In most patients, both upward and downward gaze are impaired, but pretectal lesions can cause isolated upward gaze palsy. Vertical gaze palsy is one of the clinical features of progressive supranuclear palsy (p. 130).

Internuclear Ophthalmoplegia

This condition is caused by a **lesion of the medial longitudinal fasciculus (MLF)**. When the patient attempts to look away from the side of the lesion, the ipsilateral (adducting) eye cannot fully adduct, and the contralateral (abducting) eye exhibits end-gaze nystagmus. The inability of the ipsilateral eye to adduct is not due to a lesion of the oculomotor n. nucleus, as is demonstrated by a preserved ability to adduct (converge) in the near reflex. Internuclear ophthalmoplegia (INO) can also be bilateral if the MLF is damaged on both sides.

The diagram in Fig. 11.6 illustrates the clinical findings in internuclear ophthalmoplegia with total loss of ad-

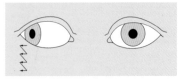

right   left

gaze straight ahead

rightward gaze:
in left eye, impaired
adduction; in right
eye, normal
abduction and
nystagmus

Fig. 11.**6 Internuclear ophthalmoplegia** (INO), left (diagram). When the patient looks straight ahead, the eyes are parallel. On attempted rightward gaze, the left medial rectus m. fails to contract (no adduction of the left eye) and there is nystagmus of the abducted right eye.

duction of the left eye. Fig. 11.**7** shows a more common type of INO, in which the inward movement of the adducting eye is merely delayed and eventually takes place with slow, horizontal saccades. This type of INO is particularly common in multiple sclerosis.

One-and-a-Half Syndrome

This name is given to the combination of horizontal gaze paresis to one side ("one") with internuclear ophthalmoplegia on attempted gaze to the other side ("half"). As one might expect, it is due to **combined lesions** of the **PPRF or abducens n. nucleus** on one side and of the **ipsilateral MLF**. The single horizontal eye movement that remains possible is abduction of the contralateral eye on attempted contralateral gaze.

Oculomotor Disturbances of Cerebellar Origin

These disturbances are listed in Table 11.**3**.

Other Supranuclear Disturbances of Eye Movement

Another disturbance worth mentioning here is **oculomotor apraxia**. In the congenital form (**Cogan syndrome**), the patient is unable, for example, to direct his or her gaze voluntarily to the beginning of a line of text while reading. Instead, the entire head must be moved into position so that the beginning of the line lands in the center of the visual field. Once this is done, the head can be moved back to its original position without loss of fixation on the text.

Lesions of the Nerves to the Eye Muscles and Their Brainstem Nuclei

Lesions of this type, like lesions of the eye muscles themselves, cause deviation of the axis of *one eye*, i.e., paralytic strabismus.

Oculomotor Nerve Palsy

An infranuclear lesion of the third cranial nerve causes paralysis of the medial, superior, and inferior rectus

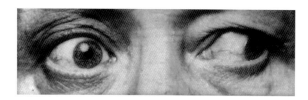

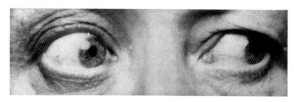

Fig. 11.**7 Right internuclear ophthalmoplegia in a patient with multiple sclerosis.** In the initial phase of leftward gaze (upper photograph), only the left eye is abducted. The right eye follows, after a delay (lower photograph).

Table 11.**3 Oculomotor disturbances due to cerebellar dysfunction**

- saccadic pursuit
- diminished optokinetic nystagmus
- gaze-deviation nystagmus
- dysmetric saccades (under and overshoot)
- inability to suppress the oculovestibular reflex by fixation
- overshooting oculovestibular reflex
- special types of nystagmus, such as upbeat nystagmus, downbeat nystagmus, rebound nystagmus, periodically alternating nystagmus, acquired pendular nystagmus, central positional nystagmus, other types
- skew deviation
- unilateral cerebellar lesions produce nystagmus to the ipsilateral side (as in spontaneous vestibular nystagmus)

muscles, the inferior oblique mm., and the levator palpebrae m. (**external ophthalmoplegia**). In addition, the smooth muscle of the pupillary sphincter is paralyzed: the pupil is "fixed and dilated," i.e., it is enlarged and responds neither to light, nor to convergence (**internal ophthalmoplegia**). The typical clinical aspect of oculomotor nerve palsy is thus immediately recognizable when the patient looks straight ahead (Fig. 11.**8**). The diagrams in Fig. 11.**9** illustrate the typical findings in

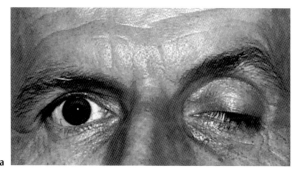

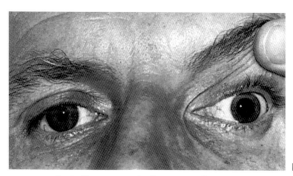

a

b

Fig. 11.**8 Complete left oculomotor palsy. a** Severe ptosis of the left eye, which is also mildly abducted (predominant effect of lateral rectus m., innervated by the abducens n.). **b** The examiner lifts the ptotic eyelid to reveal the fixed (unreactive) pupil (paralysis of the parasympathetically innervated sphincter pupillae m.). (From: Mumenthaler, M.: *Didaktischer Atlas der klinischen Neurologie*. 2nd edn, Springer, Heidelberg 1986)

straight-ahead gaze (= primary position)

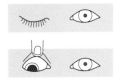

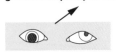

greatest disparity of images

compensatory head position:

none if ptosis is present, because there is no diplopia

fixed, dilated pupil in total CN III palsy

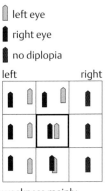

left eye

right eye

no diplopia

weakness mainly of the medial rectus muscle

Fig. 11.**9 Right oculomotor nerve palsy.** Note the position of the eyes and the position of the two visual images (diplopia) depending on the direction of gaze.

Table 11.**4   Localization and etiology of oculomotor nerve palsy**

Site of lesion	Clinical features	Etiology
Nuclear	oculomotor nerve palsy, bilateral vertical gaze palsy, bilateral ptosis	infarct, hemorrhage, trauma, tumor, multiple sclerosis, inflammation, congenital hypoplasia
Fascicular (nerve fibers within the brainstem)	oculomotor nerve palsy, contralateral hemiparesis, ataxia or rubral tremor (differential diagnosis: transtentorial herniation)	infarct, hemorrhage, multiple sclerosis
Subarachnoid space	isolated oculomotor nerve palsy	aneurysm (internal carotid a., rarely other arteries such as the basilar a.), basilar meningitis, cranial polyradiculitis, intracranial hypertension, trauma, neurosurgical complication, tumor of the oculomotor n., transtentorial herniation
Cavernous sinus, superior orbital fissure, or orbit	oculomotor nerve palsy accompanied by dysfunction of CN IV, V/1, and VI in varying combinations	aneurysm (internal carotid a.), carotid–cavernous fistula, cavernous sinus thrombosis, parasellar tumor or pituitary tumor with parasellar extension, sphenoid sinusitis, Tolosa–Hunt syndrome, herpes zoster
Orbital apex	oculomotor nerve palsy accompanied by dysfunction of CN II, IV, V/1, and VI in varying combinations	see lists of causes above and below (cavernous sinus, orbit)
Orbit	ptosis and superior rectus palsy (superior branch of CN III) or palsy of inferior and medial recti and inferior oblique mm. (inferior branch of CN III)	trauma, orbital tumor, orbital pseudotumor, infection, mucocele
No localizing significance	isolated external ophthalmoplegia (i. e., pupillary sparing)	diabetes, hypertension, arteritis, migraine

primary position and in the position of greatest deviation, as well as the positions of the two visual images depending on the patient's direction of gaze.

The third cranial nerve can be affected by a lesion at its nucleus in the brainstem (**nuclear lesion**), at various points along its course within the brainstem (**fascicular lesion**), or in the periphery (**peripheral nerve lesion**). There are many possible causes and the corresponding neurological deficits are correspondingly varied. Typical symptom constellations involving oculomotor nerve palsy and various other findings, depending on the location and etiology of the lesion, are presented in Table 11.**4**. Lesions of the oculomotor n nucleus also cause bilateral ptosis and upward gaze paresis.

Trochlear Nerve Palsy

Lesions of the fourth cranial nerve cause **paralysis of the superior oblique m.** The patient can no longer depress the affected eye in adduction, or internally rotate it in abduction. The resulting diplopia arises when the patient looks down; the images are vertically displaced and slightly tilted. The typical clinical situation is shown schematically in Fig. 11.**10**. The two images can be brought together again by tilting the head to the normal side; the distance between the images increases if the head is tilted to the affected side (*Bielschowsky phenomenon*).

Fig. 11.**10 Right trochlear nerve palsy.** Note the position of the eyes, the compensatory head tilt, and the position of the two visual images depending on the direction of gaze.

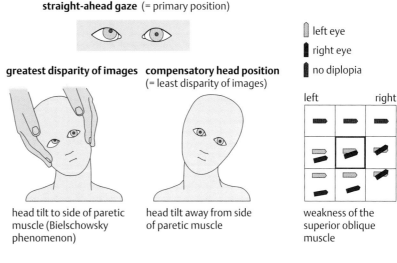

straight-ahead gaze (= primary position)

greatest disparity of images   **compensatory head position**
(= least disparity of images)

head tilt to side of paretic muscle (Bielschowsky phenomenon)

head tilt away from side of paretic muscle

left   right

weakness of the superior oblique muscle

left eye
right eye
no diplopia

Fig. 11.**11 Right abducens nerve palsy.** Note the position of the eyes, the compensatory rotation of the head, and the position of the two visual images depending on the direction of gaze.

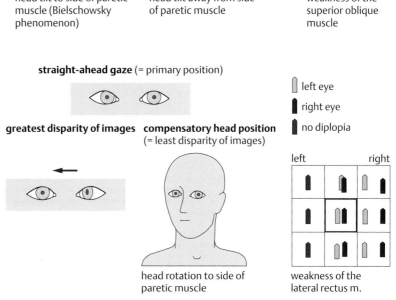

straight-ahead gaze (= primary position)

greatest disparity of images   **compensatory head position**
(= least disparity of images)

head rotation to side of paretic muscle

left   right

weakness of the lateral rectus m.

left eye
right eye
no diplopia

Diseases of the Cranial Nerves

11

Causes. The more common causes of trochlear nerve palsy are:
- congenital aplasia,
- trauma,
- midbrain hemorrhage,
- multiple sclerosis,
- ischemic neuropathy of the nerve, e. g., in diabetes mellitus,
- pathological processes in the cavernous sinus
- or in the orbit.

Pathological processes affecting the superior oblique m. The tendon of the superior oblique m. changes direction in the trochlea, sliding within it in the manner of a pulley. The tendon can sometimes be caught in the ring of the trochlea, thus becoming "stuck" in the middle of a movement. This causes intermittent vertical diplopia, typically when the patient looks up just after looking down, and typically only lasting for a very short time (*Brown syndrome*). *Myokymia of the superior oblique muscle* may occur as a sequela of a trochlear nerve palsy, or independently. Its typical clinical sign is mono-

cular, high-frequency nystagmus with oscillopsia and diplopia.

Abducens Nerve Palsy

Paralysis of the abducens m. caused by a lesion of the sixth cranial nerve causes inward strabismus of the affected eye. Horizontal diplopia is sometimes present even in the primary position of gaze and worsens as the patient looks toward the affected side. The findings are presented schematically in Fig. 11.**11** and the more common causes are listed in Table 11.**5**.

Combined Lesions of Multiple Cranial Nerves Innervating the Muscles of Eye Movement, and Other Disorders in the Differential Diagnosis of Diplopia

If multiple cranial nerves innervating the muscles of eye movement on one side are affected, the lesion usually lies *in the cavernous sinus, at the orbital apex, or in the orbit itself*. Bilateral, multiple palsies of the muscles of

Table 11.**5**   Localization and etiology of abducens nerve palsy

Site of lesion	Clinical features	Etiology
Nuclear, pontine paramedian reticular formation	gaze palsy, often combined with peripheral or nuclear facial nerve palsy	infarct, hemorrhage, tumor, multiple sclerosis, inflammation, trauma, congenital aplasia
Fascicular	abducens palsy with contralateral hemiparesis, occasional also trigeminal deficit	infarct, hemorrhage, multiple sclerosis
Subarachnoid space	isolated abducens nerve palsy	intracranial hypertension, intracranial hypotension, aneurysm (AICA, PICA, basilar a.), subarachnoid hemorrhage, basilar meningitis, cranial polyradiculitis, trauma, neurosurgical complication, tumor of the abducens n., clivus tumor
Petrous apex, petrous bone	deficits of CN V and VI, sometimes also VII and VIII	extradural infection in otitis media
Cavernous sinus, superior orbital fissure	abducens nerve palsy accompanied by dysfunction of CN III, IV, and V/1 in varying combinations	aneurysm (internal carotid a.), carotid–cavernous fistula, cavernous sinus thrombosis, parasellar tumor or pituitary tumor with parasellar extension, sphenoid sinusitis, Tolosa–Hunt syndrome, herpes zoster
Orbital apex	abducens palsy accompanied by dysfunction of CN III, IV, and V/1 in varying combinations	see lists of causes above and below (cavernous sinus, orbit)
Orbit	isolated lateral rectus palsy, or combined with other deficits	trauma, orbital tumor, orbital pseudotumor, endocrine ophthalmopathy, infection, mucocele
No localizing significance	isolated lateral rectus (abducens nerve) palsy	diabetes, hypertension, arteritis, migraine

eye movement are often due to *brainstem processes*; the differential diagnosis includes the entire spectrum of *supranuclear oculomotor disturbances*. In addition, *disorders of neuromuscular transmission*, such as myasthenia gravis (p. 275), and *diseases of the eye muscles themselves* must be considered, including myositis of the eye muscles (rare), mitochondrial myopathy (Kearns–Sayre syndrome), or endocrine ophthalmopathy in hyperthyroidism.

Ptosis

Ptosis is present when the upper lid covers the upper border of the pupil. The cause of ptosis can be **myogenic**, **neurogenic**, or **mechanical** (e. g., dehiscence of the levator aponeurosis).

The eyelid is actively elevated mainly by the action of the striated **levator palpebrae m.**, which is innervated by the oculomotor n. Paralysis of this muscle causes ptosis that is most evident when the patient looks up. The eyelid is also held up, however, by the sympathetically innervated, smooth **superior tarsal m.** It follows that ptosis can be produced by lesions either of the oculomotor n. or of the sympathetic innervation of the eye. The causes of ptosis are listed in Table 11.**6**.

Horner syndrome is caused by loss of the sympathetic innervation of the eye and consists of:
- ptosis (paralysis of the sympathetically innervated superior tarsal m.), most evident when the patient looks slightly downward;
- miosis (paralysis of the sympathetically innervated dilator pupillae m.);

Table 11.**6**   Causes of ptosis

Pathogenesis	Causes (examples)
Mechanical factors	connective tissue defect (e. g., dehiscence of levator aponeurosis) local orbital change microphthalmia
Muscle disease	progressive external ophthalmoplegia Steinert myotonic dystrophy
Neuromuscular transmission disorder	myasthenia gravis botulism
Neurogenic: loss of innervation	oculomotor nerve lesion midbrain infarction cortical lesion sympathetic lesion (central or peripheral)
Neurogenic: excessively strong innervation	blepharospasm faulty regeneration after facial nerve palsy hemifacial spasm

- **mild enophthalmos** (paralysis of Müller muscle, a smooth muscle in the orbit); and
- **conjunctival hyperemia** (loss of the constrictive effect of the sympathetic nervous system on the conjunctival vessels).

When Horner syndrome is not accompanied by a loss of sweating in one-half of the face, the responsible lesion is located in the (ventral) roots of C8 through T2 proximal to their joining with the sympathetic chain. If it is accompanied by a loss of sweating in the face, neck, and arm on one side, then the lesion is at the stellate ganglion, or at a more cranial level of the sympathetic plexus in the neck. A lesion of the sympathetic chain immediately below the stellate ganglion impairs sweating in the ipsilateral upper quarter of the body without producing Horner syndrome. (It is worth noting that thoracic sympathectomy is sometimes performed at this site for the treatment of hyperhidrosis.)

Pupillary Disturbances

Pupillary motility is regulated by the *parasympathetic portion of the oculomotor n.* (sphincter pupillae m.) and by the *sympathetic nervous system* (ciliary m. = dilator pupillae m.). The constrictor and dilator muscles of the pupil are both smooth muscles; the parasympathetic nervous system constricts the pupil and the sympathetic nervous system dilates it. A lesion of the oculomotor n. thus produces a wide pupil, while a lesion of the sympathetic supply (e. g., in Horner syndrome) produces a narrow pupil.

Abnormalities of the Size and Shape of the Pupil

In **pupillary ectopia**, the pupil occupies an eccentric position in the iris. This may be due to a congenital malformation, an inflammatory disorder of the iris, or incomplete nerve regeneration after prior oculomotor nerve palsy. **Abnormally shaped pupils** are usually due to a congenital malformation. Mild **inequality of pupillary size** is a common, normal finding, but marked asymmetry is generally pathological. Inequality of the pupils is called **anisocoria**; its causes include Horner syndrome and Adie syndrome (see below) and others.

Abnormalities of the Pupillary Reflexes

Impairment of the direct and consensual pupillary light reflexes (p. 20) may be caused by any of the following:

- **Local affections of the eye**, such as glaucoma or posterior synechiae.
- The **Marcus Gunn phenomenon** is an impairment of the direct pupillary response to light on the side of a prior episode of retrobulbar neuritis.
- **Adie pupil** (= pupillotonia) is usually unilateral, at least at first. The pupil is wider on the affected side and constricts very slowly in response to light, but promptly and completely on convergence. The subsequent widening of the pupil is slow (tonic). Women are more commonly affected than men; often, but not always, individual intrinsic muscle reflexes are absent. The pathogenesis of this condition is poorly understood. The underlying lesion is thought to lie either in the midbrain or in the ciliary ganglion.
- **Acute ciliary ganglionitis** (after an infection or trauma) renders the pupil unresponsive to light or convergence.
- **Reflex pupillary rigidity** (= Argyll Robertson pupil) is a typical finding in late neurosyphilis. The pupils are generally narrow, usually oblong, and unresponsive to light, but they constrict on convergence. It should be emphasized, however, that fixed and dilated pupils can also be seen in neurosyphilis.
- The presence of a normal pupillary light reflex in a patient who is totally blind indicates bilateral damage to the visual pathway at some point between the lateral geniculate body and the visual cortex of the occipital lobe. The usual cause is bilateral infarction of the visual cortex. The light reflex is preserved because the nerve fibers subserving this reflex branch off the visual pathway proximal to the lateral geniculate body and travel to the pretectal area to innervate their target nuclei.
- **Hippus**, a rhythmic fluctuation of pupillary width, is usually physiological.

The major abnormalities of pupillary size and responsiveness are summarized in Fig. 11.**12**.

Diseases of the Cranial Nerves

11

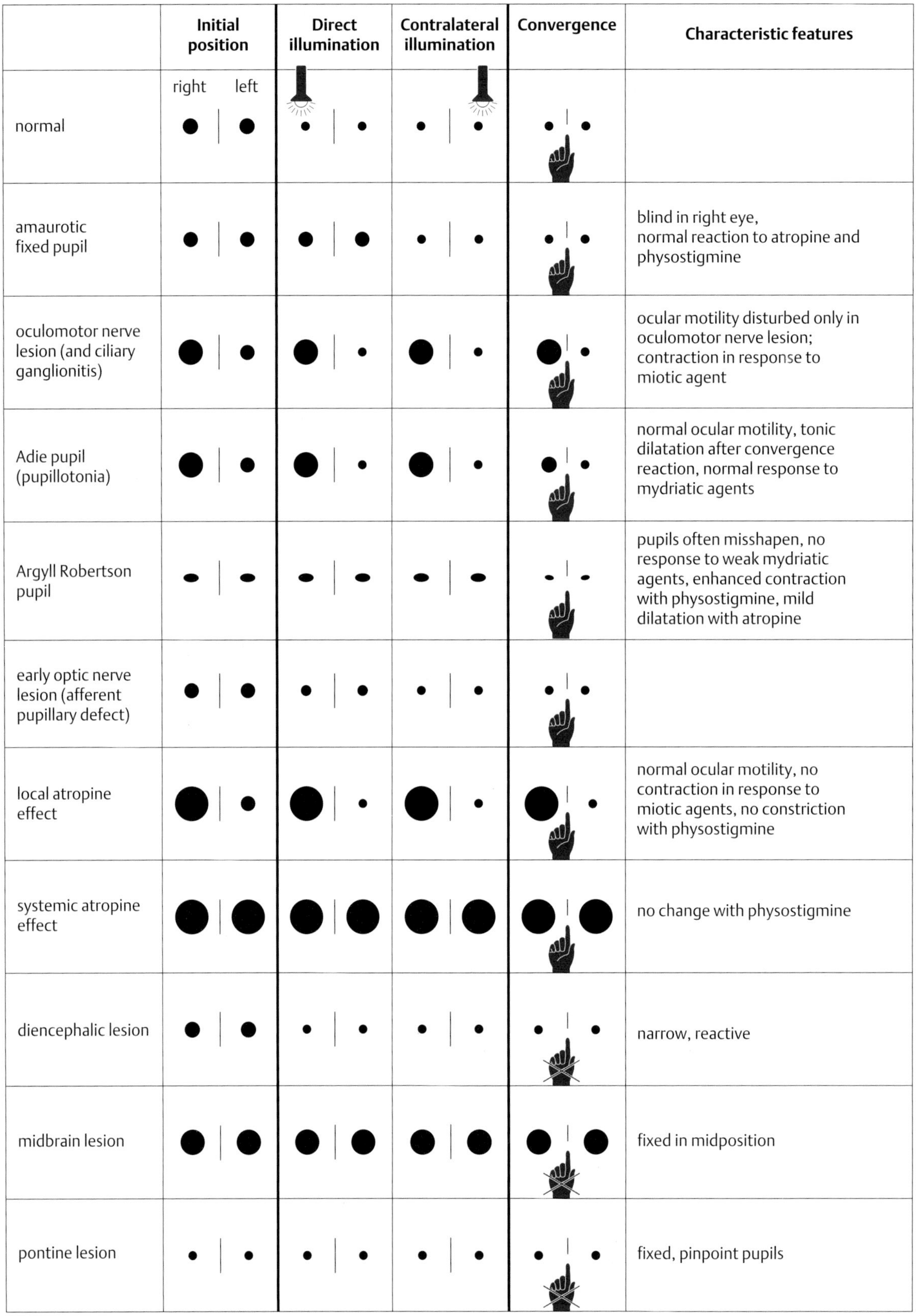

	Initial position		Direct illumination		Contralateral illumination		Convergence		Characteristic features
	right	left							
normal	●	●	●·	·	·	·●	·	·	
amaurotic fixed pupil	●	●	●	●	·	·	·	·	blind in right eye, normal reaction to atropine and physostigmine
oculomotor nerve lesion (and ciliary ganglionitis)	⬤	·	⬤	·	⬤	·	⬤	·	ocular motility disturbed only in oculomotor nerve lesion; contraction in response to miotic agent
Adie pupil (pupillotonia)	⬤	·	⬤	·	⬤	·	⬤	·	normal ocular motility, tonic dilatation after convergence reaction, normal response to mydriatic agents
Argyll Robertson pupil	▬	▬	▬	▬	▬	▬	▬	▬	pupils often misshapen, no response to weak mydriatic agents, enhanced contraction with physostigmine, mild dilatation with atropine
early optic nerve lesion (afferent pupillary defect)	·	●	·	·	·	·	·	·	
local atrophine effect	⬤	·	⬤	·	⬤	·	⬤	·	normal ocular motility, no contraction in response to miotic agents, no constriction with physostigmine
systemic atrophine effect	⬤	⬤	⬤	⬤	⬤	⬤	⬤	⬤	no change with physostigmine
diencephalic lesion	●	●	·	·	·	·	·	·	narrow, reactive
midbrain lesion	●	●	●	●	●	●	●	●	fixed in midposition
pontine lesion	·	·	·	·	·	·	·	·	fixed, pinpoint pupils

Fig. 11.**12 Abnormalities of the pupillary reflexes** (right side abnormal).

Lesions of the Trigeminal Nerve

> The trigeminal n. is responsible for the somatosensory innervation of the skin of the face and forehead and of many of the mucous membranes of the face and head. It also carries motor fibers innervating the muscles of mastication. Lesions of this nerve thus produce **sensory deficits** and **paralysis of the muscles of mastication**.

The anatomical course and distribution of the trigeminal n. are shown in Fig. 3.**10**, p. 23 and the technique of clinical examination is presented on p. 22.

Clinical manifestations. Trigeminal lesions produce **sensory deficits in the face and head**. The somatosensory distribution of the three branches of the trigeminal n. are shown in Fig. 11.**13**. A lesion of the motor portion of the third branch causes **paralysis of the muscles of mastication**. The examiner can usually easily feel the diminished contraction of the masseter m. on one side. When the mouth is opened, the jaw deviates toward the paralyzed side because of weakness of the pterygoid mm. (Fig. 11.**14**).

Causes. Nuclear lesions of the trigeminal n. are located in the pons or medulla and are usually due to vascular processes, encephalitis, a focus of multiple sclerosis, or a space-occupying lesion (glioma, syringobulbia). The nerve can also be affected in its **peripheral** course by mass lesions, toxic influences, or mechanical (iatrogenic) factors. The trigeminal n. can also be affected as a component of cranial polyradiculitis. Occasionally, no clear cause can be found (idiopathic trigeminal neuropathy, which is usually unilateral). Trigeminal neuralgia is discussed below on p. 253.

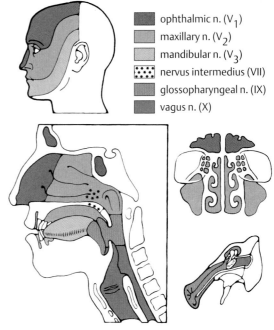

■	ophthalmic n. (V$_1$)
■	maxillary n. (V$_2$)
■	mandibular n. (V$_3$)
✳	nervus intermedius (VII)
■	glossopharyngeal n. (IX)
■	vagus n. (X)

Fig. 11.**13** **Sensory innervation of the face and the mucous membranes of the head.**

Fig. 11.**14** **Lesion of the motor portion of the left trigeminal nerve. a** Atrophy of the left temporalis and masseter muscles. **b** Deviation of the jaw to the left on opening.

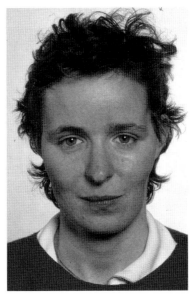

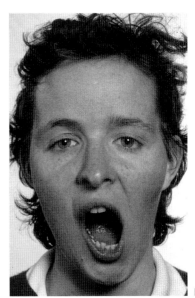

a

b

Diseases of the Cranial Nerves

11

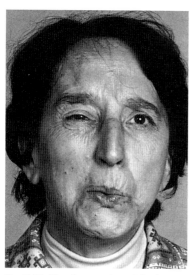

Fig. 11.17 Mass innervation of the face after right peripheral facial nerve palsy. Because of faulty redirection of regenerating motor axons to their muscular targets, the active contraction of a muscle group in the face can be accompanied by involuntary contraction of other muscle groups. In the patient shown, whistling is accompanied by involuntary eye closure. (From: Mumenthaler, M.: *Didaktischer Atlas der klinischen Neurologie.* 2nd edn, Springer, Heidelberg 1986)

Differential diagnosis. Facial weakness of central origin must be distinguished from peripheral facial nerve palsy. In central weakness, the lesion lies above the level of the facial nerve nucleus, i. e., in the portion of the motor cortex subserving facial movements, or along the course of the corticobulbar efferent fibers. With meticulous clinical examination, one can always distinguish central from peripheral facial weakness; the criteria for making the distinction are summarized in Table 11.7. The most important one is the *lesser involvement of the forehead and periocular musculature,* compared with the remainder of the facial muscles, in central facial palsy.

The explanation is that the neurons in the superior portion of the facial nerve nucleus in the pons receive impulses from both cerebral hemispheres; therefore, a unilateral lesion of the motor cortex or corticobulbar tract can usually be compensated for by the corresponding, intact pathway on the opposite side (cf. Fig. 11.15). The caudal portion of the facial nerve nucleus, on the other hand, is "controlled" only by the contralateral hemisphere.

In addition, central facial palsy is often accompanied by *weakness elsewhere in the body* in areas not inner-

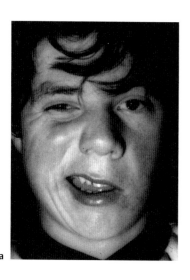
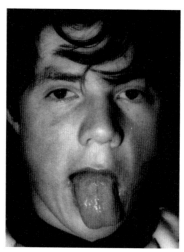

a   b

Fig. 11.18 Left central facial palsy. a Impaired innervation of the lower portion of the face is evident when the patient tries to show his teeth. **b** As part of the central hemiparesis, the motor innervation of the left side of the tongue is also impaired, and the tongue therefore deviates to the left on protrusion.

Table 11.7 Differentiation of central and peripheral facial palsy

	Central facial palsy	Peripheral facial palsy
History	Usually seen in elderly persons as a sudden, acute event; usually accompanied by hemiparesis mainly affecting the upper limb	May occur at any age; often accompanied by retroauricular pain; weakness develops over the course of one or two days, rather than suddenly
Facial appearance at rest	Usually normal	Often normal; blinking may be less frequent; the affected side of the face is flaccid in longstanding, complete peripheral facial palsy
Examination of facial musculature	The globe is always completely covered when the patient closes the eyes; the frontal branch is always much less affected	If the palsy is complete, the patient can never completely close the affected eye (though this is still possible in partial lesions of CN VII); the frontal branch is affected to the same extent as the rest of the nerve (Fig. 11.16)
Additional findings	There may be accompanying, ipsilateral weakness of the tongue, or central hemiparesis of the ipsilateral limbs	In the cryptogenic form, the sense of taste is lost on the ipsilateral side of the anterior two-thirds of the tongue; diminished lacrimation and salivation; electromyography reveals denervation

vated by the facial n., e. g., in the tongue. If the tongue is weak on one side, it deviates, when protruded, to the side of the lesion (Fig. 11.**18**).

Hemifacial Spasm

This condition is characterized by synchronous, irregular, rapid, brief contractions of all of the muscles of facial expression supplied by the facial n. on one side of the face, particularly including the platysma. On close observation, hemifacial spasm is readily distinguishable from a facial tic (Fig. 11.**19**). It rarely arises in the aftermath of a peripheral facial nerve palsy. The usual cause is *irritation of the facial nerve root by a looping blood vessel just distal to its point of exit from the pons*; this explains why neurosurgical intervention ("microvascular decompression") is usually successful. It is very rare for hemifacial spasm to be caused by a brainstem glioma. The condition can be treated symptomatically with anticonvulsants such as carbamazepine, or with injections of botulinus toxin.

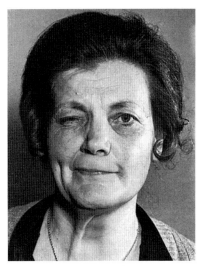

Fig. 11.**19 Right hemifacial spasm** in a 47-year-old patient. All of the muscles innervated by the facial nerve, including the platysma, contract repeatedly, synchronously, and involuntarily.

Disturbances of Hearing and Balance; Vertigo

Lesions of the vestibulocochlear n. can impair hearing, balance, or both. A lesion of its cochlear portion produces **sensorineural hearing loss** (impairment of sound perception), which must always be differentiated from **conductive hearing loss** (impairment of sound conduction, usually due to blockage of the external auditory canal by cerumen, or to a disease process in the middle ear). A lesion of the vestibular portion causes **disequilibrium** and **vertigo**. Vestibular vertigo usually occurs in a particular direction and is accompanied by autonomic symptoms and nystagmus. Common vestibular disorders causing vertigo include **vestibular neuritis** and **benign paroxysmal positioning vertigo**. A vestibular lesion, however, is only one possible cause of vertigo; many other disorders must be included in the differential diagnosis.

The eighth cranial nerve (vestibulocochlear n.) conducts auditory and vestibular information to the central nervous system.
● Auditory impulses arise in the organ of Corti in the cochlea and travel by way of the cochlear n. to the cochlear nuclei of the brainstem and then onward in the auditory pathway to the auditory cortex in the temporal lobe.
● Vestibular impulses arise in the ampullae and in the macula statica of the saccule and utricle, the organ of equilibrium; they then travel by way of the vestibular n. to the vestibular nuclei, from which they are conducted to multiple areas of the brain, including the cerebellum.

These anatomical relations are depicted in Fig. 3.**11** and discussed on p. 24.

Neurological Disturbances of Hearing

The differentiation of sensorineural from conductive hearing loss helps determine whether the underlying cause is located in the middle ear or external auditory canal (more common sites, conductive hearing loss) or in the sensory cells of the inner ear or the neural apparatus of hearing (less common sites, sensorineural hearing loss). The method of examination and typical findings are summarized above on p. 22. The diagnosis and treatment of conductive hearing loss and of disorders of the cochlea are the responsibility of the otologist.

Neurological disturbances of hearing. Hearing loss due to a lesion of the inner ear or the vestibulocochlear n. may be unilateral or bilateral and its development may be more or less rapid:

Unilateral hearing loss, if **acute**, is usually due to an infectious process, e. g., mumps or other viral infection. If it is **slowly progressive**, the physician should suspect a mass lesion compressing the eighth cranial n., such as an acoustic neuroma or a meningioma in the cerebellopontine angle (Fig. 11.**20**). Larger masses in the cerebellopontine angle can affect not only the eighth cranial nerve, but also the facial and trigeminal nn.

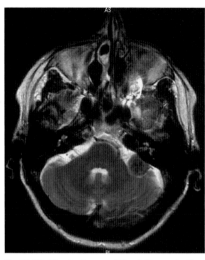

Fig. 11.**20 Meningioma of the left cerebellopontine angle** seen by MRI. The hazelnut-sized, spherical tumor is based on the pyramid of the petrous bone.

Bilateral hearing loss, if acute, is also most commonly due to a viral or other infection; bacterial meningitis is a rare cause. *Progressive bilateral hearing loss*, whether it is slow or rapid, should prompt suspicion of, e.g., chronic basilar meningitis (e.g., in tuberculosis), carcinomatous meningitis, an infectious disease (syphilis, toxoplasmosis), or an intoxication. Very slowly progressive, bilateral hearing loss may be due to a metabolic disorder, e.g., Refsum disease or one of the collagenoses.

A number of diseases that can produce hearing loss as their most prominent manifestation are listed in Table 11.**8**.

Tinnitus. Noises in one or both ears are a common complaint. They are usually *subjective*, i.e., audible only by the patient. They are termed *objective* when the examiner, too, can hear them with the stethoscope.

The most common variety of **subjective tinnitus** involves a noise heard continually in both ears. The patient usually finds it most disturbing in quiet surroundings, particularly in bed at night. The cause is un-

Table 11.**8** **Diseases causing prominent hearing loss**

Category	Disease	Remarks
Hereditary congenital malformations of the inner ear	isolated hereditary deafness Mondini syndrome Alport syndrome Klein–Waardenburg syndrome Usher syndrome Laurence–Moon–Biedl syndrome mitochondrial encephalomyopathies	Most of these malformations are genetically transmitted in an autosomal recessive pattern, while a few are dominant or X-chromosomal. The inheritance pattern of mitochondrial encephalomyopathies is nearly always strictly maternal, as these diseases are transmitted in mitochondrial DNA
Nonhereditary congenital malformations of the inner ear	thalidomide dysplasia measles embryopathy hyperbilirubinemia (kernicterus) perinatal asphyxia cretinism congenital syphilis toxoplasmosis	In thalidomide dysplasia and measles embryopathy, the ear anomalies are often accompanied by other anomalies elsewhere in the body. Kernicterus often causes athetosis; cretinism causes feeblemindedness
Infections	viral: herpes, mumps, measles, mononucleosis, HIV, and other neurotropic viruses bacterial meningitis otitis media and malignant otitis chronic otitis media, cholesteatoma syphilis, borreliosis	Hearing loss is a common late sequela of bacterial meningitis; otitis media causes conductive (not sensorineural) hearing loss; otoscopic examination is mandatory
Polyneuropathies combined with hearing loss	Refsum disease hereditary neuropathy (Charcot–Marie–Tooth)	Retinitis pigmentosa in Refsum disease
Tumors	acoustic neuroma glomus tympanicum tumor paraneoplastic	Acoustic neuroma occurs sporadically or as a component of neurofibromatosis, type I or II. The presenting symptom of a glomus tympanicum tumor is often pulsatile tinnitus
Cerebrovascular disorders	infarct in the territory of the labyrinthine a. migraine	
Autoimmune disorders	collagen diseases Susac syndrome Cogan syndrome	Various types of autoantibody can be demonstrated in these conditions
Trauma	transverse fracture of petrous bone labyrinthine contusion acoustic trauma chronic exposure to noise barotrauma	The clinical history leads to the diagnosis
Toxic/iatrogenic	aminoglycosides, cytostatic agents	Usually bilateral, often with a bilateral vestibular deficit

Continued →

Table 11.**8** **Diseases causing prominent hearing loss** (Continued)

Category	Disease	Remarks
Specific ear diseases	Ménière disease Lermoyez syndrome otosclerosis acute hearing loss perilymph fistula	In these conditions, vestibular symptoms are often present in combination (or in alternation) with hearing loss
Miscellaneous	superficial hemosiderosis of the CNS	Progressive hearing loss and ataxia

known and the problem can resolve spontaneously. Various therapeutic measures have been proposed, including perfusion-enhancing medications and oxygen, but are of questionable benefit.

Pulsatile tinnitus is rare in comparison to continual tinnitus. It is caused by a pulsating blood vessel near the petrous bone and must be taken very seriously. The examiner, too, can often hear the pulse-synchronous bruit through a stethoscope (sometimes even without one). Some possible causes are listed in Table 11.**9**.

Table 11.**9** **Diseases that can present with pulsatile tinnitus**

- Carotid dissection
- Fibromuscular dysplasia
- High-lying carotid stenosis due to atheromatous plaque
- Arteriovenous malformation
- Retromastoid dural fistula
- Carotid–cavernous fistula
- Glomus tumor (glomus jugulare or glomus tympanicum)
- Tumor in or near petrous bone
- Infection in or near petrous bone
- Intracranial hypertension
- Pseudotumor cerebri

Disequilibrium and Vertigo

The vestibular organ (semicircular canals, saccule, and utricle) plays a central role in the regulation of balance. Disturbances of the vestibular apparatus (composed of the vestibular organ, the vestibulocochlear n., and the vestibular nuclei of the brainstem) cause dysequilibrium, the main symptom of which is vertigo. It must be emphasized, however, that vestibular disturbances are just *one* cause of vertigo (see below) and not even the most common one.

Regulation of equilibrium. Equilibrium (balance), i. e., the optimal static and dynamic mechanical stability of the human being in space, is maintained by the following neural processes:

- *impulses from the vestibular apparatus* concerning the position, movement, and acceleration of the individual in space;
- *impulses from the visual system* concerning the body's relation to visual space;
- *impulses from the exteroceptive pathways* concerning the body's contact with underlying surfaces (floor, mattress, etc.);
- *impulses from the proprioceptive pathways* concerning the positions of the joints and the spatial relations of the parts of the body to each other;
- impulses concerning movements in the process of being executed, from the pyramidal, extrapyramidal, and cerebellar systems;
- conscious (cognitive) and unconscious (emotional) influences;
- finally, the integration of all of these signals in the brainstem.

The various components of the regulation of balance are depicted schematically in Fig. 11.**21**.

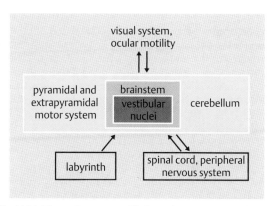

Fig. 11.**21 The maintenance of balance by integration of information from multiple channels**

Disturbances of the regulation of equilibrium. Vertigo arises if individual informational and/or control components of the regulatory system are lost (see below), if the information coming through different sensory channels seems to be incompatible (so-called *multisensory mismatch*, e. g., in seasickness), or the sensory input is highly unusual (e. g., uncommon visual input from a great height). So many different structures play a role in the maintenance of equilibrium and their interactions are so complex, that the causes of vertigo are, understandably, highly varied. Different types of vertigo result from lesions at different sites.

Types of vertigo. Directional vertigo (vestibular vertigo) is characteristic of lesions of the peripheral portion of the vestibular apparatus, i. e., the vestibular organ and/or the vestibulocochlear n. The patient *perceives the*

Table 11.10   Differentiation of peripheral vestibular, central vestibular, and nonvestibular vertigo

Signs and symptoms	Type of vertigo		
	peripheral vestibular (labyrinth, nerve)	central vestibular	nonvestibular
Nausea, vomiting, diaphoresis	severe	moderate	mild
Vertigo—intensity	marked	moderate	mild
Vertigo—type	in a specific direction	directional to some degree	not in any specific direction
Nystagmus	spontaneous nystagmus of vestibular type	spontaneous nystagmus of vestibular type	nonvestibular nystagmus, or no pathological nystagmus
Hearing loss, tinnitus	usual	unusual	absent
Other neurological deficits	unusual	usually present	the neurological examination may or may not yield positive findings

environment *as if it were in motion* (= *oscillopsia*), e. g., rotating or heaving up and down like the deck of a boat. Vestibular vertigo is often accompanied by *autonomic manifestations*, such as nausea and vomiting, and by *nystagmus.* Central vestibular lesions (i. e., lesions of the vestibular nuclei in the brainstem) also cause directional vertigo, which is generally less intense than that due to peripheral lesions. The autonomic manifestations, too, tend to be milder or absent.

Nonvestibular vertigo is nondirectional and often difficult for the patient to describe. The patient may report a woozy feeling, emptiness in the head, or darkness before the eyes. Oscillopsia is absent and there are usually no autonomic manifestations. Central nervous lesions can cause pathological nystagmus, as listed in Tables 11.1, 11.2. Nonvestibular vertigo is caused either by a lesion of the nonvestibular parts of the regulatory system for balance, or else by faulty information processing within the central nervous system (e. g., because of a cerebellar lesion). Pathological processes outside the central nervous system, such as orthostatic hypotension or aortic stenosis, can also cause nonvestibular vertigo.

The characteristic features of peripheral and central vestibular vertigo and of nonvestibular vertigo are summarized in Table 11.10.

Special aspects of history taking and diagnostic evaluation. The clinician should be able to tell whether the patient is suffering from *vestibular* or *nonvestibular vertigo* based on a meticulously elicited clinical history alone. It is also important to determine whether the vertigo is *episodic* or *continuous* and to ask about any *precipitating factors* (e. g., changes of position or particular situations that make the vertigo worse). If the vertigo worsens in the dark or when the patient's eyes are closed, the cause is likely to be a disturbance of proprioception (polyneuropathy, posterior column disease) or a bilateral vestibulopathy. The examiner should also always ask about *accompanying symptoms* (in particular, autonomic symptoms, tinnitus, hearing loss, and prior illnesses and infections). The history combined with the physical findings (nystagmus, results of balance tests, any other neurological abnormalities) usually allows localization of the functional disturbance. Further testing

(e. g., caloric testing of the vestibular organ, ENT consultation, neuroimaging of the head) mainly serves to determine the etiology.

We will now describe the main neurological causes of vertigo, particularly vestibular disturbances, in greater detail.

Vestibular Vertigo

Acute loss of vestibular function is also called vestibular neuritis, acute vestibular neuropathy, or an acute vestibular crisis. It can be produced by a variety of pathogenetic mechanisms, the most common of which is a viral infection. The patient suddenly experiences *acute rotatory vertigo with nausea, vomiting,* and *falling to the side of the diseased vestibular organ.* Every movement of the head makes the vertigo worse; therefore the patient, noting this, lies perfectly still. Examination reveals *horizontally beating, spontaneous nystagmus* in the direction opposite the side of the lesion, with a rotatory component. The nystagmus is more intense when the patient lies on the affected side; it can be diminished by visual fixation. The affected vestibular organ is *less responsive than normal to caloric stimulation.* Vertigo usually resolves fully within a few days, rarely within a few hours. Often a so-called "trigger labyrinth" remains as a residual phenomenon, i. e., vertigo on acceleration or rapid movements of the head. The condition may relapse.

Positional and positioning vertigo. These types of vertigo arise only with certain positions or positioning movements of the head and manifest themselves as *brief attacks of vertigo* that diminish in intensity if they are provoked in rapid succession. These conditions have a number of different causes.

Benign paroxysmal positioning vertigo is the most common type of positioning vertigo. It is provoked by *changes in the position of the head,* usually involving lying down rapidly, bending forward, turning in bed, or rapidly sitting up. It manifests itself as very brief (15–30 seconds) and very severe *attacks of rotatory vertigo and nausea.*

Fig. 11.**22 Hallpike positional testing** for the demonstration of benign paroxysmal positioning vertigo. See text.

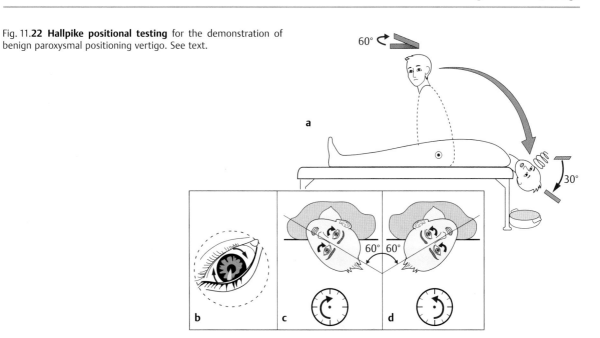

With respect to the *pathogenesis* of this condition, it is thought that small pieces of the otolith membranes of the saccule and utricle can break off and float freely in the endolymph—usually in the posterior semicircular canal, less commonly in the horizontal one. When the head is moved, these free particles move together with the endolymph and slide over the hair cells of the cupula, even after the movement is completed. The abnormally prolonged activation of the hair cells induces acute rotatory vertigo. The condition is also termed *cupulolithiasis* or *canalolithiasis*.

The *Hallpike positioning maneuver* can be used as a diagnostic test (Fig. 11.**22**). The patient is rapidly taken from an upright sitting position into the supine position with the head held down 30° below the level of the examining table and turned 60° to the right or left. Within a few seconds, the examiner should be able to observe rotatory nystagmus, which then disappears after 5–30 seconds. This is easiest to see if the patient is wearing Frenzel goggles. If the head is turned to the right, the nystagmus is counterclockwise; if to the left, clockwise.

Certain positioning maneuvers, e.g., those of Epley and Semont, have been shown to be useful as *treatment* for this condition. These maneuvers work by flushing the floating otoliths out of the affected semicircular canal.

Central positional vertigo is a rarer type of positionally dependent vertigo appearing with certain tilted positions of the head. The nystagmus usually beats to the uppermost ear and does not habituate on repeated provocation. The vertigo is generally not very severe.

Ménière disease is a common cause of acute vestibular vertigo. It is caused by *endolymphatic hydrops* and manifests itself clinically in *episodes of acute rotatory vertigo*, a tendency to fall to the affected side, and horizontal, directional, *spontaneous nystagmus*, accompanied by *nausea*, *vomiting*, and *tinnitus*. Slowly progressive *hearing loss* is worse after each attack.

Bilateral vestibular deficits. While *unilateral* dysfunction of the vestibular apparatus can either recover or be compensated for by the intact opposite side within a matter of weeks, *bilateral* dysfunction deprives the regulatory system for balance of all incoming vestibular information. Consequently, the patient's gait becomes very unsteady in the dark (i.e., when visual input, too, is inoperative), or when the patient must walk on an uneven or soft surface (i.e., when the incoming proprioceptive information is difficult to interpret). Subjectively, the patient suffers from oscillopsia (apparent movement of the external world), particularly when walking, because the vestibulo-ocular reflex (p. 186) is inoperative and visual fixation is, therefore, unstable.

Nonvestibular Vertigo

Dysfunction of the nonvestibular components of the regulatory system for balance can also cause vertigo.
- **Visually induced vertigo** occurs, e.g., when an individual looks down from a great height, or when the incoming proprioceptive information is inconsistent with the visual information (*polysensory mismatch*). The vertigo of seasickness is a type of visually induced vertigo.
- **Impaired proprioception**, e.g., in polyneuropathy or posterior column disease, can also cause vertigo.
- **Cervical vertigo** is thought to be due to faulty proprioceptive information arising in diseased cervical intervertebral joints or the adjacent soft tissues, which is then transmitted to the integrating apparatus for balance in the brainstem. This type of vertigo worsens in the dark. Its existence is debated.

Diseases of the Cranial Nerves

11

- **Pathological processes affecting the central motor structures** (e. g., paralysis, cerebellar or extrapyramidal disease, brainstem disorders) impair the patient's motor adaptation to changes in position, or cause oculomotor disturbances that can give rise to "dizziness."
- **Partial impairment of consciousness**, e. g., in presyncope or certain types of epilepsy (particularly temporal lobe epilepsy and absence seizures), is often experienced by the patient as "dizziness."

- Another frequent occurrence is **psychogenic vertigo**, particularly due to phobias, in the setting of depression, neurotic conflict situations, and panic attacks.
- Finally, any **general medical conditions** that can temporarily diminish blood flow to the brain must be included in the differential diagnosis of "dizziness" and vertigo, e. g., arterial hypotension and heart disease.

The Lower Cranial Nerves

Here we consider the clinical presentations of dysfunction of cranial nerves IX–XII. Lesions of the glossopharyngeal and vagus nn. produce **dysphagia**, **hoarseness**, and **dysphonia**. Lesions of the accessory n., depending on their level, produce **weakness of the sternocleidomastoid m. and trapezius m.** Lesions of the hypoglossal n. produce ipsilateral **weakness of the tongue**.

Lesions of the Glossopharyngeal and Vagus Nerves

Anatomy. The anatomical course and distribution of these nerves is described above on p. 18.

Typical deficits. A unilateral lesion of the glossopharyngeal and vagus nn. causes ipsilateral weakness of the soft palate and posterior pharyngeal wall, which is evident as the *curtain sign* (Fig. 11.**23**, see also Fig. 3.**13**, p. 26). The associated sensory deficit causes *dysphagia and* unilateral paralysis of the vocal cord causes *hoarseness*. The patient usually does not notice the loss of sensation in the external auditory canal or the loss of taste on the posterior third of the tongue.

Causes. Palsy affecting the ninth and tenth cranial nerves can be caused by *infarction* of the corresponding *brainstem nuclei* (e. g., in Wallenberg syndrome, p. ■■). *Lesions of the peripheral nerve trunks* can be caused by a mass in the posterior fossa or by a bony fracture impinging on the nerves at their site of exit from the jugular foramen. In the latter case, the injury involves not only these nerves, but also the accessory n. (Siebenmann syndrome). Finally, isolated neuritis of these nerves can occur, e. g., in the setting of herpes zoster, or as a cryptogenic event.

Accessory Nerve Palsy

The anatomy and method of examination of the accessory n. are described above.

Typical deficits. *A lesion of the purely motor main trunk of the accessory n.* causes paralysis of the sternocleidomastoid m. and of the upper portion of the trapezius m. (Fig. 11.**24**). *Lesions of the accessory n. in the lateral triangle of the neck*, however, are much more common. These spare the sternocleidomastoid m. and weaken only the upper portion of the trapezius m., causing a shoulder droop and an externally rotated position of the scapula (i. e., tilting of the caudal angle of the scapula

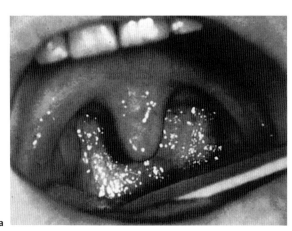

a

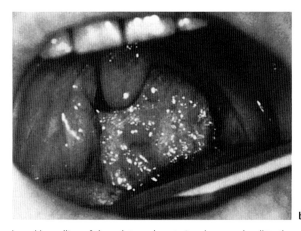

b

Fig. 11.**23 Curtain sign** revealing left-sided palatopharyngeal weakness in a 36-year-old patient with Wallenberg syndrome. **a** Normal appearance at rest. **b** Elicitation of the gag reflex is followed by pulling of the palate and posterior pharyngeal wall to the unaffected right side. (From: Mumenthaler M.: *Didaktischer Atlas der klinischen Neurologie*. 2nd edn, Springer, Heidelberg 1986.)

toward the midline). This condition is depicted in Fig. 11.**25**.

Causes. *Dysfunction of the main trunk of the accessory n.* is caused by mass lesions in the posterior fossa or at the base of the skull (Siebenmann syndrome, see above). Accessory nerve palsy due to *interruption of the nerve in the lateral triangle of the neck* is practically always iatrogenic, e. g., as a complication of lymph node biopsy at the posterior border of the sternocleidomastoid m.

Hypoglossal Nerve Palsy

The anatomy and technique of examination of the hypoglossal n. are described above on p. 27.

Typical deficits. The ipsilateral half of the tongue is *paretic* and, in the course of time, becomes *atrophic*. When the tongue is protruded, it deviates to the paretic side. This condition is illustrated in Fig. 3.**16**, p. 27.

Causes. Unilateral hypoglossal nerve palsy is usually due to a bony fracture or a mass lesion—rarely, a congenital malformation—in the posterior cranial fossa. Carotid dissection is another possible cause. Rarely, isolated hypoglossal nerve palsy arises as a postinfectious or cryptogenic event.

Differential diagnosis. Unilateral tongue weakness can also be of *central* origin, i. e., due to a lesion of the corticobulbar pathway to the hypoglossal nerve nucleus (Fig. 11.**18**). Central weakness is unaccompanied by atrophy.

Bilateral tongue weakness and atrophy in the setting of *true bulbar palsy* (p. 80, p. 155) is due to progressive loss of motor neurons in the nucleus of the hypoglossal nerve on both sides of the medulla. The observable abnormalities are slowly progressive and accompanied by fasciculations of the tongue.

Tongue weakness in *pseudobulbar palsy* (p. 80) is due to bilateral, usually ischemic damage of the central corticobulbar pathways. Because the lesion is central, no atrophy or fasciculations are seen. Examination reveals dysarthria, dysphagia, and abnormal prominence of the perioral reflexes.

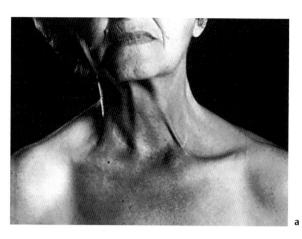
a

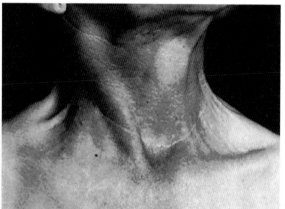
b

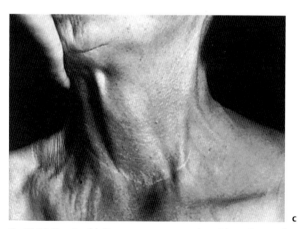
c

Fig. 11.**24 Proximal left accessory nerve palsy** with weakness of both the sternocleidomastoid m. and the trapezius m. **a** Even in the resting position, the upper edge of the trapezius m. is visibly thinner than on the right side, and the left sternocleidomastoid m. is barely discernible. **b** When the patient turns her head to the left, the intact right sternocleidomastoid m. is clearly seen. **c** When the head is turned to the right, there is only faint contraction of the left sternocleidomastoid m. (From: Mumenthaler M.: *Didaktischer Atlas der klinischen Neurologie.* 2nd edn, Springer, Heidelberg 1986.)

Diseases of the Cranial Nerves

11

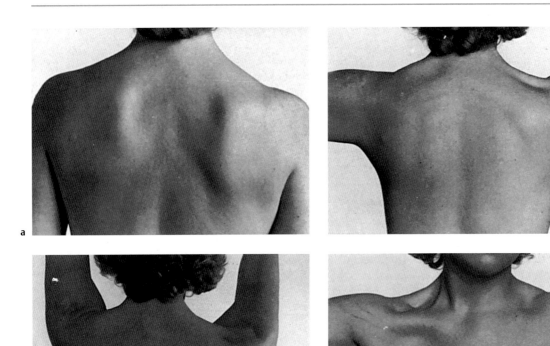

Fig. 11.**25 Lesion of the right accessory n. in the lateral triangle of the neck. a** At rest, the right shoulder is somewhat lower, and the right scapula is somewhat farther from the midline. **b** When the arms are raised horizontally, the contour of the levator scapulae m. is easily seen below the atrophic edge of the trapezius m. **c** When the arms are raised vertically, the scapula tilts and the shoulder is low. **d** The atrophic upper edge of the trapezius m. is clearly seen in this frontal view. (From: Mumenthaler M.: *Didaktischer Atlas der klinischen Neurologie.* 2nd edn, Springer, Heidelberg 1986.)

Multiple Cranial Nerve Deficits

Lesions affecting more than one cranial nerve at a time are seen in various typical combinations:

- Progressive involvement of multiple lower cranial nerves (*Garcin syndrome*) is usually due to a tumor at the base of the skull. *Chronic basilar meningitis*, e. g., in tuberculosis, causes multiple cranial nerve palsies in varying combinations.
- *Cranial polyradiculitis* affects the cranial nerves symmetrically; the most prominent manifestation is bilateral facial nerve palsy.
- *Further causes* of multiple, and possibly recurrent, cranial nerve palsies include sarcoidosis, paraproteinemia, Wegener granulomatosis, malignant otitis, and others.

12 Diseases of the Spinal Nerve Roots and Peripheral Nerves

Fundamentals

Lesions of the peripheral nervous system cause flaccid weakness, sensory deficits, and autonomic disturbances in variable distributions and combinations depending on their localization and extent. They can be classified as lesions of the spinal nerve roots (**radicular lesions**), **plexus lesions**, or **lesions of individual peripheral nerve trunks or branches**.

Spinal Radicular Syndromes

> Radicular lesions are usually due to **mechanical compression**; less commonly, they may be infectious/inflammatory or traumatic. Their main clinical manifestation is **pain**, usually accompanied by a **sensory deficit** in the dermatome of the affected nerve root. Depending on the severity of the lesion, there may also be **flaccid weakness** and **areflexia** in the muscle(s) innervated by the nerve root.

Preliminary anatomical remarks. The spinal nerve roots constitute the initial segment of the peripheral nervous system. The **anterior (ventral) nerve roots** contain **efferent fibers**, while the **posterior (dorsal) nerve roots** contain **afferent fibers**. The motor roots from T2 to L2 or L3 also contain the efferent fibers of the sympathetic nervous system. The anterior and posterior roots at a single level of the spinal cord on one side join to form the **spinal nerve** at that level, which then passes out of the spinal canal through the corresponding intervertebral foramen. At this point, the nerve roots are in close proximity to the intervertebral disk and the intervertebral (facet) joint (Fig. 12.**1**).

In their further course, the fibers of the spinal nerve roots of multiple segments form plexuses, from which they are then distributed to the peripheral nerves. The areas innervated by the nerve roots thus differ from those innervated by the peripheral nerves.

The sensory component of a spinal nerve root innervates a characteristic segmental area of skin, which is called a **dermatome**. The efferent fibers of a spinal nerve root, after redistribution into various peripheral nerves, innervate multiple muscles (the "**myotome**" of the nerve root at that level). Each muscle, therefore, obtains motor impulses from *more than one* nerve root, even if it is only innervated by a *single* peripheral nerve.

Fig. 12.**1 View of a cervical vertebra and intervertebral disk.** The normal anatomy of the intervertebral (neural) foramen is shown on the left side of the figure; narrowing of the foramen by uncarthrosis is shown on the right. 1 Facets of the intervertebral joint; 2 root with spinal ganglion; 3 lateral/medial intervertebral disk herniation; 4 vertebral arteries; 5 uncarthrosis; 6 dorsal spondylosis; 7 ventral spondylosis; 8 spinal dura mater. (Modified from Mumenthaler M.: *Der Schulter–Arm–Schmerz*, 2nd edn, Huber, Bern 1982.)

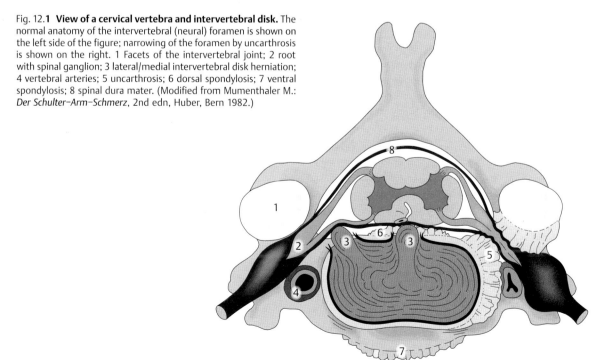

12

Table 12.**1** **Synopsis of radicular syndromes**

Segment	Sensory deficit	Motor deficit	Reflex deficit	Remarks
C3/4	pain and hypalgesia in shoulder region	diaphragmatic paresis or plegia	none detectable	partial diaphragmatic paresis is more ventral in C3 lesions, more dorsal in C4 lesions
C5	pain and hypalgesia on lateral aspect of shoulder over deltoid m.	deltoid and biceps paresis	diminished biceps reflex	
C6	radial side of arm and forearm down to thumb	biceps and brachioradialis paresis	diminished or absent biceps reflex	
C7	dorsolateral to C6 dermatome down to 2nd, 3rd, and 4th fingers	triceps, pronator teres, and (occas.) finger flexor paresis; thenar eminence often visibly atrophic	diminished or absent triceps reflex	triceps reflex key to differential diagnosis vs. carpal tunnel syndrome
C8	dorsal to C7 dermatome, down to little finger	intrinsic hand muscles visibly atrophic, particularly on hypothenar eminence	diminished triceps reflex	triceps reflex key to differential diagnosis vs. ulnar nerve palsy
L3	from greater trochanter crossing over the anterior aspect to the medial aspect of the thigh and knee	quadriceps paresis	weakness of quadriceps (knee-jerk) reflex	differential diagnosis vs. femoral nerve palsy: sensation intact in distribution of saphenous n.
L4	from lateral thigh across patella to upper inner quadrant of calf and down to medial edge of foot	quadriceps and tibialis anterior paresis	weakness of quadriceps reflex	differential diagnosis vs. femoral nerve palsy: involvement of tibialis anterior m.
L5	from lateral condyle above knee across the upper outer quadrant of the calf to the great toe	paresis and atrophy of extensor hallucis longus m., often also of extensor digitorum brevis m.; paresis of tibialis posterior m. and of hip abduction	absent tibialis posterior reflex (of diagnostic value only when clearly elicitable on opposite, unaffected side)	differential diagnosis vs. peroneal nerve palsy: in the latter, tibialis posterior and hip abduction are preserved
S1	from posterior thigh over posterior upper quadrant of calf and lateral malleolus to little toe	paresis of the peronei, often also of the gastrocnemius and soleus mm.	absent gastrocnemius reflex (ankle-jerk or Achilles reflex)	
Combined L4, L5	combination of L4 and L5 dermatomes	paresis of all foot and toe extensors and of quadriceps m.	diminished quadriceps reflex, absent tibialis posterior reflex	differential diagnosis vs. peroneal nerve palsy: peronei spared. Note reflex findings
Combined L5, S1	combination of L5 and S1 dermatomes	paresis of toe extensors, peronei, occasional also gastrocnemius and soleus mm.	absent tibialis posterior and gastrocnemius reflexes	differential diagnosis vs. peroneal nerve palsy: tibialis anterior spared. Note reflex findings

Table 12.**1** lists the muscles that are often affected by radicular lesions in a way that is easily revealed by clinical neurological examination. The muscles that derive most of their innervation from a single nerve root are known as "**root-indicating muscles**."

Causes of radicular syndromes. In most patients, the cause is **compression** of the nerve root by a *space-occupying lesion*, most often a herniated intervertebral disk, but sometimes a tumor, abscess, or other mass. In the cervical segments, *spondylotic narrowing of the in-*

tervertebral foramina, is a further common cause of radicular pain and brachialgia (Fig. 12.**2**). **Infectious and inflammatory processes** can cause monoradicular deficits, e.g., *herpes zoster* and *borreliosis* (Lyme disease, p. 117). **Diabetes mellitus**, too, can cause monoradiculopathy with pain and weakness. Finally, **traumatic lesions**, e.g., bony fractures, can affect individual nerve roots (Fig. 12.**3**).

> **!** *Radiculopathy is often due to a mechanical injury or irritation of a nerve root by degenerative disease of the spine, particularly intervertebral disk herniation. A radicular deficit, however, should never simply be assumed to be due to disk herniation. Other etiologies (see above) must always be considered.*

General clinical manifestations of radicular lesions.
Regardless of the etiology, the following symptoms and neurological findings are characteristic:

● **pain** in the distribution of the affected nerve root;
● a **sensory deficit** and irritative sensory phenomena (paresthesia, dysesthesia) in the dermatome of the affected nerve root; in monoradicular lesions, these are easier to bring out by testing with noxious (painful) stimuli, rather than with ordinary somatosensory stimuli;

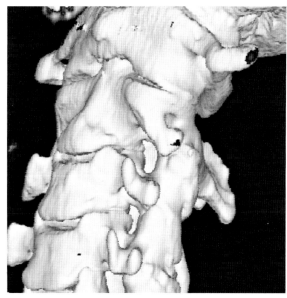

Fig. 12.**2 Stenosis of the left C3/4 intervertebral foramen** (3D CT reconstruction).

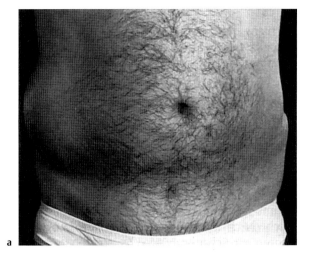

a

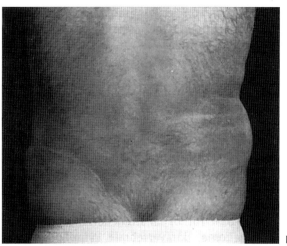

b

Fig. 12.**3 Weakness of the abdominal wall musculature on the right** in a 33-year-old man, 7 months after spinal and pelvic trauma. The muscle weakness is evident both from the front (**a**) and from the back (**b**). The CT scan (**c**) reveals a fracture of the right transverse process of a vertebra, which is the cause of the lesion of the motor spinal nerve roots.

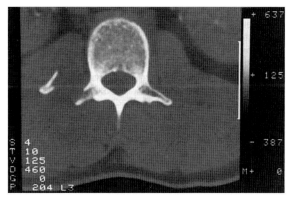

c

12

Diseases of the Spinal Nerve Roots and Peripheral Nerves

- **paresis** of the muscle(s) supplied by the affected nerve root, generally less marked than the paresis caused by a peripheral nerve lesion (no plegia!) because of the polyradicular innervation of most muscles, but possibly severe in the root-indicating muscles;
- **muscle atrophy** is common, but usually less severe than in peripheral nerve lesions, while chronic radicular lesions can, rarely, cause fasciculations;
- **impaired reflexes** in the segment corresponding to the affected nerve root.

The characteristic syndromes of the individual nerve roots supplying the upper and lower limbs are summarized in Table 12.**1**.

Differential diagnosis. Radicular syndromes must be differentiated from lesions in more distal components of the peripheral nervous system (plexuses, peripheral nerves). This can usually be done by careful clinical examination alone, but electromyography may be required for unambiguous confirmation. The *lack of an autonomic deficit* may be a useful clinical criterion in the differential diagnosis of radicular lesions that affect the *limbs*, because sympathetic fibers travel in the spinal nerve roots only at levels T12 through L2 (see above); therefore, an autonomic deficit in a limb always indicates a lesion distal to the nerve root. Some of the conditions that enter into the differential diagnosis of various radicular and peripheral nerve syndromes are listed in Table 12.**1**.

When there is a purely motor deficit, unaccompanied by a sensory deficit or pain, a **lesion of the spinal motor neurons** (e. g., spinal muscular atrophy or amyotrophic lateral sclerosis) should be suspected, rather than a radicular lesion. If the patient complains only of pain radiating into the periphery, in the absence of any demonstrable sensory deficit or weakness, the clinician should think of **pseudoradicular pain** (p. 261) due to mechanical overuse or other pathology of the musculoskeletal apparatus.

Radicular Syndromes Due to Intervertebral Disk Herniation

The proximity of the spinal nerve root to the intervertebral disk at the level of the intervertebral foramen carries with it the danger of root compression by disk herniation. The nerve root can be compressed either by a merely bulging disk or by a disk herniation in the truest sense, i. e., a prolapse of nucleus pulposus material (which is usually soft) through a hole in the annulus fibrosus.

General clinical manifestations. The typical manifestations of acute radiculopathy due to intervertebral disk herniation are the following:
- **local pain** in the corresponding area of the spine, with painful restriction of movement and, sometimes, a compensatory, abnormal posture of the spine (scoliosis, flattening of lordosis).
- usually, after a few hours or days, **radiation of pain** into the cutaneous area of distribution (dermatome) of the affected nerve root.

- **pain on extension** (in the lower limb, a positive Lasègue sign).
- exacerbation of pain by coughing, abdominal pressing (Valsalva maneuvers), and sneezing.
- objectifiable **neurological deficits** (hyporeflexia or areflexia, paresis, sensory deficit, atrophy in the late stage; see above) depending on the severity of the root lesion.

Cervical Disk Herniation

Cervical disk herniation is a common cause of acute torticollis and of acute (cervico) brachialgia.

Etiology. Cervical disk herniation may occur as the result of nuchal trauma, a twisting injury of the cervical spine, an excessively rapid movement, or mechanical overload.

Clinical manifestations. The most commonly affected segments are C6, C7, and C8. *Subjectively*, patients usually complain of pain in the neck and upper limb, and sometimes of a sensory deficit, which does not necessarily cover the entire zone of innervation of the affected root.

Diagnostic evaluation. The *clinical history* and *physical examination* should already enable identification of the affected nerve root. The objectively observable *neurological deficits* are listed in Table 12.**1**. The *Spurling* test can provide further evidence of irritation of a cervical nerve root: the head is leaned backward and the face is turned to the side of the lesion. Carefully titrated axial compression by the examiner's hand may induce pain radiating in a radicular distribution (Fig. 12.**4**). *Imaging studies* (CT and/or MRI) are indispensable for the demonstration of nerve root compression by a herniated intervertebral disk. These are sometimes supplemented by *neurography* (i. e., measurement of nerve conduction velocities) and *electromyography*. One should not forget, however, that a mere disk protrusion without any detectable nerve root compression is a common radiological finding in asymptomatic persons.

Treatment. *Temporary rest* and *physical therapy*, with the addition of appropriate exercises as soon as the patient can tolerate them, usually suffice as treatment. Sufficient *analgesic medication* must also be provided, to prevent the chronification of the pain syndrome through the maintenance of an abnormal, antalgic posture (persistent fixation of the affected spinal segments by muscle spasm) and through nonphysiological stress on other muscle groups. If *operative treatment* is necessary (e. g., because of intractable pain, persistent, severe or progressive paresis, or signs of compression of the spinal cord), then the appropriate treatment is *fenestration* of the intervertebral space at the appropriate level for exposure of the nerve root and disk, widening of the bony intervertebral foramen (*foraminotomy*), then *diskectomy*, and, under some circumstances, *spondylodesis* (fusion) if there is thought to be a risk of spinal instability afterward. Fusion should be performed in such a way as to distract the vertebrae above and below and thereby maintain the patency of the intervertebral foramen.

Lumbar Disk Herniation

Lumbar disk herniation is one of the more common causes of acute low back pain and sciatica. The anatomical relationship of the lumbar roots to the intervertebral disks (both normal and herniated) is shown schematically in Fig. 12.**5**.

Clinical manifestations. A first bout of lumbar disk herniation (and often the first or second recurrence as well) may present with no more than *acute low back pain* (lumbago). The event may be *precipitated* by a relatively banal movement in the wrong direction; in particular, the lumbar spine may suddenly freeze in a twisted position as the unfortunate individual attempts to lift a heavy load while the upper body is turned to one side. Any further movement of the lumbar spine is blocked by muscle spasm, a reflex response to the pain. Even the smallest movement is painful, as are coughing and abdominal pressing (Valsalva maneuvers). The pain usually resolves after a few days of bed rest. It is usually only when the herniation recurs later that the patient experiences pain radiating into the leg, i. e., *sciatica*, and possibly in combination with typical *radicular neurological deficits*.

In our experience, *motor deficits* generally arise only later in the course of this syndrome. The patient must be examined carefully to determine whether a deficit is present. The L5 root is most commonly affected, usually by an L4–5 disk herniation, and the S1 root is the next most commonly affected after that, usually by an L5–S1 disk herniation. The corresponding clinical findings are listed in Table 12.**1**.

Diagnostic evaluation. As in cervical disk herniation, the level of the nerve root that is affected can generally be determined from the pattern of referred pain and any motor, sensory, and reflex deficits that may be present. The peripheral nerve trunk containing the axons whose more proximal portions are located in the affected root is often sensitive to pressure (at the *Valleix pressure points*) and stretching of the nerve is often painful. The latter can be tested by passive raising of the supine patient's leg, extended at the knee (the *Lasègue test*). Pain caused by elevation of the leg on the side opposite the sciatica (the *crossed Lasègue sign*) usually indicates a large, prolapsed disk herniation. If a higher lumbar root (L3 or L4) is affected, one should look for the reverse Lasègue sign, i. e., test for pain on *extension* of the leg in the *prone* patient, which stretches the femoral n. rather than the sciatic n. (*reverse Lasègue test*). If the herniation is lateral or extraforaminal, pain will also be inducible by lateral bending of the trunk.

Imaging studies are not absolutely essential if the clinical picture is sufficiently characteristic, but they should be performed if there is any doubt as to the etiology of nerve root compression, or if the situation requires operative intervention. *CT* is the method of choice if the segmental level of the suspected disk herniation is clinically unambiguous; the main advantage of CT is that it can clearly demonstrate a far lateral disk herniation, if this turns out to be present (Fig. 12.**6**). It can also reveal bony deformities of the spinal canal and nerve root impingement by spondylotic changes, if present

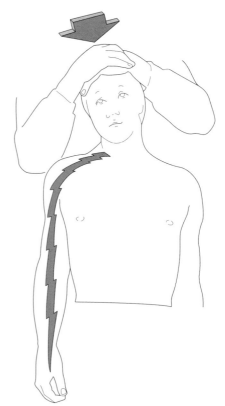

Fig. 12.**4 Spurling cervical compression test** for the provocation of radicular pain in cervical disk herniation (after Mumenthaler M.: *Der Schulter–Arm–Schmerz*, 2nd edn, Huber, Bern 1982.) Pain can often be elicited by reclination and rotation of the head toward the affected side even without compression.

(Fig. 12.**7**). MRI is to be preferred over CT, however, if the level of the lesion is not fully clear on clinical grounds. The images should always be interpreted critically and in consideration of the associated clinical findings.

Neurography and electromyography are sometimes worth performing as supplementary tests.

Treatment. The initial treatment is *conservative* in practically all patients and is along the same lines as described above for cervical disk herniation. *Operative* treatment should be considered only if conservative treatment fails.

An incipient *cauda equina syndrome* (bladder and bowel dysfunction, saddle hypesthesia, bilateral pareses, and impairment of the anal reflex, cf. p. 144) is an absolute indication for urgent surgery.

> **!** When the clinical signs of cauda equina syndrome are present because of lumbar intervertebral disk herniation, an emergency neurosurgical procedure must be performed immediately.

Further indications for operative treatment are set forth in Fig. 12.**8**. At operation, the *herniated disk tissue is removed*, and, if there is a danger of postoperative instability at the level being operated on, a fusion (*spondylodesis*) is performed as well. This is more likely to be the

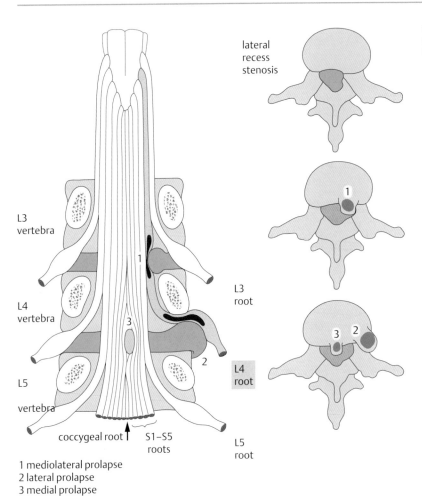

Fig. 12.**5 Anatomical relationships of the lumbar intervertebral disks to the exiting nerve roots.**

L3 vertebra

L4 vertebra

L5 vertebra

lateral recess stenosis

L3 root

L4 root

L5 root

coccygeal root

S1–S5 roots

1 mediolateral prolapse
2 lateral prolapse
3 medial prolapse

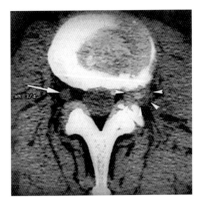

Fig. 12.**6 Lateral L3/4 disk herniation** (arrowheads), CT image. The normal spinal ganglion on the right side is visible in the intervertebral foramen (arrow).

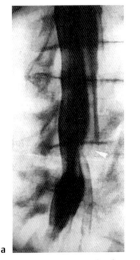

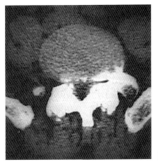

Fig. 12.**7 Left S1 radicular compression** in a 40-year-old man. **Myelography** (**a**) reveals a broadened and shortened left S1 nerve root (arrowhead) and an indentation of the dural sack from the right at this level. **CT** (**b**) reveals high-grade spondyloarthrosis and bilateral stenosis of the lateral recesses.

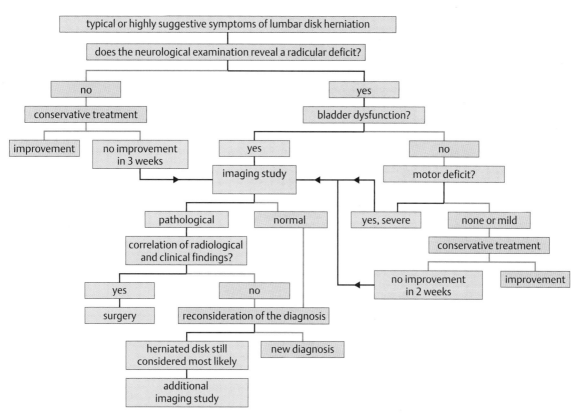

Fig. 12.**8 Diagnostic and therapeutic flowchart in lumbar disk herniation.**

case in older patients and when the intervertebral disk degeneration is very advanced. As in cervical disk procedures, spondylodesis must be performed in such a way as to keep the vertebral bodies above and below the disk a sufficient distance apart (in distraction), so that *the intervertebral foramina are held open.*

Radicular Syndromes Due to Spinal Stenosis

Slowly progressive mechanical compression of the intraspinal neural structures is usually seen in older patients in whom congenital narrowness of spinal canal has been accentuated by further, progressive, degenerative osteochondrotic and reactive-spondylogenic changes.

Cervical Spinal Stenosis

A narrow cervical spinal canal can compress not only the cervical nerve roots, but also the spinal cord itself, producing a myelopathy. **Cervical spondylogenic myelopathy** is discussed in detail above on p. 147.

Lumbar Spinal Stenosis

For anatomical reasons, a narrow lumbar spinal canal causes an entirely different clinical syndrome than cervical spinal stenosis:

Clinical manifestations. In addition to low back pain, which is usually chronic, **neurogenic intermittent claudication** is the most characteristic symptom: as the patient walks, sciatica-like pain arises on the posterior aspect of one or, usually, both lower limbs and then becomes progressively severe. The pain appears earlier if the patient is walking downhill, because of the additional lumbar lordosis that downhill walking induces. This historical feature differentiates neurogenic from vasogenic intermittent claudication, in which the pain tends to be more severe when the patient walks uphill. A further differentiating feature of neurogenic, as opposed to vasogenic, intermittent claudication is that standing still will not, by itself, cause the pain to go away. The patient must additionally bend forward, sit down, or crouch—these maneuvers induce kyphosis of the lumbar spine and thereby decompress its neural contents.

Diagnostic evaluation. Nowadays, the definitive diagnostic study is *MRI*, though radiculography and myelographic CT are still sometimes needed (Fig. 12.**9**).

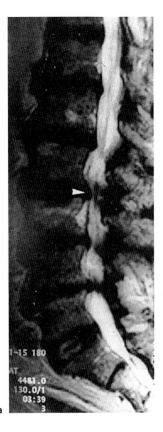
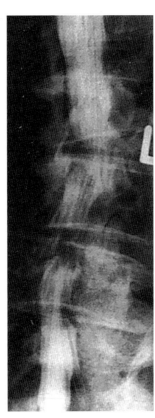

a   b

Fig. 12.**9 Lumbar disk herniation** in a 70-year-old man with neurogenic intermittent claudication due to degenerative lumbar spinal canal stenosis. The MRI (**a**) and myelogram (**b**) reveal compression of the dural sac and the nerve roots at the L2–3 (arrow) and L3–4 disk levels, as well as at L4–5 (less severe).

Treatment. If the symptoms are very severe, and the neurological deficits are progressive, then a treatment option to be considered is *operative decompression* of the affected segments by opening of the narrowed lateral recesses, possibly in combination with a stabilizing spondylodesis (fusion).

Radicular Syndromes Due to Space-Occupying Lesions

The term "space-occupying lesion," in its narrowest sense, refers to a **tumor**. *Neurinoma* (Fig. 12.**10**) and *meningioma* are the most common types of intraspinal

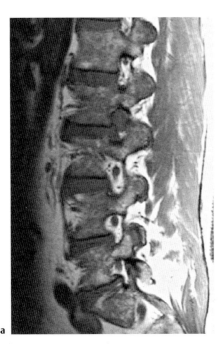
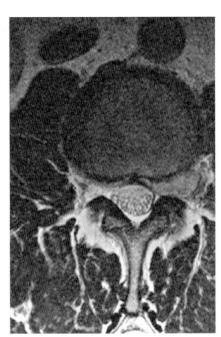

a   b

Fig. 12.**10 Nerve root neurinoma filling the left L3/4 intervertebral foramen** (MR images). Normal nerve roots, free of compression, are seen in the intervertebral foramina above and below the level of the lesion (**a**). The axial section (**b**) reveals an hourglass-shaped neurinoma, lying partly within and partly outside the spinal canal.

primary tumor, while *ependymoma* (Fig. 12.**11**), *glioma* (usually astrocytoma), and *vascular tumors* are rarer. Nerve root lesions can also be caused by a *primary destructive process* affecting a spinal vertebra (Fig. 12.**12**), particularly *metastatic carcinoma*. Finally, **infectious and inflammatory processes** of the vertebrae and intervertebral disks (e. g., spondylodiscitis), as well as **spinal abscesses and empyema**, can cause radicular or spinal cord compression.

Clinical manifestations. The patient usually complains of pain radiating into the periphery; if the lesion is at a thoracic level, the pain tends to be in a bandlike distribution around the chest. Motor or sensory deficits may also be clinically detectable, depending on the level of the lesion. A space-occupying lesion within the lower lumbar canal can produce cauda equina syndrome, which may be of greater or lesser severity.

Diagnostic evaluation. *Imaging studies* are indispensable for diagnosis. If the underlying lesion is a nerve root neurinoma, plain films may already reveal the characteristic, widened intervertebral foramen, e. g., in the cervical region (Fig. 12.**13**). Nonetheless, CT or MRI (Fig. 12.**14**) is always necessary to demonstrate the full extent of the tumor.

Treatment. *Operative treatment* (resection of the lesion) is needed in most patients. Depending on the underlying illness, further treatment may be required (radiotherapy, antineoplastic chemotherapy, or antibiotics after the removal of an abscess or empyema).

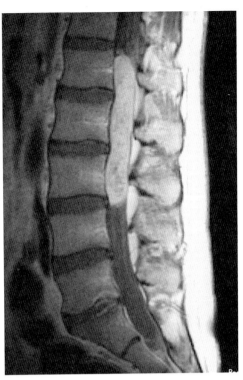

Fig. 12.**11** Sausage-shaped **cystic ependymoma** filling the spinal canal from L1 to L3 and compressing the cauda equina (MR image).

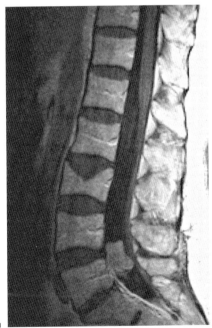

a

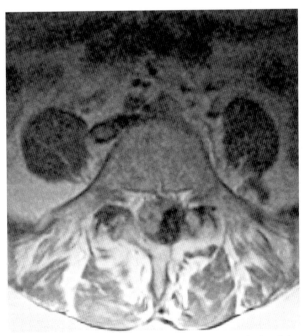

b

Fig. 12.**12** **Metastatic melanoma** in the lumbosacral spinal canal, 8 years after resection of the primary tumor: sagittal (**a**) and axial (**b**) MR images. The patient presented with cauda equina syndrome. The nerve roots of the cauda equina are displaced dorsally and to the left by the compressive lesion.

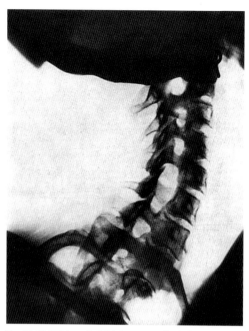

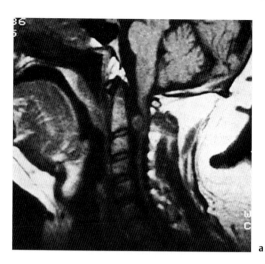

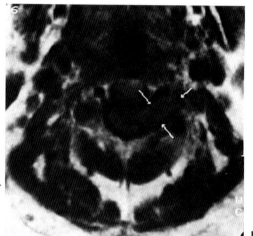

Fig. 12.**13 Widened C5/6 intervertebral foramen** caused by a neurinoma of the C6 root. The C5/6 foramen has opened up into the C6/7 foramen below it.

Fig. 12.**14 Left C3 root neurinoma.** The sagittal MR image (**a**) ▷ reveals a compressive lesion anterior to the spinal cord. The axial image (**b**) shows the deformed cervical spinal cord posterior to the dens. The arrows indicate the left C3 root, which is expanded by the tumor.

Peripheral Nerve Lesions

Fundamentals

When we speak here of the "peripheral nerves," we are referring to the **nerve plexuses** formed by the junction and regrouping of fibers derived from the spinal nerve roots, as well as to the more distally lying **peripheral nerve trunks and branches**. The plexuses always contain **mixed fiber types** and the peripheral nerve trunks nearly always do, i. e., somatic motor, somatosensory, and often also autonomic (particularly sympathetic) fibers. The individual peripheral nerve trunks bear an anatomically invariant relationship to the muscles and cutaneous zones that they innervate. This pattern of innervation is fundamentally different from that of the spinal nerve roots, because, as we recall, the nerve root fibers undergo reassortment in the plexuses. This fact enables the clinical examiner to distinguish a peripheral nerve lesion from a radicular lesion based on the observed pattern of neurological deficits. The main clinical manifestations of peripheral nerve lesions are **marked paresis, extensive sensory deficits**, and **diminished sweating** in the zone of innervation of the affected nerve or nerve branch. Pain can be produced by either a radicular lesion or a peripheral nerve lesion and is thus not a distinguishing feature of either.

Preliminary anatomical remarks. A peripheral nerve is a cablelike bundle of **nerve fibers** of different functional types (see p. 3). The nerve fiber is the smallest "building block" of a peripheral nerve; it consists of an axon and an encasing myelin sheath (if present), which is the membrane of a Schwann cell wrapped around the axon numerous times. Individual nerve fibers are surrounded by a delicate connective tissue called **endoneurium**. The nerve fibers and the endoneurium are then bundled together into larger fascicles, each of which is surrounded by a tough **perineurium**. Along the length of the nerve, the individual fascicles make many plexus-like interconnections with one another; they are held together as a single peripheral nerve by an encompassing layer of epineurium. The epineurium is not a tough husk around the nerve, but rather a loose, lipid-rich layer of connective tissue, reinforced by transversely and longitudinally oriented collagen fibers. It contains not only the nerve fascicles, but also the *vasa nervorum*. The nerve trunks are fixed to the adjacent connective tissue at only a few points, at which they are especially vulnerable to mechanical damage. Larger nerve trunks are often found together with arteries and veins in so-called **neurovascular bundles** surrounded by a common connective tissue sheath. These bundles form an anatomical unit that is clearly demarcated from the surrounding structures.

Causes of peripheral nerve lesions. Most lesions of the nerve plexuses or the peripheral nerve trunks are either **traumatic** (caused by excessive traction, stab wounds, cuts, bony fractures, etc.), or else due to **prolonged compression**, which may occur through *external influences*, at *anatomical bottlenecks*, or because of *space-occupying lesions* in the vicinity of the nerve (especially tumors and hematomas). Less commonly, plexus and nerve lesions can be caused by **infection and/or inflammation**, e. g., neuralgic shoulder amyotrophy, which is probably an autoimmune disorder affecting the brachial plexus (p. 222). Nearly all lesions affecting a single peripheral nerve trunk or branch (*mononeuropathy*) are of mechanical origin; in contrast, most polyneuropathies (cf. Chapter 10) are of toxic, infectious/inflammatory, or paraneoplastic origin.

General clinical manifestations of peripheral nerve lesions. Depending on the particular segment of plexus or peripheral nerve trunk/branch that is affected, there may be a motor, sensory, autonomic, or (usually) mixed neurological deficit:

- **flaccid paresis** of the muscle(s) innervated by the affected nerve;
- usually marked **atrophy** of the affected muscle(s);
- the corresponding **reflex deficits**;
- **diminished sensation** and possibly also **pain and paresthesia** in the cutaneous area innervated by the nerve, though the pain is often felt beyond this area as well; all sensory modalities are affected to a comparable extent; in contrast to a radicular lesion, the affected area of skin is more easily demarcated by testing the sense of touch than by testing nociception;
- because the sudomotor fibers travel together with the somatosensory components of the peripheral nerves, **diminished sweating** is often found in the hypesthetic area of skin and autonomic abnormalities of other kinds may also be present in the distribution of the affected nerve; radicular lesions affecting the limbs, in contrast, generally leave sweating intact (an important criterion for differential diagnosis);
- fasciculations only in exceptional cases; these are much more common in anterior horn disease.

Grades of severity of peripheral nerve lesions. A peripheral nerve can be damaged more or less severely, with corresponding implications for treatment and prognosis. The traditional, clinically useful threefold distinction is as follows:

- **Neurapraxia:** the nerve is dysfunctional, but its anatomical components are still in continuity (e. g., nerve dysfunction due to pressure on the nerve when the individual has slept for a prolonged period in an unusual posture); the functional deficit is completely reversible.
- **Axonotmesis:** the axons within the nerve are interrupted, but the external structure of the nerve and its internal connective tissue sheaths remain intact; the full clinical picture of a peripheral nerve lesion results; under optimal conditions, full recovery may still be possible.
- **Neurotmesis:** the axons and all surrounding structures are interrupted and the nerve is no longer in continuity (e. g., because of tearing or sharp transection of the nerve); a surgical procedure is needed to restore nerve integrity and the prognosis for recovery is uncertain.

Diseases of the Brachial Plexus

Anatomy of the brachial plexus. In the brachial plexus, the axons derived from the nerve roots of C4 to T1 (or T2) are regrouped and distributed to the various nerves that innervate the upper limb (Fig. 12.**15**). The brachial plexus passes through three anatomical bottlenecks on its way to the upper arm; the first two are the *scalene hiatus*, where it is accompanied by the subclavian a., and the *costoclavicular space* between the first rib and the clavicle. At this location, the caudal portion of the plexus is in close proximity to the apex of the lung. A bit further distally, the brachial plexus is covered by the pectoralis minor m., which originates from the *coracoid process* of the scapula, and it can be compressed at this location when the arm is elevated. These bottlenecks are sketched in Fig. 12.**16**.

General clinical manifestations of brachial plexus lesions. The complex structure of the brachial plexus and the redistribution of individual radicular elements within it make it very difficult to localize brachial plexus lesions exactly based on the neurological findings alone. Nonetheless, detailed functional testing of the affected muscles can reveal the root levels that are involved and this, in turn, permits localization of the lesion within the plexus with a fair degree of precision. The information provided in Fig. 12.**17** will be helpful in this regard.

Classification of brachial plexus lesions. In addition to total paralysis of the entire upper limb, there are three types of partial lesion in the customary, **topically oriented** classification, namely, upper and lower brachial plexus lesions and C7 lesions. An alternative (or additional) classification is by **etiology**: traumatic, compressive, or infectious/inflammatory.

Topical Classification of Brachial Plexus Lesions

Upper brachial plexus lesion (Erb–Duchenne palsy). This type of lesion involves the fibers originating in the C5 and C6 nerve roots. The affected muscles are the abductors and external rotators of the shoulder joint, the flexor muscles of the upper arm, the supinator m., and

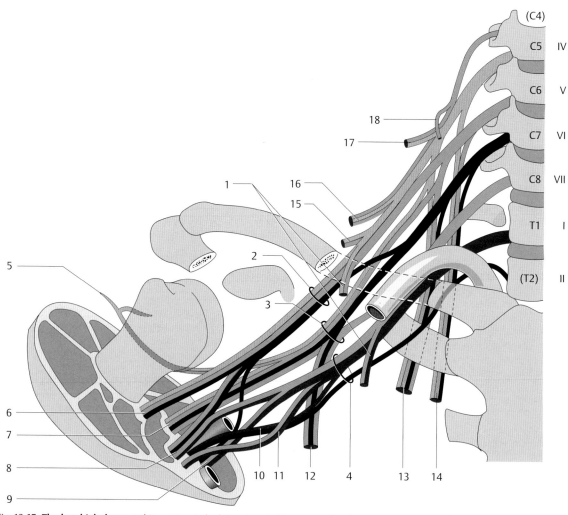

Fig. 12.15 The brachial plexus and its anatomical relationships to the surrounding bony structures.

1   **pectoral nn.** (med./lat.) C5–T1
     pectoralis major & minor mm.
2   lateral cord
3   dorsal (posterior) cord
4   medial cord
5   **axillary n.** C5, 6
     deltoid m. C5, 6
     teres minor m. C5, 6
6   **musculocutaneous n.** C5–7
     biceps brachii m. C5, 6
     coracobrachialis m. C6, 7
     brachialis m. C5, 6
7   **radial n.** C5–T1
     triceps brachii m. C7–T1
     anconeus m. C7, 8
     brachioradialis m. C5, 6
     extensor carpi rad. long./brev. mm. C6–8
     extensor digit. m. C7, 8
     extensor indicis m. C7, 8
     extensor digiti minimi m. C7, 8

ext. poll. long./brev. mm. C7, 8
abd. poll. long. m. C7, 8
8   **median n.** C5–T1
     pronator teres m. C6, 7
     flexor carpi radialis m. C6–8
     palmaris longus m. C7, 8
     flexor digit. superf. m. C7–T1
     flexor digit. prof. m. (radial side, II/III)
     C7–T1
     pronator quadratus m. C7–T1
     opponens pollicis m. C7, 8
     abductor poll. brev. m. C7, 8
     superf. head of flex. poll. brev. m. C6–8
     lumbrical mm. I & II C8–T1
9   **ulnar n.** (C7) C8–T1
     flexor carpi uln. m. C8–T1
     flexor digit. prof. m. (ulnar side, IV/V)
     C8–T1
     palm./dors. interossei mm. C8–T1
     lumbrical mm. III & IV C8–T1
     adductor pollicis m. C8–T1

deep head of flex. poll. brev. m. C8–T1
palmaris brevis m. C8–T1
10   **medial brachial cutaneous n.** C8–T1
11   **medial antebrachial cutaneous n.**
     C8–T1
12   **thoracodorsal n.** C6–8
     latissimus dorsi m.
13   **subscapular nn.** C5–8
     subscapular m. C5–7
     teres major m. C5–6
14   **long thoracic n.** C5–7
     serratus anterior m.
15   **nerve to the subclavius m.** C5, 6
     subclavius m.
16   **suprascapular n.** C4–6
     supraspinatus m. C4–6
     infraspinatus m. C4–6
17   **dorsal scapular n.** C3–5
     levator scapulae m. C4–6
     rhomboid mm. C4–6
18   **phrenic n.** C3, 4

Fig. 12.**16 Anatomical bottlenecks in the shoulder region,** at which nerves and/or blood vessels can be compressed.

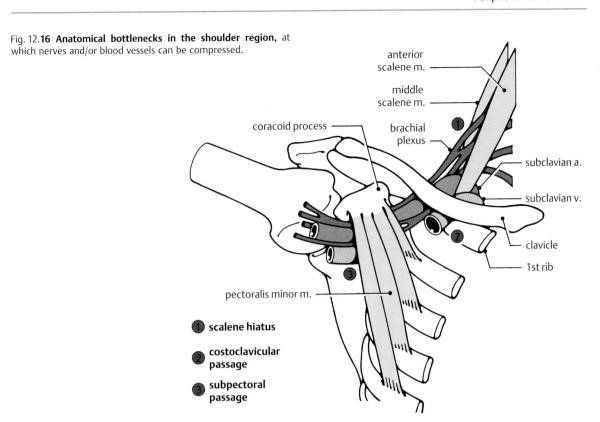

Diseases of the Spinal Nerve Roots and Peripheral Nerves

12

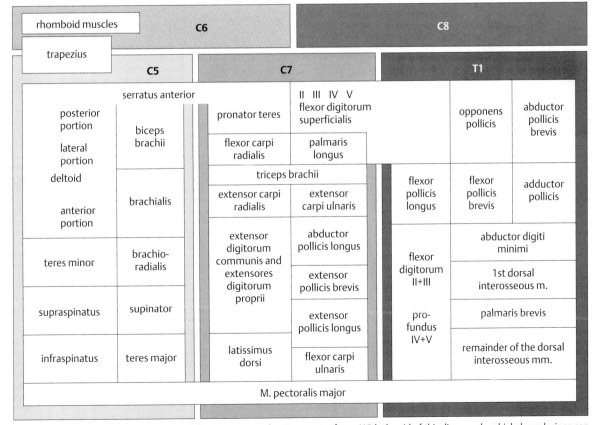

Fig. 12.**17 Muscles of the upper limb and the nerve roots that innervate them.** With the aid of this diagram, brachial plexus lesions can be localized from the pattern of muscle weakness that they cause.

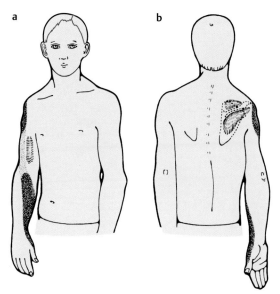

Fig. 12.**18 Upper limb posture and sensory deficit in right upper brachial plexus palsy** (diagram). The deltoid, biceps, and supra- and infraspinatus mm. are atrophic, the arm is internally rotated, and the palm of the hand points posteriorly.

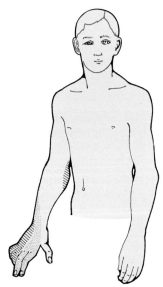

Fig. 12.**19 Upper limb posture and sensory deficit in right lower brachial plexus palsy** (diagram). The intrinsic muscles of the hand are atrophic, the sensory deficit corresponds to the C7 and C8 dermatomes, and there is an accompanying Horner syndrome.

sometimes the elbow extensors and the extensors of the hand. A sensory deficit is not necessarily present; if there is one, it is located in the area of the shoulder, on the outer surface of the upper arm, or on the radial edge of the forearm (Fig. 12.**18**).

Lower brachial plexus lesion (*Dejerine–Klumpke palsy*). This type of lesion involves the fibers originating in the C8 and T1 roots. Its prominent findings include weakness of the intrinsic muscles of the hand, some-

times also of the long flexors of the fingers, and rarely of the wrist flexors. The triceps brachii m. usually remains intact. The mechanism of the precipitating accident, and the anatomical relationships in this area, often lead to an accompanying dysfunction of the cervical sympathetic supply, resulting in Horner syndrome with impaired sweating. On the basis of these findings, a lesion of the T1 root is presumed to be present, proximal to the origin of its branch to the sympathetic chain. There is always a sensory deficit involving the ulnar edge of the forearm, hand, and fingers (Fig. 12.**19**).

C7 palsy. In the present context, we are speaking not of a lesion of the C7 root itself, but rather of the fibers derived from it that make up the C7 portion of the brachial plexus. This type of palsy involves deficits in the distribution of the radial n. (p. 226), while the function of the brachioradialis m. is preserved.

Etiologic Classification of Brachial Plexus Lesions

Traumatic Lesions

Traumatic lesions of the brachial plexus are usually due to motor vehicle accidents; rarer causes include occupational injury and direct stab or gunshot wounds. The initial clinical finding is not uncommonly a total upper limb paralysis (Fig. 12.**20**), which may later improve until it resembles one of the types of localized brachial plexus lesion described above. The *prognosis* is generally better for upper brachial plexus lesions; bloody CSF obtainable by lumbar puncture and, later, clinical evidence of myelopathy are poor prognostic signs indicating probable nerve root avulsion. In such patients, MRI may reveal empty nerve root pouches (Fig. 12.**21**). The *treatment* consists of the fitting of an abduction splint and the performance of passive exercises to prevent freezing of the shoulder joint. Brachial plexus surgery is highly complex and demanding and is occasionally resorted to in cases of upper brachial plexus injury.

Brachial plexus palsy caused by trauma during delivery is the result of obstetrical complications, such as breech delivery. When the damaged axons regenerate, they may reconnect to the "wrong" muscles and/or muscle groups, leading to pathological accessory movements and abnormal motor patterns.

Compressive Lesions of the Brachial Plexus

External compression can injure the brachial plexus in persons who carry heavy loads on their shoulders or wear heavy *backpacks*. Lesions of this type usually affect the upper brachial plexus and sometimes only individual branches of it. The long thoracic n. is most frequently involved (p. 224).

Compression at anatomical bottlenecks. The collective designation **"thoracic outlet syndrome" (TOS)** is commonly used for these conditions, usually in nonspecific fashion, and often, unfortunately, as a vague term for brachialgia of as yet undetermined origin, or for other unexplained symptoms relating to the brachial plexus. **Scalene syndrome** is usually due to the

Fig. 12.**20 Complete right brachial plexus palsy.** Atrophy of all muscles of the upper limb, internal rotation of the arm.

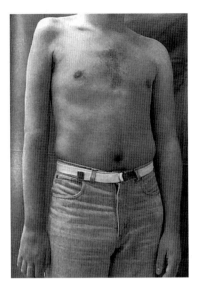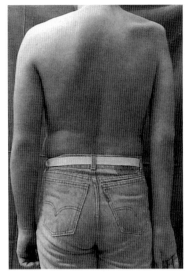

anomalous presence of a **cervical rib**, a fibrous band (which may be visible in a CT scan), or some other type of structural anomaly in the scalene hiatus. The typical manifestations of scalene syndrome include: clinical evidence of a lower brachial plexus lesion, worsening of symptoms on lowering of the arm, and fixed or motion-induced circulatory insufficiency of the subclavian a. (as revealed by a vascular bruit, and/or by disappearance of the radial pulse when certain maneuvers are performed, e.g., the Adson maneuver—turning the chin to the side of the lesion, with simultaneous backward bending of the head).

Costoclavicular syndrome. This syndrome, like the scalene syndrome, should be diagnosed only if a causative anatomical anomaly and objectifiable neurological deficits (usually, a lower brachial plexus palsy) can be found. An arteriogram is occasionally helpful in establishing the diagnosis, as it may demonstrate motion-dependent compression of the subclavian artery or vein (Fig. 12.**22**).

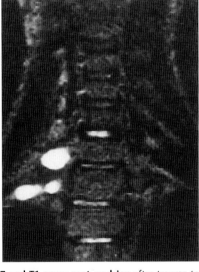

Fig. 12.**21 Right C7 and T1 nerve root avulsion** after trauma to the brachial plexus. The T2-weighted coronal MR image reveals the empty nerve root sleeves containing only cerebrospinal fluid.

Fig. 12.**22 Costoclavicular syndrome** in a 24-year-old patient with clinical evidence of a lower brachial plexus lesion. An arteriogram of the brachial a. reveals free passage of contrast medium (**a**) when the arm is dependent. When the arm is elevated, however, (**b**) the subclavian a. is compressed between the clavicle and the first rib.

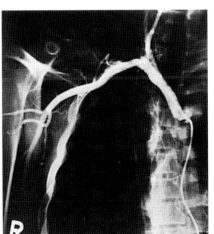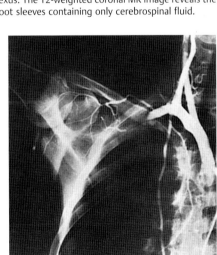

a   b

Treatment of compression syndromes. Both the scalene syndrome and costoclavicular syndrome should be treated conservatively at first, once their diagnosis has been definitively established. Special exercises are used to strengthen the shoulder-elevating muscles. Surgical treatment is reserved for the small minority of patients with objectifiable, severe neurological deficits. A supra- or transclavicular approach gives the surgeon optimal access to the anatomical structures.

Neuralgic Shoulder Amyotrophy

Pathogenesis. This disorder is presumed to be due to an inflammatory/allergic affection of the brachial plexus. It usually arises spontaneously, but is sometimes seen in the aftermath of an infectious disease, or after the administration of serum (brachial plexus neuritis).

Clinical manifestations. This disease affects men more often than women and is usually located in the right arm. It always begins with intense local pain in the shoulder, which generally lasts for a few days. Rarely, the pain will persist at a milder intensity for a longer period. Once the pain subsides, motor weakness of the muscles of the shoulder girdle and/or of the arm develops. The weakness can, in principle, affect any muscle group of the upper limb, but it tends to affect the muscles innervated by the upper portion of the brachial plexus. Paresis of the serratus anterior m. is particularly common. There may be no objectifiable sensory deficit.

Treatment. No specific treatment is required beyond analgesic medication in the initial, painful phase.

Prognosis. The prognosis is generally good, but it may take many months for the weakness to resolve completely.

Other Causes of Brachial Plexus Lesions

Radiation-induced brachial plexus lesions usually appear with a *latency* of one or more years after radiotherapy, usually in women who have been treated with surgery and radiotherapy for breast cancer. In 15% of patients, *pain* is the main symptom; it can increase over the course of several years. The *differentiation* of radiation-induced brachial plexopathy from a recurrent malignant tumor is not always easy; a short interval between the completion of radiotherapy and the onset of pain (except when a very high radiation dose was given) and very intense pain, both tend to suggest a recurrent tumor rather than radiation injury as the cause. Imaging studies are helpful, but even these cannot always reliably distinguish scarring from new tumor tissue.

Pancoast tumors of the apex of the lung usually cause a lower brachial plexus palsy accompanied by severe pain. The sympathetic chain is usually involved as well; thus, Horner syndrome and diminished sweating in the upper body on the affected side are typical findings (Fig. 12.**23**).

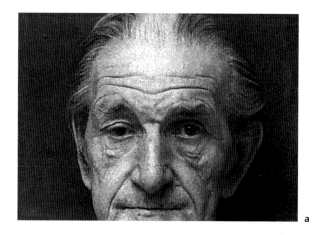

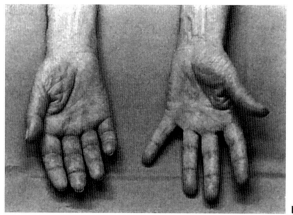

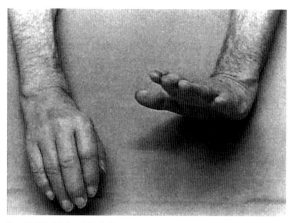

Fig. 12.**23 Right-sided Pancoast tumor** in a 68-year-old man. There is clinical evidence of compression of the lower brachial plexus and of the sympathetic chain. **a** Right Horner syndrome. **b** Atrophy of the intrinsic muscles of the right hand, especially the thenar muscles. **c** Weakness of the wrist and finger extensors on the right.

Other causes of brachial plexus palsy, some of which are very rare, are usually diagnosable only by the specialist: acute palsy due to *occlusion of a small artery supplying the plexus*, after *medical procedures*, in *heroin addicts*, in *familial brachial plexus neuritis*, *parainfectious* and *serogenic forms*, etc.

Differential Diagnosis of Brachial Plexus Lesions

A precise clinical and, if necessary, electrophysiological examination of the patient should always permit a reliable differentiation between brachial plexus lesions and lesions affecting *multiple nerve roots* or a *peripheral nerve*. Experience suggests, however, that it is not always easy to distinguish a lower brachial plexus lesion (affecting fibers derived from C8 and T1) from an ulnar nerve lesion (p. 231). The same can be said for the distinction between a (traumatic) upper brachial plexus lesion and a lesion of the axillary n. or a rotator cuff injury.

Diseases of the Peripheral Nerves of the Upper Limbs

Suprascapular N. (C4–C6)

Anatomy. This nerve innervates the *supraspinatus and infraspinatus mm.* It reaches them after passing through the scapular notch and then running dorsally. It receives sensory branches from the shoulder joint, but not from the skin.

Typical deficits. A lesion of the suprascapular n. produces weakness and atrophy of the two muscles on the dorsal surface of the scapula (Fig. 12.**24**). The first 15° of lateral elevation of the arm are weak (supraspinatus m.), as is external rotation of the arm at the shoulder joint (infraspinatus m.) (Fig. 12.**25**).

Causes. Overuse of the arm can lead to mechanical compromise of the nerve in the scapular notch. Other causes include trauma and a ganglion lying in the notch.

Axillary N. (C5–C6)

Anatomy. This nerve provides motor innervation to the *deltoid* and *teres minor mm.* and sensory innervation to a palm-sized patch of skin on the proximal, lateral surface of the upper arm (*superior lateral brachial cutaneous n.*) (Fig. 12.**26**).

Typical deficits. Axillary nerve palsy manifests itself as marked weakness of lateral abduction and forward elevation of the arm. The normal roundness of the shoulder is flattened. External rotation of the arm at the shoulder joint is lessened at rest, so that the dependent arm is held in mild internal rotation (Fig. 12.**27**).

Causes. The most common cause of axillary n. palsy is *dislocation of the shoulder* (forward and downward). The prognosis in such patients is favorable.

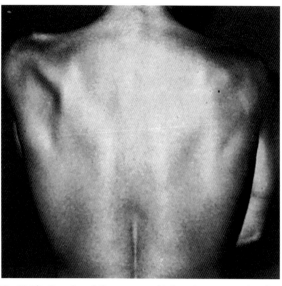

Fig. 12.**24 Atrophy of the supra and infraspinatus muscles due to a lesion of the left suprascapular n.** in a 25-year old man. The etiology remained unclear in this case.

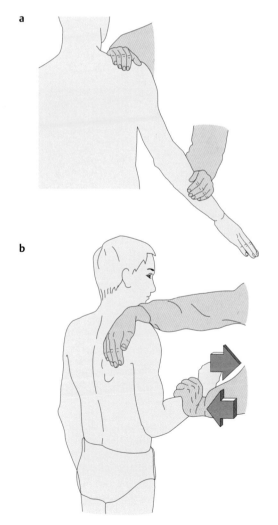

Fig. 12.**25 Testing of the muscles innervated by the suprascapular n. a** Weakness of the supraspinatus m. is most evident in the first 15° of lateral elevation of the arm. **b** Weakness of the infraspinatus m. is evident when the arm is externally rotated at the shoulder joint.

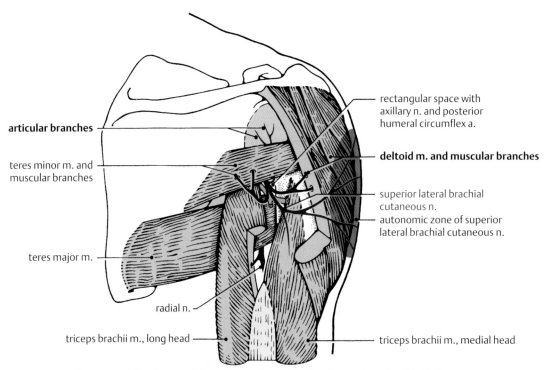

articular branches

teres minor m. and
muscular branches

teres major m.

radial n.

triceps brachii m., long head

rectangular space with
axillary n. and posterior
humeral circumflex a.

deltoid m. and muscular branches

superior lateral brachial
cutaneous n.
autonomic zone of superior
lateral brachial cutaneous n.

triceps brachii m., medial head

Fig. 12.**26 Anatomical course and distribution of the axillary n.** Sensory (red) and motor branches (black). The autonomous sensory area of the superior lateral brachial cutaneous n. is shaded in red.

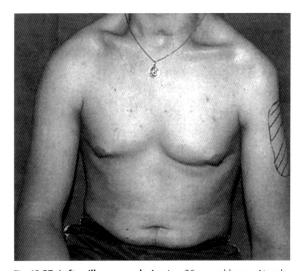

Fig. 12.**27 Left axillary nerve lesion** in a 26-year-old man. Atrophy of the left deltoid m. with "pointed" shoulder contour. The sensory deficit in the territory of the superior lateral brachial cutaneous n. is indicated.

Differential diagnosis of axillary nerve palsy includes complex *brachial plexus lesions* affecting the upper portion of the plexus, *rotator cuff lesions*, and restriction of movement by pain in *humeroscapular periarthropathy*.

Long Thoracic N. (C5–C7)

Anatomy. This nerve is the longest branch of the brachial plexus. It is a purely motor nerve supplying the *serratus anterior m.*

Typical deficits. A long thoracic nerve palsy causes winging of the scapula, which is particularly evident when the arms are held high, or when the patient extends the arms and presses with the palms of the hands against a wall (Fig. 12.**28**).

Causes. Lesions of the long thoracic n. are usually due to *excessive mechanical strain on the shoulder* (carrying heavy loads) or to *neuralgic shoulder amyotrophy* (p. 222). Cryptogenic cases also occur.

Musculocutaneous N. (C5–C7)

Anatomy. This nerve innervates the *biceps brachii and coracobrachialis mm.* and a portion of the *brachialis m.* Its sensory terminal branch, the *lateral antebrachial cutaneous n.*, innervates the skin on the radial side of the forearm (Fig. 12.**29**).

Typical deficits. Lesions of the musculocutaneous n. cause marked weakness of elbow flexion. This must be tested with the forearm in the supinated position, because, if the forearm is pronated or in neutral position, the elbow can still be flexed by the powerful brachioradialis m., which is innervated by the radial n.

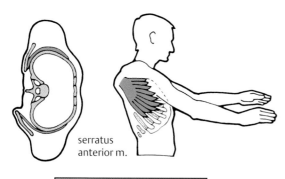

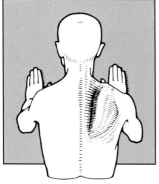

serratus
anterior m.

Fig. 12.**28 Lesion of the right long thoracic n.** Weakness of the serratus anterior m. causes winging of the scapula, which is particularly evident when the patient extends the arms forward and pushes against a wall.

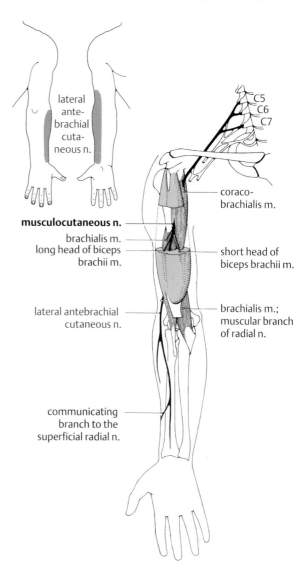

Fig. 12.**29 Anatomical course and distribution of the musculocutaneous n.**

Causes. The usual cause is *trauma*, in which case further signs of an upper brachial plexus lesion may be present. *Cryptogenic* lesions of the musculocutaneous n. and palsy of this nerve in the setting of *neuralgic shoulder amyotrophy*, are rarer events.

Differential diagnosis. *A tear of the long tendon of the biceps brachialis m.* only rarely causes weakness of elbow flexion when the forearm is held in the supinated position. This condition is easy to differentiate from musculocutaneous nerve palsy for two further reasons: one is the typical appearance of the belly of the muscle on the volar surface of the forearm; the other is the absence of a sensory deficit.

Radial N. (C5–C8)

Anatomy. The anatomy of the radial n. is depicted in Fig. 12.30. It provides motor innervation to the *triceps brachii, brachioradialis,* and *supinator mm.,* as well as all of the *extensors of the wrist, thumb, and finger joints.* Its sensory innervation is to the dorsal skin of the upper arm and forearm as well as the dorsum of the hand, with an autonomic zone located between the first and second metacarpal bones.

Typical deficits. The clinical manifestations of radial nerve palsy depend on the level of the lesion:
- **Lesion in the upper arm:** the radial n. is particularly vulnerable to injury in the radial nerve canal of the humerus, because it lies directly on the bone at this location. The corresponding, readily apparent neuro-

logical deficit is a **wrist drop** (Fig. 12.31), attributable to loss of action of the wrist and finger extensors. In addition, sensation is diminished on the radial portion of the dorsum of the hand.
- **"High radial nerve lesion":** if the nerve is injured more proximally in the upper arm or in the axilla, the triceps brachii m. is also weak and the elbow can no longer be actively extended against resistance.
- **Supinator canal syndrome:** if the radial n. is compromised at the site of its passage through the supinator m., only its deeply penetrating *motor terminal branch* is affected. The resulting deficit is purely motor. The branch to the extensor carpi radialis m. and the brachioradialis m., which leaves the nerve proximal to its passage through the supinator m., is unaffected, but all of the other forearm muscles innervated by the radial n. are paretic. Finger extension is impaired, but wrist extension is preserved, particularly on the radial side (Fig. 12.**32**).

Diseases of the Spinal Nerve Roots and Peripheral Nerves

12

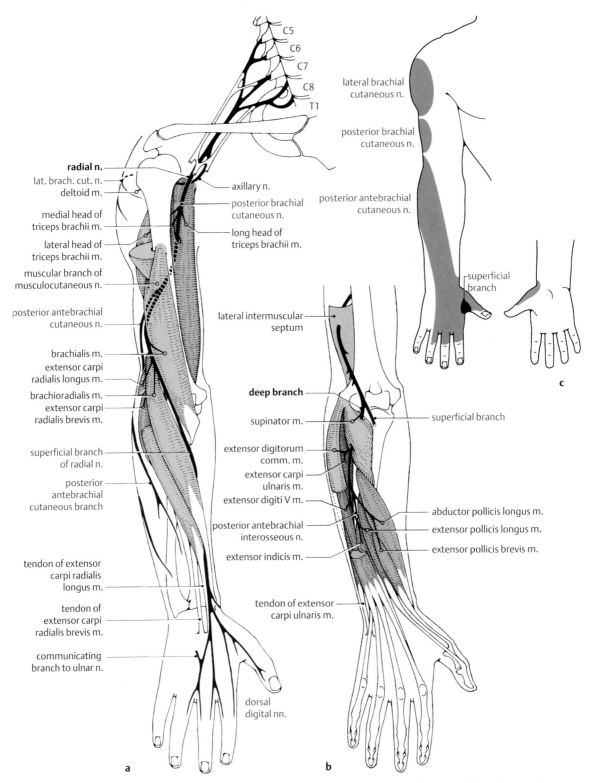

Fig. 12.30 Anatomical course and distribution of the radial n. a Proximal muscle branches (black) and course of the sensory superficial branch (red). **b** Course of the motor deep branch. **c** Zones of cutaneous innervation of the branches of the radial n. and sensory autonomous area of the superficial branch.

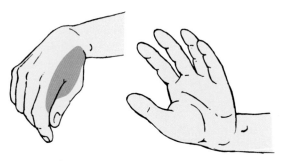

Fig. 12.**31** **Right wrist drop** due to a radial nerve lesion. The shading indicates the sensory autonomous area in the distribution of the superficial branch of the radial n.

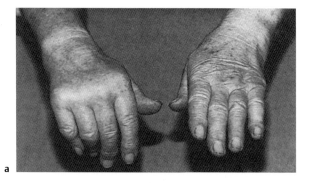

a

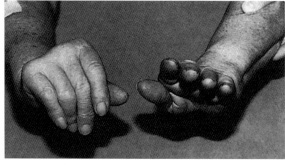

b

Fig. 12.**32** **Right supinator tunnel syndrome** in a 71-year-old woman. Marked weakness of the finger extensors (**a**) with preservation of wrist extension (**b**), particularly on the radial side of the wrist.

Causes. Radial nerve lesions can be produced by *trauma* and by *pressure*, e. g., by the use of crutches that press in the axilla, or by external pressure on the upper arm (humerus). The supinator canal syndrome is an anatomical bottleneck (*entrapment*) syndrome.

Differential diagnosis of radial nerve palsy must include *predominantly distal weakness of central origin*, which can also present with a wrist drop. The flexor weakness and enhanced intrinsic muscle reflexes that are present in central weakness serve to differentiate this condition from radial nerve palsy. Spinal muscular atrophy can, in rare cases, affect the wrist extensors on one side only. Steinert myotonic dystrophy (p. 268) commonly produces a bilateral wrist drop.

Median N. (C5–T1)

Anatomy. The anatomy of the median n. is shown in Fig. 12.**33**. All of the muscles innervated by this nerve are distal to the elbow. In the forearm, these include most of the *long flexors of the fingers* (with the exception of the deep flexors of the fourth and fifth fingers, which are innervated by the ulnar n.), as well as the *flexor carpi radialis*, *pronator teres*, and *pronator quadratus mm.* After the nerve passes through the carpal tunnel together with the long flexor tendons (see below), it innervates most of the *thenar muscles* (abductor pollicis brevis and opponens pollicis m. and the superficial head of the flexor pollicis brevis m.), as well as the *first and second lumbrical mm.* Its sensory innervation is to the radial side of the palm, the volar surface of the fingers from the thumb to the radial half of the fourth finger, and the dorsal surface of the terminal phalanges of these fingers.

Typical deficits. In median nerve lesions, too, the clinical manifestations depend on the level of the lesion:

- **Median nerve lesion in the upper arm** (i. e., proximal to the origin of its motor branches to the forearm flexors): the typical clinical appearance is that of the "pope's blessing hand," as depicted in Fig. 12.**34**, caused by weakness of the radial finger flexors.
- **Median nerve lesion at the wrist.** A lesion of the median n. in the carpal tunnel causes weakness of the thenar muscles. Clinically, pain and paresthesia are the most prominent symptoms. Carpal tunnel syndrome is discussed separately, in detail, because of its special clinical importance (see below).
- **Kiloh–Nevin syndrome.** An *isolated lesion of the anterior interosseous n.* is a rare event. This nerve is the motor terminal branch of the median n., which innervates the flexor pollicis longus m., the radial portion of the flexor digitorum profundus m. (flexion of the terminal phalanges of the 2nd and 3rd fingers), and the pronator quadratus m. A lesion of this terminal branch—due either to trauma or, occasionally, to entrapment—mainly impairs flexion of the terminal phalanges of the thumb and index finger. The patient can no longer form an "O" with these two fingers.

Causes. The median n. is the nerve most frequently injured by *direct trauma*, often by a cut in the wrist. *Pressure palsies* of the median n. also occur, both in the upper arm (due to prolonged maintenance of an awkward position, or to an Esmarch tourniquet) or in the palm of the hand (e. g., in occupational injuries). *Compression at anatomical bottlenecks* (entrapment) is a further cause of median nerve lesions. In many individuals, a bony spur is present just above the medial epicondyle of the humerus (the *supracondylar process*). A fibrous band (of Struther) may run from this spur to the medial epicondyle, forming a tunnel through which the median n. passes. The nerve can be compressed either by the supracondylar process or by the fibrous band. Further compression syndromes affecting the median n. are the *Kiloh–Nevin syndrome* (see above) and the *carpal tunnel syndrome*, which is described below.

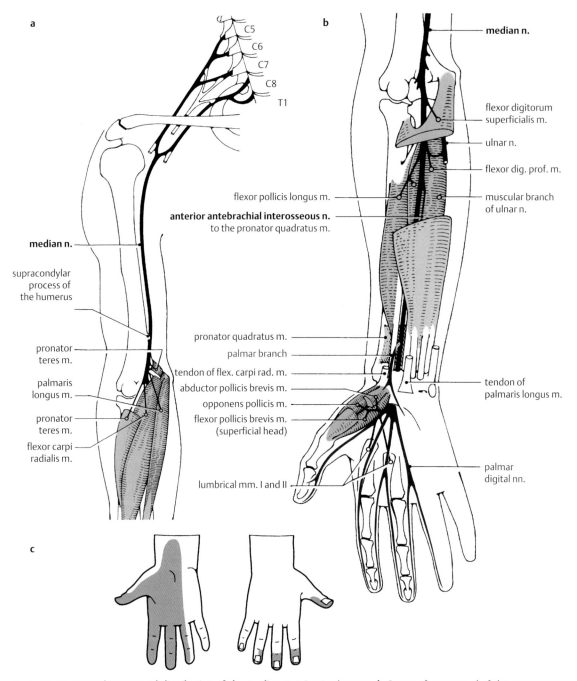

a

C5
C6
C7
C8
T1

median n.

supracondylar
process of
the humerus

pronator
teres m.

palmaris
longus m.

pronator
teres m.

flexor carpi
radialis m.

flexor pollicis longus m.

anterior antebrachial interosseous n.
to the pronator quadratus m.

pronator quadratus m.
palmar branch
tendon of flex. carpi rad. m.
abductor pollicis brevis m.
opponens pollicis m.
flexor pollicis brevis m.
(superficial head)

lumbrical mm. I and II

b

median n.

flexor digitorum
superficialis m.

ulnar n.

flexor dig. prof. m.

muscular branch
of ulnar n.

tendon of
palmaris longus m.

palmar
digital nn.

Fig. 12.**33 Anatomical course and distribution of the median n. a** Proximal course. **b** Course after traversal of the pronator teres m.
c Zones of cutaneous innervation in the hand.

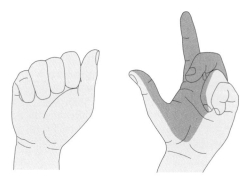

Carpal Tunnel Syndrome

The carpal tunnel syndrome (CTS) is caused by (mechanical) compression of the median n. as it passes through the carpal tunnel. It is considerably more common in women than in men and tends to develop around the time of the menopause. It usually affects the dominant hand, but it may affect the nondominant hand, or both. Factors that promote or precipitate the

◁ Fig. 12.**34 "Preacher's hand" due to a proximal left median nerve lesion.** The hypesthetic area is shaded dark red.

development of CTS include hormonal changes (menopause, pregnancy), weight gain, hypothyroidism, diabetes mellitus, and others.

Typical deficits. CTS is characterized by the following manifestations:
- in the first stage, which lasts several months or years, the manifestations are subjective: dull pain in the arm at night (*brachialgia paresthetica nocturna*),
- which is felt not merely in the hand, but in the whole upper limb up to the shoulder,
- wakes the patient from sleep and can be relieved by shaking and massaging the arms,
- the fingers are stiff and uncoordinated for a short time after the patient arises in the morning,
- in the more advanced stage, abnormal sensations (paresthesiae) develop and the sense of touch is impaired, mainly in the thumb and index finger,
- careful clinical examination is needed to reveal objectifiable sensory and/or motor deficits.

Examination and diagnostic evaluation. An occasional objective finding is point tenderness to pressure at the root of the thenar muscles, or a positive *Tinel sign* (paresthesiae in the radial portion of the palm and the radial fingers induced by a tap on the transverse carpal ligament). Paresthesiae in the fingers can sometimes be induced by sustained passive hyperflexion or hyperextension of the wrist (*Phalen sign*). Only later in the course of CTS can one find a discrete impairment of the sense of touch, particularly in the index finger (e. g., a worsening of two-point discrimination to > 5 mm). The major finding, however, is an inability to abduct the thumb fully, particularly when compared with the normal, opposite side, because of weakness of the abductor pollicis brevis m. This can be demonstrated by having the patient grasp a cylindrical object; a "*positive bottle sign*" is seen (Fig. 12.**35**). Impaired opposition of the thumb is more difficult to observe clinically (Fig. 12.**36**).

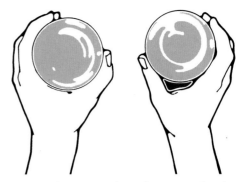

Fig. 12.**35** **"Bottle" sign in right median nerve palsy.** The thumb cannot be adequately abducted and opposed.

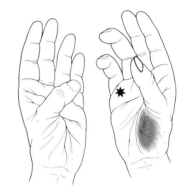

Fig. 12.**36** **Inadequate opposition and pronation of the thumb in a patient with a right median nerve lesion.** Because the thumb is insufficiently rotated, the thumbnail is seen tangentially rather than head on.

Overt CTS is unequivocally demonstrated by a finding of impaired conduction in the median n. across the carpal tunnel, as revealed by *electroneurography* (Fig. 12.**37**). This study should always be done before any operation is performed. Diminished conduction velocity alone, in

Fig. 12.**37** **Motor median neurography in right carpal tunnel syndrome.** The recording is performed over the abductor pollicis m. The distal motor latency is prolonged (9.2 ms, compared to normal 3.9 ms). The nerve conduction velocities in the arm and forearm are normal.

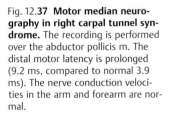

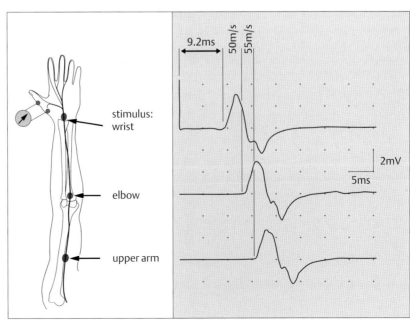

stimulus: wrist

9.2 ms

50 m/s

55 m/s

2 mV

5 ms

elbow

upper arm

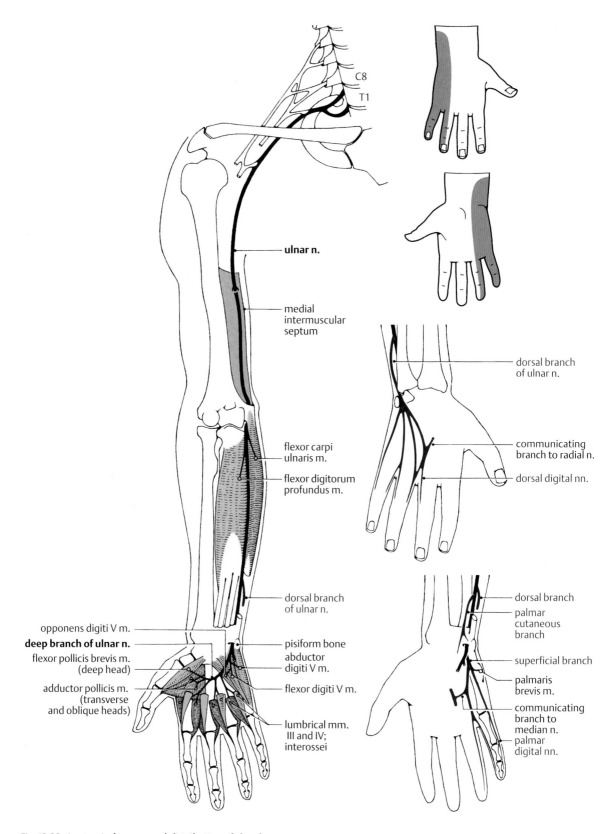

ulnar n.

medial intermuscular septum

flexor carpi ulnaris m.

flexor digitorum profundus m.

dorsal branch of ulnar n.

opponens digiti V m.

deep branch of ulnar n.

flexor pollicis brevis m. (deep head)

adductor pollicis m. (transverse and oblique heads)

pisiform bone abductor digiti V m.

flexor digiti V m.

lumbrical mm. III and IV; interossei

C8

T1

dorsal branch of ulnar n.

communicating branch to radial n.

dorsal digital nn.

dorsal branch

palmar cutaneous branch

superficial branch

palmaris brevis m.

communicating branch to median n.

palmar digital nn.

Fig. 12.**38 Anatomical course and distribution of the ulnar n.**

the absence of characteristic symptoms, is not an indication for surgery.

Treatment. *Keeping the hand in the neutral position at night* with a well-padded volar splint often brings relief. If it does not, or if objectifiable neurological deficits are already present, there should be no hesitation in proceeding to surgery. Operative *carpal tunnel release* involves splitting of the flexor retinaculum with an open or endoscopic technique (generally performed either by a neurosurgeon or by a hand surgeon).

Ulnar N. (C8–T1)

Anatomy. The anatomy of the ulnar n. is shown in Fig. 12.**38**. Among the muscles innervated by this nerve, the ulnar flexors of the wrist and fingers (the flexor carpi ulnaris m. and the ulnar portion of the flexor digitorum profundus m.) are functionally much less important than the ulnar-innervated intrinsic *muscles of the hand.* The ulnar n. is, indeed, the most important nerve for finger function: it innervates not only the *hypothenar mm.,* but also all of the *interossei,* the *3rd and 4th lumbrical mm.,* and, in the thenar region, the *adductor pollicis m.* and the *deep head of the flexor pollicis brevis m.* It provides sensory innervation to the ulnar edge of the hand, the volar surface of the fifth finger, and ulnar half of the fourth finger. A sensory branch arising from the ulnar n. in the distal third of the forearm innervates the skin on the ulnar side of the dorsum of the hand, as well as on the dorsal surface of the fifth finger and the ulnar half of the fourth finger.

Typical deficits. The typical clinical picture of ulnar nerve palsy is a **claw hand** (Fig. 12.**39**): because the interossei and lumbrical muscles cannot contract, the ulnar digits are hyperextended at the metacarpophalangeal joints, while the remaining digits are flexed at these joints. The long fingers can no longer be fully adducted against one another, the fingers cannot be strongly spread apart, and the patient cannot flick the middle finger against the examiner's palm with full, normal strength. A key finding is that, when the patient grasps a flat object (such as a piece of paper) between the thumb and the index finger, weakness of the adductor pollicis m. (ulnar n.) leads to functional substitution by the flexor pollicis longus m. (median n.), and therefore to flexion of the thumb on the affected side at the interphalangeal joint. This finding, called *Froment sign,* is highly characteristic of ulnar nerve palsy (Fig. 12.**40**).

In addition to these general clinical manifestations of ulnar nerve palsy, there are other specific findings that depend on the level of the lesion:

- If the lesion is **proximal** (at the elbow or higher), it will also affect the ulnar portion of the flexor digitorum profundus m., thereby impairing flexion of the distal phalanx of the fourth and fifth digits (Fig. 12.**41**).

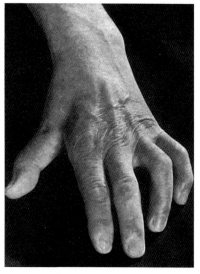

Fig. 12.**39 Claw hand due to a right ulnar nerve lesion at the elbow.** Typical features include hyperextension at the metacarpophalangeal joints and hyperflexion at the interphalangeal joints, particularly on the ulnar side of the hand. There is marked atrophy of the interossei and of the hypothenar muscles.

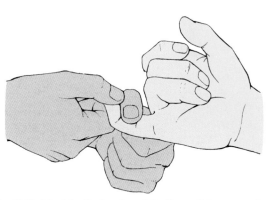

Fig. 12.**41 A test for the function of the flexor digitorum profundus m. of the little finger** (ulnar n.). Flexion of the little finger at the distal interphalangeal joint.

Fig. 12.**40 Froment sign in right ulnar nerve palsy.** Flexion of the interphalangeal joint of the thumb when the patient pulls on a flat object (piece of paper).

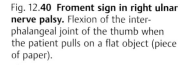

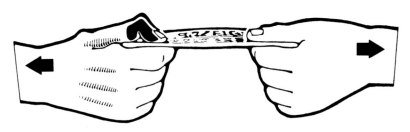

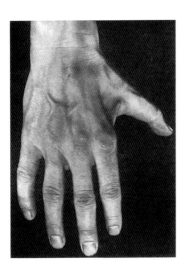

Fig. 12.**42 Typical appearance of the hand in a lesion of the deep branch of the ulnar nerve at the wrist.** Marked muscle atrophy in the first interosseous space, with preservation of the hypothenar musculature. Sensation was intact in this case.

Causes. Ulnar nerve palsy is often of *traumatic* origin. The nerve can be chronically *dislocated* at the elbow, where it can slip out of the ulnar groove on the medial epicondyle of the humerus; it is also vulnerable to *external compression* at this point (the "funny bone"), as well as to compression due to *anatomical variations of the ulnar groove* (sulcus ulnaris syndrome, **cubital tunnel syndrome**). Similarly, the ulnar n. can be damaged in the palm of the hand (e. g., by occupational tools), or by anatomical variations at the wrist (syndrome of the "loge de Guyon").

Treatment. The treatment depends on the cause and location of the lesion. Chronic compression of the nerve is treated by removal of the source of compression. This may involve splinting or padding of the elbow, or even operative relocation of the nerve from a more dorsal to a more volar position.

Diseases of the Nerves of the Trunk

Anatomy. The peripheral nerves supplying the thoracic and abdominal wall are derived from nerve roots T2 through T12. Each peripheral nerve in this region contains fibers that are (nearly) exclusively derived from a single nerve root. We recall that this is not the case in the limbs, where there is an intervening plexus between the nerve roots and the peripheral nerves, in which the nerve fibers are reassorted. The clinical manifestations of a peripheral nerve lesion in the trunk are thus very similar to those of a nerve root lesion.

Typical deficits. The most characteristic neurological syndrome due to nerve dysfunction in this area is **intercostal neuralgia**, i. e., bandlike, usually burning pain radiating around the trunk from back to front, at a single dermatomal level.

Causes. The nerves of the trunk can be damaged by viral infection (e. g., herpes zoster), by mass lesions, or by a diabetic or infectious mononeuritis (e. g., borreliosis). Mononeuritis can produce unilateral weakness of the musculature of the abdominal wall; the corresponding segment of the abdominal wall becomes flaccid and pouches visibly outward (Fig. 12.**43**). Sensation in this area is diminished, too, and the abdominal skin reflex is absent at the corresponding level.

Rarely, painful *entrapment neuropathy* may affect individual sensory terminal branches of the nerves of the trunk. *Notalgia paraesthetica* is a neuropathy of this kind causing pain in the back: one of the dorsal rami of the thoracic spinal nerve roots becomes stuck in a small gap in the fascia, producing hypesthesia in a coin-sized, paravertebral area of skin, as well as pain. There are comparable entrapment syndromes of the ventral rami, causing, e. g., the so-called *rectus abdominis syndrome*.

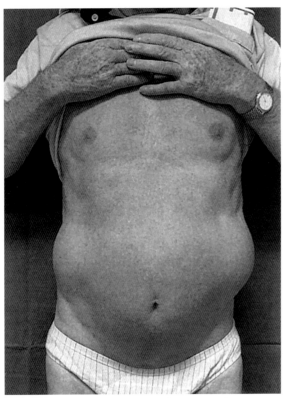

Fig. 12.**43 Weakness of the abdominal wall musculature,** worse on the left side, due to neuroborreliosis affecting the caudal thoracic nerve roots.

- If the lesion is **at the wrist**, it can be precisely localized by the involvement or noninvolvement of the palmaris brevis m. and the spatial configuration of the sensory deficit. The flexor muscles of the forearm that are innervated by the ulnar n. remain intact.
- An isolated lesion of the purely motor terminal branch of the ulnar n. (its *deep branch*) causes weakness of the interossei, while the hypothenar and lumbrical mm. and the muscles of the forearm innervated by the ulnar n. are spared. There is usually no sensory deficit (Fig. 12.**42**).

Diseases of the Lumbosacral Plexus

Anatomy. The structure of the **lumbosacral plexus** is illustrated in Fig. 12.**44**. It lies in a well-protected location in the posterior wall of the pelvis. Its cranial portion (the

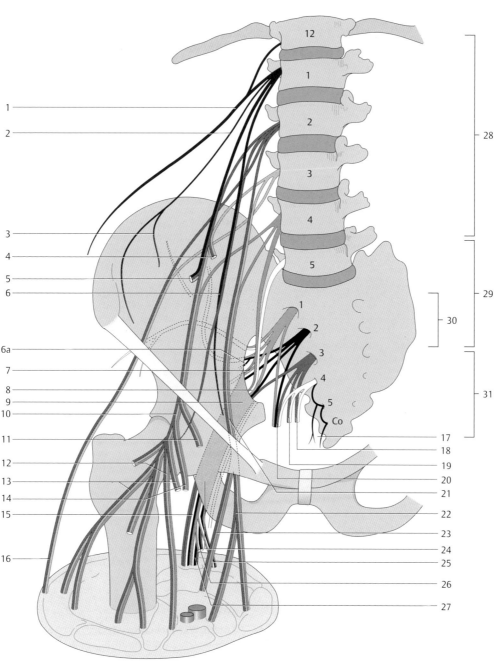

Fig. 12.**44 Anatomy of the lumbosacral plexus.**

1 **iliohypogastric n.** L1 (T12)
  lower abdominal wall muscles
2 **ilioinguinal n.** L1
  lower abdominal wall muscles
3 branch to iliacus m.
4 (femoral n., see 10, below)
  branch to psoas m.
5 branch to iliacus m.
6 **genitofemoral n.** L1, 2
  genital branch L2
  cutaneous branch L1
  (= femoral branch)
6a N. cutaneus femoris
  posterior S1–S3
7 **superior gluteal n.** L4–S1
  gluteus medius m.
  gluteus minimus m.
  tensor fasciae latae m.

8 **inferior gluteal n.** L5–S2
  gluteus maximus m.
9 **sciatic n.** L4–S3
  common fibular
  (peroneal) n. L4-S2
  tibial n. L4–S3
10 **femoral n.** L1–4
  psoas m. L1–3
  iliacus m. L1–3
11 pectineus m. L2–4
12 sartorius m. L2–3
13 quadriceps m. L2–4
14 saphenous n. L2–4
15 **common fibular
  (peroneal) n.** L2–S2
  biceps m. (short head)
  L5–S2
  fibularis (peroneus)
  longus m. L5-S2

fibularis (peroneus) brevis
  m. S1
  tibialis anterior m. L4-5
  extensor dig. long. m. L4-S1
  extensor hallucis long. m. L4-5
16 **lat. femoral cutaneous n.** L2–3
17 anococcygeal nn.
18 coccygeus m.
19 levator ani m.
20 **pudendal n.** S1–4
21 **obturator n.** L2–4
22 ant. branch/add. brev. m. L2–4
  ant. branch/add. long./gracilis
23 post. branch/add. min.
  & magn. mm. L3–4
24 **tibial n.** L4–S3
25 common flexor head
  semitendinosus m. S1–2

26 add. magnus m. L4–5
  semimembranosus m. L4-S1
27 long head of biceps m.
  gastrocnemius m. S1–2
  popliteus m. L4–S1
  soleus m. L5–S2
  flexor dig. long. m. L5-S1
  tibialis post. m. L5-S1
  flex. hall. long. m. L5–S2
  plant. ped. mm., abductors,
  adductors, interossei,
  lumbricals, etc., L5–S2
28 lumbar plexus
29 sacral plexus
30 "pudendal plexus"
31 coccygeal plexus

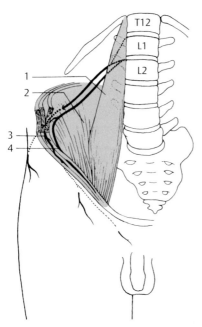

Fig. 12.**45 Anatomical course of the iliohypogastric and ilioinguinal nn. 1** Psoas major m. **2** Iliacus m. **3** Iliohypogastric n. **4** Ilioinguinal n.

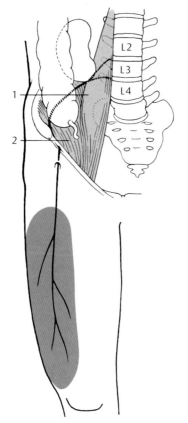

Fig. 12.**46 Anatomical course and distribution of the lateral femoral cutaneous n.** The nerve turns from a nearly horizontal to a nearly vertical course (in the standing patient) at the point where it traverses the inguinal ligament. **1** Psoas major m. **2** Iliacus m.

lumbar plexus, L1–L4) gives off, as its main branches, the *ilioinguinal, iliohypogastric, femoral,* and *obturator nn.* These nerves innervate most of the hip flexors and knee extensors. The caudal portion of the lumbosacral plexus (the **sacral plexus**, L5–S3) gives off the *superior* and *inferior gluteal nn.* for the gluteal muscles, as well as the *sciatic n.,* which supplies the knee flexors and all muscles of the lower leg and foot.

Typical deficits. The clinical manifestations of a lumbosacral plexus lesion depend on its location; in general, one finds a combination of the deficits seen in lesions of the individual peripheral nerve trunks lying distal to the plexus lesion.

Causes. Lumbosacral plexus palsy is usually due to a local *mass,* but it may also be due to prior *radiation therapy* or to an autoimmune disorder known as *chronic, progressive lumbosacral plexopathy.*

Diagnostic evaluation. Ancillary testing, primarily with CT or MRI, is generally needed to identify the etiology of a lumbosacral plexopathy. These imaging studies can demonstrate the presence of a mass.

Diseases of the Peripheral Nerves of the Lower Limbs

Genitofemoral and Ilioinguinal Nn. (L1–L2)

Anatomy. The course of these two (almost) monoradicular, mixed nerves is depicted in Fig. 12.**45**.

Typical deficits. Lesions of these nerves cause local pain in the groin (*ilioinguinal nerve syndrome*), a sensory deficit in the corresponding zone(s) of cutaneous innervation, and sometimes, in men, loss of the cremaster reflex (because the afferent arm of the reflex loop is interrupted). The associated motor deficit only affects oblique muscles of the abdominal wall and is hardly noticeable.

Lateral Femoral Cutaneous N. (L2–L3)

Anatomy. This purely sensory nerve passes through the three layers of the abdominal wall and then penetrates the inguinal ligament, usually at a point three finger breadths medial to the anterior superior iliac spine, to emerge onto the anterior fascia of the thigh. It provides sensory innervation to a palm-sized area of skin on the *anterolateral surface of the thigh* (Fig. 12.**46**).

Typical deficits. The lateral femoral cutaneous n. is vulnerable to injury at the point where it penetrates the inguinal ligament. The resulting clinical disturbance is an entrapment neuropathy called **meralgia paresthetica**, characterized by *burning pain in the cutaneous distribution of the nerve.* The pain is better when the hip is flexed, e. g., when the patient raises the ipsilateral foot onto a low stool; it is worse on hyperextension of the leg (*reverse Lasègue sign*). The site where the nerve passes through the inguinal ligament is often tender to light pressure. Most patients find the symptoms bearable and need only be reassured that the condition is benign. Surgery is only rarely necessary; the goal of the operation is to widen the aperture in the ligament through which the nerve passes, relieving compression.

Causes. Meralgia paresthetica may be due to marked weight gain or pregnancy. It can also arise after prolonged, continuous extension of the hip joint (supine position). Some cases have no apparent cause.

Differential diagnosis. Meralgia paresthetica must be distinguished from an *L3 nerve root lesion.* L3 root lesions impair the quadriceps reflex; they also produce a more extensive sensory deficit, which, unlike that of meralgia paraesthetica, crosses over the midline of the thigh onto its anteromedial surface.

Femoral N. (L1–L4)

Anatomy. The femoral n. provides motor innervation to the *hip flexors* (iliacus and psoas major mm.) and the *knee extensors* (quadriceps femoris m.). It provides sensory innervation by way of *anterior cutaneous branches* to the anterior surface of the thigh, and, through its terminal branch, the *saphenous n.,* to the medial quadrant of the anterior surface of the lower leg. Its anatomical course is shown in Fig. 12.**47**.

Typical deficits. A lesion of the femoral n. impairs *hip flexion and knee extension.* The hip flexors are examined with the patient sitting up and the knee extensors are examined with the patient supine (Fig. 12.**48**). In the standing patient, a *low-lying patella* is seen on the side of the lesion. The *quadriceps reflex* (patellar tendon re-

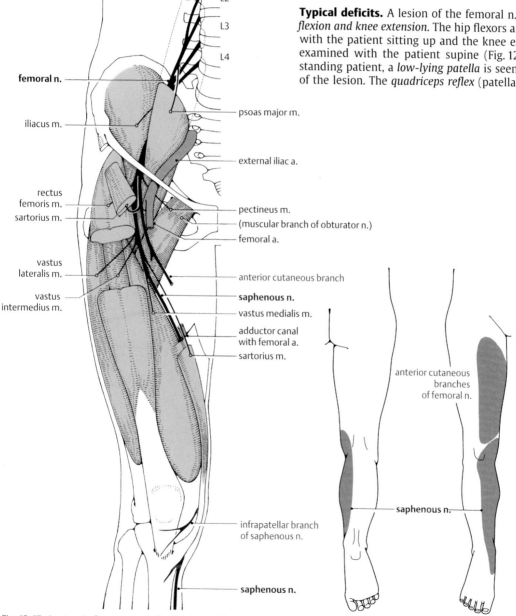

Fig. 12.**47 Anatomical course and distribution of the femoral n.**

femoral n.

iliacus m.

rectus
femoris m.
sartorius m.

vastus
lateralis m.

vastus
intermedius m.

L1
L2
L3
L4

psoas major m.

external iliac a.

pectineus m.
(muscular branch of obturator n.)
femoral a.

anterior cutaneous branch

saphenous n.
vastus medialis m.

adductor canal
with femoral a.
sartorius m.

infrapatellar branch
of saphenous n.

saphenous n.

anterior cutaneous
branches
of femoral n.

saphenous n.

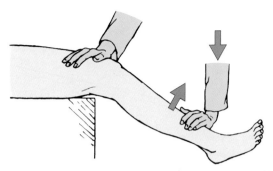

Fig. 12.48 Testing of knee extensors in the supine patient (the leg is able to hang freely downward). This testing position permits optimal use of the knee extensors that originate at the pelvis and thus span two joints, the hip joint and the knee joint (i. e., the rectus femoris and sartorius mm.).

flex) *is absent*. The patient cannot climb stairs with the affected leg and keeps it in a hyperextended position while walking (Fig. 3.**2**, p. 15). Sensation is diminished in the territory of the sensory terminal branches (anteromedial surface of the thigh and medial surface of the lower leg, Fig. 12.**47**).

Causes. Lesions of the femoral n. are commonly *traumatic* or *iatrogenic* (surgery). The nerve can also be involved by a pelvic *tumor* or, acutely, by a *hematoma in the psoas sheath*, e. g., in an anticoagulated patient.

Obturator N. (L3–L4)

Anatomy. The obturator n. supplies the *thigh adductors* (Fig. 12.**49**). Its sensory innervation is to a small area of skin just above the medial aspect of the knee.

Typical deficits. A lesion of the obturator n. impairs *thigh adduction*. The examining technique needed to demonstrate this is shown in Fig. 12.**50**. The adductor reflex, elicited by a tap on the medial condyle of the femur, is diminished and there is a small area of hypesthesia on the medial aspect of the thigh, just above the knee. Sometimes, irritation of the obturator nerve trunk can produce pain in this area as the sole clinical manifestation. This is called the *Howship–Romberg phenomenon*.

Causes. *Masses* in the pelvis or the obturator foramen are the usual causes; an obturator hernia is rarer.

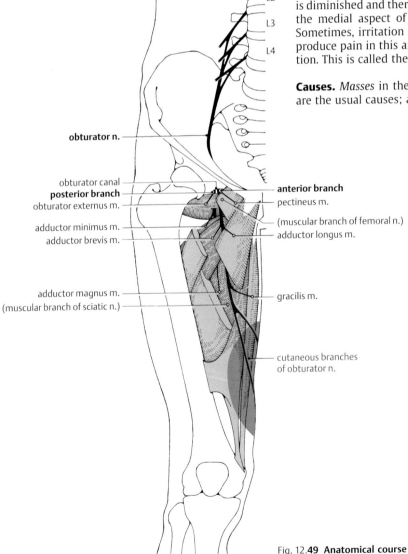

Fig. 12.49 Anatomical course and distribution of the obturator n. The area of cutaneous sensory innervation is shaded dark red.

Gluteal Nn. (L4–S2)

Anatomy. The gluteal nn. are purely motor. They innervate the hip abductors and extensors. The course of the two gluteal nn. is shown in Fig. 12.**51**.

Lesions of the superior gluteal n. produce weakness of the hip abductors (gluteus medius and minimus mm. and tensor fasciae latae m.). This impairs the stability of the pelvis on the side of the stationary leg when the patient walks; the pelvis tilts to the side of the swinging leg (so-called *Trendelenburg gait*). In an incomplete superior gluteal n. palsy, the patient barely manages to prevent tilting of the pelvis by inclining the trunk to the side of the stationary leg, thus displacing the body's center of gravity laterally (so-called *Duchenne gait*; cf. Fig. 3.**2**, p. 15 and Fig. 14.**3**, p. 266).

Lesions of the inferior gluteal n. (L5–S2) produce weakness of the gluteus maximus m., impairing hip extension. This makes it difficult for the patient to climb stairs (for example). Atrophy of the gluteus maximus m. is usually difficult to see because of the overlying fatty tissue, but, when the gluteus maximus mm. on either side are simultaneously and actively contracted, the lack of muscle tone on the affected side is easily appreciated by palpation. The natal fold is lower on the affected side.

Causes. The gluteal nn. are often injured by intramuscular injections with faulty technique.

Differential diagnosis. Trendelenburg gait can be observed in many diseases of the hip, e. g., in *congenital hip dislocation*. Weakness of the gluteus maximus m. can be caused by an *S1 nerve root lesion* (Fig. 12.**52**), while

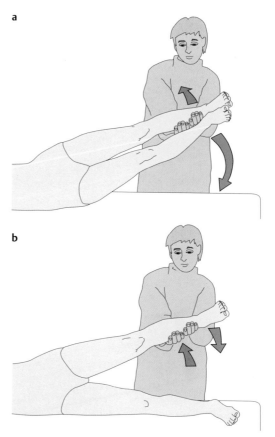

Fig. 12.50 Functional testing of the thigh adductors. a A patient lying in the lateral decubitus position can normally lift the lower leg off the examining table when the examiner lifts the upper leg. **b** A patient with adductor weakness cannot do this.

Fig. 12.**51 Anatomical course and distribution** ▷ **of the superior and inferior gluteal nn.**

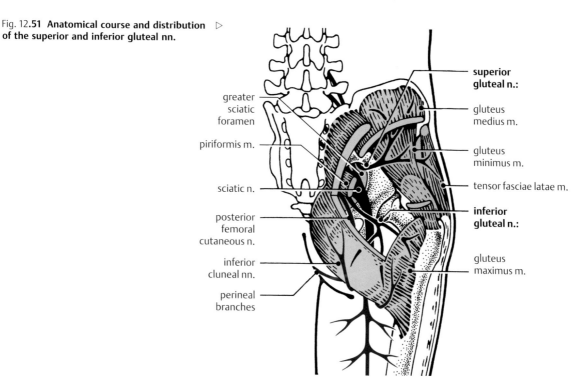

greater sciatic foramen

piriformis m.

sciatic n.

posterior femoral cutaneous n.

inferior cluneal nn.

perineal branches

superior gluteal n.:

gluteus medius m.

gluteus minimus m.

tensor fasciae latae m.

inferior gluteal n.:

gluteus maximus m.

Diseases of the Spinal Nerve Roots and Peripheral Nerves

12

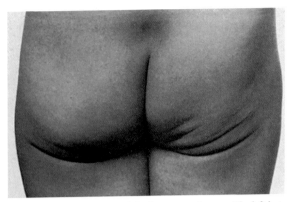

Fig. 12.**52 Weakness of the left gluteus maximus m.** The left buttock, on active contraction, is less voluminous than the right, and the left gluteal fold hangs lower.

weakness of the gluteus minimus and gluteus medius mm. can be caused by an *L5 nerve root lesion*. Bilateral weakness of the hip abductors is found, for example, in muscular dystrophy.

Sciatic N. (L4–S3)

Anatomy. The sciatic n. is the common trunk of the fibular (= peroneal or common peroneal) and tibial nn. It is the longest and thickest nerve in the human body. Its anatomy is shown in Fig. 12.**53**. The portions of the sciatic n. that are destined to become the fibular and tibial nn. are already clearly distinct from one another in the sciatic n. just distal to its exit from the pelvis, but they are usually ensheathed in a common epineurium nearly all the way down to the level of the popliteal fossa. The sciatic nerve trunk, in its proximal portion, gives off cu-

Fig. 12.**53 Anatomical course and distribution of the sciatic n.**

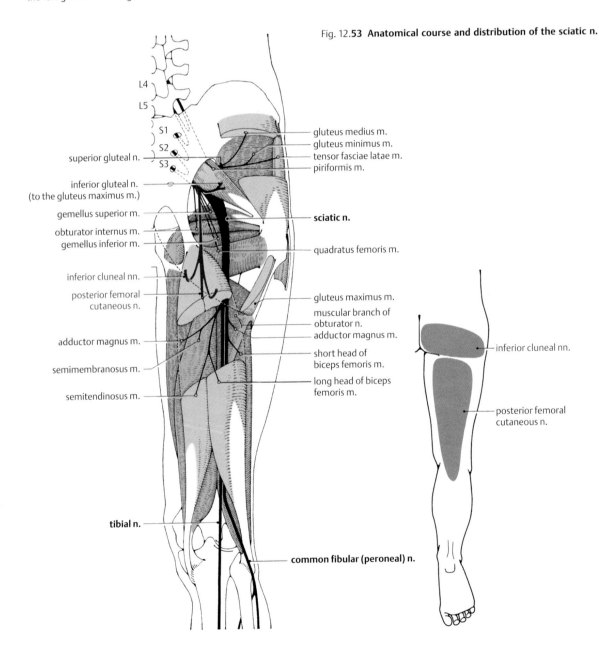

13 Painful Syndromes

Fundamentals

Many conditions whose most prominent, or sole, symptom is pain lie within the neurologist's area of expertise. In this chapter, we will discuss painful syndromes by location: **headache, shoulder–arm pain, pain in the trunk**, and **pain in the lower limb**. The etiological differential diagnosis of a painful syndrome cannot be restricted to neurological conditions but must always include diseases of nonneurological origin.

The generation and perception of pain. Pain is a type of unpleasant sensation. In terms of **pathophysiology**, it arises when specialized sensory end organs are excited by certain mechanical, thermal, or chemical stimuli of a potentially damaging ("noxious") nature. The pain-related ("nociceptive") impulses are conducted centrally, mainly by way of thin, poorly myelinated fibers, through the posterior root and into the spinal cord. The nociceptive fibers cross the midline in the spinal cord at their level of entry. They then ascend in the spinothalamic tract to the thalamus and onward to higher centers in the brain, through which pain can be consciously felt (cf. p. 73). **Biochemical factors** also play an important role in pain perception. In the *periphery*, the intensity of pain is increased by a variety of biogenic amines, e.g., substance P. In the *central nervous system*, the intensity of pain is modulated by the production of opioid substances in certain areas of the brain. Finally, **psychological factors**—determined both by personality and by the sociocultural environment—affect the manner in which pain is experienced and processed.

General aspects of the clinical history in patients with pain. Many painful syndromes have their origin in the nervous system and many others, in which there is no evident dysfunction of the nervous system (e. g., most kinds of headache), are nonetheless traditionally evaluated and treated by neurologists. These facts justify the inclusion of painful syndromes in a textbook of neurology for medical students. It should be emphasized, however, that the physician must not merely analyze the symptom "pain" from the narrow viewpoint of his or her particular specialty, but must, rather, apply the full range of general medical knowledge.

This purpose is best served, first, by the taking of a systematic and directed **pain history**. Some important elements of the pain history are listed in Table 13.**1**. Further, specific questions will need to be asked depending on the nature and location of pain in the partic-

ular case and ancillary diagnostic tests may be necessary.

In the remainder of this chapter, we will discuss various major painful syndromes, classifying them by location.

Table 13.**1** **Pain history**

Where is the pain?
- Precisely localized or diffuse?
- Constant or varying localization?
- Radiating?

How long has it been present?
- For what length of time?
- Since what precipitating event, if any?

Continuous or intermittent?
- If continuous: of constant or variable intensity?
- If intermittent: how long and how frequent are the episodes of pain?

Quality?
- Hammering?
- Throbbing?
- Stabbing?
- Dull?
- Burning?

Intensity?
- On a scale of 0 (no pain) to 10 (intolerable pain)

Precipitating and/or aggravating factors?
- None?
- Constant or variable factors—which, if any?
- Dependence on posture?

Alleviating factors?
- None?
- Constant or variable factors—which, if any?
- Medications—which ones, with what effect, lasting how long?

How severely is the patient impaired by the pain?
- At work?
- In the personal sphere?

Current complaints other than pain?

What is the patient's own explanation for the pain?

Other medical history?

Living situation?

Painful Syndromes of the Head And Neck

Headache can be either idiopathic or symptomatic. The most common **idiopathic** or "**primary**" types of headache are **tension-type headache**, **migraine**, and **cluster** headache. These three types of headache were once collectively designated "vasomotor headache." While migraine and cluster headache are typified by highly characteristic, usually unilateral attacks of pain, tension-type headache more commonly assumes the form of a diffuse, continuous headache of lesser intensity. **Symptomatic** headaches are, by definition, a manifestation of some other underlying condition. The possible causes include many types of neurological disease, as well as diseases of the eyes, teeth, jaw, ear, nose, and throat. Spondylogenic headache is caused by pathological processes in the cervical spine.

Headache can also include a variably significant component of **facial pain**—a typical example is cluster headache, in which the pain is felt mainly in the forehead, eye, and temple. Headache and facial pain cannot be cleanly separated from each other and are therefore considered under one heading in the IHS classification (see below and also Table 13.**2**). Nonetheless, it is pedagogically useful, for the purpose of clarity, to distinguish syndromes in which the pain is mainly in the head from others in which the pain is mainly in the face. Facial pain will accordingly be discussed in the next section.

IHS Classification of Headache

The classification of headache syndromes proposed by the *International Headache Society* (IHS) has won general acceptance and is reproduced, in highly

Table 13.**2** **Abbreviated classification of headache and facial pain based on the International Classification of Headache Disorders, 2nd edn. (ICHD-II)**, as published in *Cephalalgia* 2004;24 (suppl 1):1–160 (also available at www.i-h-s.org). Many subclassifications of the original table have been omitted here.

ICHD-II code	ICD-10NA code	Diagnosis	ICHD-II code	ICD-10NA code	Diagnosis
1.	**G43**	**Migraine**	5.2	G44.3	Chronic post-traumatic headache
1.1	G43.0	Migraine without aura	5.3	G44.841	Acute whiplash headache
1.2	G43.1	Migraine with aura	5.4	G44.841	Chronic whiplash headache
1.2.4	G43.105	Familial hemiplegic migraine	5.5	G44.88	Traumatic intracranial hematoma
1.2.6	G43.103	Basilar-type migraine	5.6	G44.88	Other head and/or neck trauma
1.3	G43.82	Childhood periodic syndromes	5.7	G44.88	Post-craniotomy headache
1.4	G43.81	Retinal migraine	**6.**	**G44.81**	**Headache attributed to cranial or cervical vascular disorder**
1.5	G43.3	Complications of migraine			
1.5.1	G43.3	Chronic migraine	6.1	G44.810	Ischemic stroke or TIA
1.5.2	G43.2	Status migrainosus	6.2	G44.810	Nontraumatic intracranial hemorrhage
1.5.4	G43.3	Migrainous infarction	6.3	G44.811	Unruptured vascular malformation
1.6	G43.83	Probable migraine	6.4	G44.812	Arteritis
2.	**G44.2**	**Tension-type headache (TTH)**	6.5	G44.810	Carotid or vertebral artery pain
2.1	G44.2	Infrequent episodic TTH	6.6	G44.810	Cerebral venous thrombosis
2.2	G44.2	Frequent episodic TTH	6.7	G44.81	Other intracranial vascular disorder
2.3	G44.2	Chronic TTH	**7.**	**G44.82**	**Headache attributed to nonvascular intracranial disorder**
2.4	G44.28	Probable TTH			
3.	**G44.0**	**Cluster headache and other trigeminal autonomic cephalalgias (TAC)**	7.1	G44.820	High CSF pressure (intracranial hypertension)
3.1	G44.0	Cluster headache	7.2	G44.820	Low CSF pressure (intracranial hypotension)
3.2	G44.03	Paroxysmal hemicrania	7.3	G44.82	Non-infectious inflammatory disease
3.3	G44.08	Short-lasting unilateral neuralgiform headache attacks with conjunctival injection and tearing (SUNCT)	7.4	G44.822	Intracranial neoplasm
			7.5	G44.824	Intrathecal injection
3.4	G44.08	Probable TAC	7.6	G44.82	Epileptic seizure
4.	**G44.80**	**Other primary headaches**	7.7	G44.82	Chiari malformation type I
4.1	G44.800	Primary stabbing headache	7.8	G44.82	Transient headache and neurological deficits with CSF lymphocytosis (HaNDL)
4.2	G44.803	Primary cough headache			
4.3	G44.804	Primary exertional headache	7.9	G44.82	Other nonvascular intracranial disorder
4.4	G44.805	Primary headache associated with sexual activity			
4.5	G44.80	Hypnic headache	**8.**	**G44.4**	**Headache attributed to a substance or its withdrawal**
4.6	G44.80	Primary thunderclap headache			
4.7	G44.80	Hemicrania continua	8.1	G44.40	Acute substance use or exposure
4.8	G44.2	New daily-persistent headache	8.2	G44.41 or .83	Medication-overuse headache (MOH)
5.	**G44.88**	**Headache attributed to head and/or neck trauma**	8.3	G44.4	Adverse effect of chronic medication
			8.4	G44.83	Substance withdrawal
5.1	G44.880	Acute post-traumatic headache			

Continued →

Table 13.**2**   (Continued)

ICHD-II code	ICD-10NA code	Diagnosis	ICHD-II code	ICD-10NA code	Diagnosis
9.		**Headache attributed to infection**	**12.**	R51	**Headache attributed to psychiatric disorder**
9.1	G44.821	Intracranial infection			
9.2	G44.881	Systemic infection	**13.**	G44.847, .848, .85	**Cranial neuralgias and central causes of facial pain**
9.3	G44.821	HIV/AIDS	13.1	G44.847	Trigeminal neuralgia
9.4	G44.821	Chronic post-infection headache	13.2	G44.847	Glossopharyngeal neuralgia
			13.3	G44.847	Nervus intermedius neuralgia
10.	G44.882	**Headache attributed to disorder of homoeostasis**	13.4	G44.847	Superior laryngeal neuralgia
10.1	G44.882	Hypoxia and/or hypercapnia	13.5	G44.847	Nasociliary neuralgia
10.2	G44.882	Dialysis headache	13.6	G44.847	Supraorbital neuralgia
10.3	G44.813	Arterial hypertension	13.7	G44.847	Other terminal branch neuralgias
10.4	G44.882	Hypothyroidism	13.8	G44.847	Occipital neuralgia
10.5	G44.882	Fasting	13.9	G44.851	Neck–tongue syndrome
10.6	G44.882	Cardiac cephalalgia	13.10	G44.801	External compression headache
10.7	G44.882	Other disorder of homoeostasis	13.11	G44.802	Cold-stimulus headache
			13.12	G44.848	Constant pain caused by compression, irritation, or distortion of cranial nerves or upper cervical roots by structural lesions
11.	G44.84	**Headache or facial pain attributed to disorder of cranium, neck, eyes, ears, nose, sinuses, teeth, mouth, or other facial or cranial structures**	13.13	G44.848	Optic neuritis
			13.14	G44.848	Ocular diabetic neuropathy
11.1	G44.840	Disorder of cranial bone	13.15	G44.881 or .847	Herpes zoster
11.2	G44.841	Disorder of neck			
11.3	G44.843	Disorder of eyes	13.16	G44.850	Tolosa-Hunt syndrome
11.4	G44.844	Disorder of ears	13.17	G43.80	Ophthalmoplegic "migraine"
11.5	G44.845	Rhinosinusitis	13.18	G44.810 or .847	Central causes of facial pain
11.6	G44.846	Disorder of teeth, jaws, or related structures			
11.7	G44.846	Disorder of temporomandibular joint (TMJ)	13.19	G44.847	Other cranial neuralgia or other centrally mediated facial pain
11.8	G44.84	Other disorder of cranial, facial, or cervical structures	**14.**	R51	**Other headache, cranial neuralgia, central or primary facial pain**
			14.1	R51	Headache not elsewhere classified

simplified form, in Table 13.**2**. The IHS has established a list of obligatory diagnostic criteria for each type of headache listed (in this book, we give the complete IHS criteria for migraine only; cf. p. 246). This highly precise approach to headache syndromes is most useful in clinical research, particularly when the results of different teams of investigators working in different countries are to be compared with each other. For example, the potential benefit of a method of treating a particular type headache can only be reliably assessed if it is definitely known that all of the research teams reporting on it are, in fact, treating the same condition. For the beginning student of neurology, however, it is more useful to gain a descriptive overview of the more common, "classic" types of headache. In particular, he or she should learn to distinguish the common *idiopathic* types of headache, i. e., those not due to any demonstrable structural lesion in the head, from *symptomatic* types. The latter are caused by organic disease of the cranial vessels or other structures in the head. 90 % of all cases of headache are idiopathic.

Approach to the Patient with Headache

The patient who goes to the doctor because of headache is suffering from pain and, often, anxiety. He or she therefore expects

- to be taken seriously,
- to be examined carefully,
- to have the cause of the problem identified and clearly explained.

The physician must take the time needed to meet these expectations fully.

The headache history. The clinical history is a vital step in the evaluation of headache (as of any other physical complaint). Some important points to be covered in the *systematic interview of the headache patient* are listed in Table 13.**3**. A carefully elicited history usually yields a clear-cut diagnosis. Nonetheless, the neurological and general physical examination (Table 13.**4**) should never be omitted, not least because these steps help the physician win the patient's confidence—an important factor for the success of treatment.

Migraine

Migraine, a type of idiopathic headache, is the second most common type of headache overall, after tension-type headache (see below). **Migraine without aura** (formerly called **simple** or **common migraine**), whose sole neurological manifestation is headache, is distinguished from **complicated migraine**, in which additional neurological manifestations are present.

Painful Syndromes

13

Table 13.**3** **Headache history**

- **Family history** of headache?
- **How long** have headaches been present?
- **Nature of headache:**
  - site?
  - continuous or episodic?
  - usual or strange quality of pain?
  - timing of onset?
  - speed of development?
  - nature of pain?
  - precipitating factors?
  - duration of episodes?
  - accompanying signs?
- **Frequency?**
- **Headache-free intervals?**
- **Intensity,** impairment of activities at home and at work?

- **Medications and other counteractive measures:**
  - frequency
  - dose
  - efficacy
- **Other symptoms besides headache:**
  - ENT, eye, or dental disease?
  - memory?
  - neurological/neuropsychological deficits?
  - epileptic seizures?
  - general symptoms (fatigue, weight loss, circulatory problems, etc.)?
- **Personality:**
  - character?
  - occupation?
  - private life?
  - conflicts?
  - alcohol, tobacco, caffeine, drugs of abuse?
  - medications?

Table 13.**4** **Examination of patients with headache**

General medical examination	Neurological examination, with particular attention to:
blood pressure	meningism
circulatory function	signs of intracranial hypertension
renal function	focal neurological signs
signs of infection	cranial nerve deficits
signs of meningitis	
signs of malignancy	**Mental status, with particular attention to:**
ENT diseases	psycho-organic syndrome
eye diseases	neuropsychological deficit
dental diseases, jaw diseases	impairment of consciousness
cervical spondylosis	psychological conflicts
	depression
	neurotic personality traits

Pathogenesis. Multiple factors contribute to the generation of a migraine attack:

- **Genetic factors** play a role; in some patients, for example, there are well-documented ion channel abnormalities. Many patients report a history of migraine in their relatives, particularly on the maternal side.
- **Abnormal neural excitation in the diencephalon**, particularly in the **thalamic zone representing the trigeminal area**, also plays a role in the pathogenesis of migraine. Events occurring in this nuclear area are responsible for the triggering of (unilateral) migraine attacks by peripheral stimuli or emotional factors.
- The pathogenetic role of so-called "**spreading depression**" is unclear. This is a phenomenon, known from animal research, in which a stimulus delivered locally to the occipital cortex induces a wave of excitation that spreads toward the frontal lobe. The excitation is then followed by reduced excitability ("depression"). It is an established fact that the speed of this disturbance, as it moves from back to front, correlates precisely with the speed of a scintillating scotoma moving across the visual field in an attack of ophthalmic migraine.
- Finally, a number of **biochemical processes** in peripheral blood vessels, modulated by the trigeminovascular reflex, are another contributing factor. These include the *secretion of serotonin and histamine* by platelets and mast cells. A rise in serotonin concentration initially induces contraction of the cerebral vessels. At the same time, serotonin and histamine act together to increase capillary permeability. Plasma kinins penetrate the vessel wall and lower the pain threshold in the periarterial tissue. The vessels then expand again and, at the moment of vasodilation, the typical throbbing pain begins. Different types of serotonin receptors in the periphery and in the brain play a role in the generation of migraine. Many of the modern pharmacologic treatments for migraine exert their effects by influencing these processes (see below).

Migraine without Aura

An attack of simple (common) migraine develops without any premonitory symptoms (aura) and is characterized by headache and accompanying autonomic manifestations. About 70% of all migraine attacks are of this type.

Epidemiology. Women suffer from migraine more commonly than men. The initial attacks usually occur in the first or second decade of life; about 5% of all schoolchildren already suffer from true migraine. The overall prevalence of migraine in the population is estimated at 10%.

Clinical manifestations. The *headache* is unilateral (*hemicranial*) in two-thirds of patients and is usually located in the temporal and parietal areas. (The word "migraine" comes from the Latin "hemicrania.") In most

Fig. 13.**1 Migraine attack:** schematic diagram.

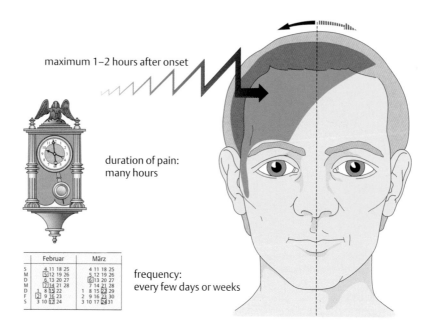

maximum 1–2 hours after onset

duration of pain: many hours

frequency: every few days or weeks

patients, the attacks tend to affect one side much more often than the other, though contralateral headaches do sometimes occur. The pain occasionally migrates from one side to the other during an attack; it is primarily bilateral in about one third of all attacks. It rises to a maximum in one hour or a few hours and then generally persists for many hours after that. The *quality of the pain* is usually described as *pulsating and throbbing*; it worsens with any kind of physical exertion, even as mild as climbing a staircase. *Accompanying symptoms* are usually present: 60% of patients complain of nausea, anorexia, and intolerance of light, sound, and (frequently) odors. Patients are often irritable and in a bad mood during the attack. The *objective findings* may include pallor, diaphoresis (common), and sometimes tachycardia, vomiting, and/or diarrhea. The *frequency* of attacks varies from a few per year to several per week. The frequency and intensity of attacks determine the degree to which migraine affects the individual patient in his or her everyday activities; the impairment may be severe.

IHS criteria. The IHS has promulgated the following defining criteria for simple migraine:
- A: At least five episodes fulfilling criteria B through D, below.
- B: The headache episodes last four to 72 hours (or, in children under 15 years of age, two to 48 hours), either when untreated or when treated unsuccessfully.
- C: The headache has at least two of the following features:
  - 1. unilateral localization,
  - 2. pulsating character,
  - 3. moderate or marked intensity (makes everyday activities difficult or impossible),
  - 4. exacerbation by climbing stairs or other habitual physical activities.
- D: At least one of the following symptoms is present during the headache:

- 1. nausea and/or vomiting,
- 2. abnormal sensitivity to light and noise.

The typical features of a migraine attack are shown schematically in Fig. 13.**1**.

Treatment. The treatment of common migraine depends on the frequency and severity of the attacks. If the attacks are rare and mild, treatment is generally not necessary.

Headaches of intermediate severity, not very prolonged duration, and low frequency (less than once per week) can be managed by **treating the individual attacks** with *analgesic medications* in adequately high doses in the early stages of each attack, e. g., 1000 mg of acetylsalicylic acid. An antiemetic should be prescribed as well, e. g., 20 mg of metoclopramide, by mouth or, if necessary, as a suppository. If these measures do not adequately treat the headache, *triptanes* are given by mouth, or, if necessary, as a nasal spray or by injection. Some patients obtain relief with *ergotamines*.

If the attacks occur more than once per week and/or severely hamper the patient's everyday activities by their severity or duration, **attack prophylaxis** can be initiated. Once begun, this must usually be maintained continuously for months or years afterward. Medications for attack prophylaxis include the beta-blocker propranolol and the tricyclic antidepressant amitriptyline, as well as valproate, dihydroergotamine, and flunarizine.

These recommendations also apply to the various types of complicated migraine described below.

Types of Complicated Migraine

About one-third of all persons with migraine have additional neurological manifestations besides the headache itself, e. g., visual disturbances, paralysis, sensory abnormalities, vertigo, or abdominal or cardiac symptoms. These manifestations may be very dramatic, sometimes

Painful Syndromes

13

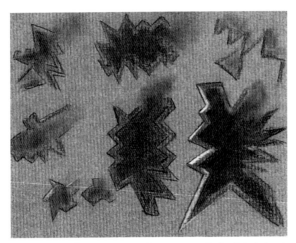

Fig. 13.**2** **Scintillating scotoma** during an attack of ophthalmic migraine: typical fortification figures.

Table 13.**5** **Manifestations of basilar migraine (according to frequency)**, after Sturzenegger and Meienberg

Bilateral visual disturbance
- scintillating scotoma or elementary hallucinations
- diffuse loss of visual acuity
- transient amaurosis
- visual field defects
- dysmorphopsias

Nausea

Impairments of consciousness
- syncope
- confusion
- stupor
- amnesia
- coma

Paresthesiae (bilateral)

Vomiting

Dizziness

Gait ataxia

Dysarthria

Limb weakness

overshadowing the headache to such an extent that the patient's illness is not immediately recognizable as migraine. We will now describe the major types of complicated migraine individually.

Ophthalmic migraine , the most common and probably best-known type of migraine, is often called "classic migraine" in the English-speaking world. (Note: clinicians in other parts of the world call *simple* migraine "classic migraine," so we will avoid confusion here by not using the term any further.) A scintillating scotoma appears 10 to 20 minutes before the headache. It begins in the center of the visual field, impairing the patient's ability to read (for example). A bright, zigzag line then travels from the center of the visual field outward in one-half of the visual field, until it "falls off the visual field" at the periphery, leaving behind a transient blurriness of vision in the corresponding hemifield. A typical scintillating scotoma or "fortification specter" (think of a crenellated medieval fortress) is shown in the diagram in Fig. 13.**2**. The scintillating scotoma is usually followed by

an attack of *hemicranial headache*. Occasionally, a scintillating scotoma may occur without subsequent headache; such events are called "*migraine sans migraine.*" So-called retinal migraine is a very rare variant involving a vertically demarcated scintillating scotoma or a monocular visual disturbance lasting a few minutes.

Migraine accompagnée is characterized by the combination of headache with hemiparesis, a hemisensory deficit, or some other type of focal neurological or neuropsychological deficit. This variant of migraine usually has its onset in childhood or adolescence. In each attack, the affected individual progressively develops, for example, weakness or numbness and paresthesia on one half of the body, over the course of a few minutes. When the migrainous process is located in the left hemisphere, the patient can often become aphasic as well. The hemiparesis is never complete (i. e., never a hemiplegia) and the patient remains conscious. The headache usually comes after the neurological disturbances, but may also accompany or precede them, and it may be on the same or the opposite side. All manifestations resolve within a few hours, or in one or two days at most. Low-grade CSF pleocytosis and a focus of δ-activity in the EEG can often be demonstrated during an attack. SPECT, too, reveals focal changes. If there is no headache, one speaks of "migraine sans migraine" here as well (just as in ophthalmic migraine without headache). With regard to *differential diagnosis*, an attack of migraine accompagnée can usually be distinguished from an acute ischemic stroke by the slow development of the neurological deficit and by the accompanying headache. In patients without headache, however, this distinction is not always easy to make, particularly in a first attack, and a thorough diagnostic evaluation is required.

Basilar migraine. In this type of migraine, the pathological process takes place in the *structures of the posterior fossa*. Basilar migraine mainly affects girls and young women. Its main manifestations are listed in Table 13.**5**: visual disturbances, symmetrical paresthesiae in the perioral region and the limbs, and impairment of consciousness. The accompanying headache is commonly felt at the back of the head.

Other types. Two special types of migraine deserve mention. **Familial hemiplegic migraine**, caused by a hereditary disease of ion channels, generally appears in childhood and may be accompanied by cerebellar ataxia. Rarely, an attack of this type of migraine can be followed by a permanent neurological deficit. The rare **alternating migraine of childhood** begins in the first year of life and is associated with progressive psychomotor retardation. Attacks of hemiparesis on alternating sides of the body last from a quarter of an hour to several hours or even days. There may also be dystonic movements, nystagmus, or tonic crises. Naloxone and flunarizine are effective in treating this disorder.

Cluster Headache

Alternative names for this disorder include "Bing–Horton neuralgia" and "erythroprosopalgia."

Fig. 13.**3 Cluster headache:** schematic diagram of an attack.

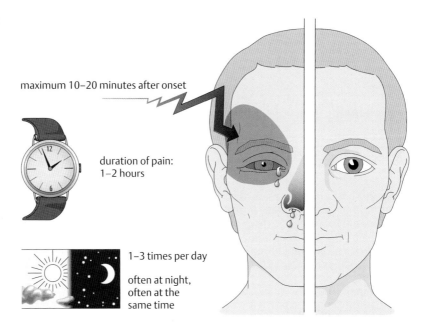

maximum 10–20 minutes after onset

duration of pain:
1–2 hours

1–3 times per day

often at night,
often at the
same time

Etiology and pathogenesis. The appearance of cluster headache attacks in a circadian rhythm seems to imply that this disorder is due to a functional disturbance of the diencephalon. It shares a number of pathophysiological and biochemical features with migraine. In addition to idiopathic cluster headache, there are also symptomatic forms, caused, e. g., by mass lesions.

Clinical manifestations. These are highly typical and are illustrated in Fig. 13.**3**.
- The *headache attacks* always occur on the same side of the head. The pain is mainly felt in the temple, eye, and forehead.
- The pain reaches its maximum in 10–20 minutes. Each attack lasts from half an hour to two hours; attacks may occur "*on schedule*" at the same time of day every day (during a cluster), particularly at night.
- *A number of attacks can occur* "*in series*" in a 24-hour period.
- The *pain* is very intense, often *pulsating and throbbing.* The patient is agitated and paces around restlessly.
- Attacks are usually accompanied by the following *objective findings*:
- *Horner syndrome* of the ipsilateral eye.
- A *red*, *teary eye* and periorbital erythema.
- A stuffed nose and/or increased nasal secretion.
- The attacks appear during periods called "clusters," lasting weeks or months; the clusters alternate with attackfree intervals lasting months or years.

Besides the **episodic form** just described, there is also a **chronic form** of cluster headache, in which the headache attacks occur every day and there are no attack-free intervals. It is not uncommon for typical migraine to be replaced by typical cluster headache (or vice versa) at some point in a patient's life. Many patients, too, have headaches bearing some of the features of both migraine and cluster headache.

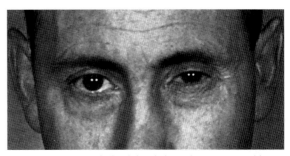

Fig. 13.**4 Cluster headache,** left-sided attack in a 45-year-old man. The left palpebral fissure is narrowed, and the conjunctiva and periorbital area are erythematous.

Diagnostic evaluation. The acute attacks, because they are brief, are only rarely observed by the physician. The diagnosis thus depends on a *precise clinical history* (as it does in nearly all types of headache). A physician who has the good fortune to observe the patient during an attack will likely see the characteristic appearance shown in Fig. 13.**4**.

Treatment. Treatment of an acute attack is difficult. *Triptanes* can be given by subcutaneous injection, or the patient can be given *pure oxygen* to breathe (7 liters per minute for 15 minutes). Medications for the **reduction of attack frequency** include *verapamil* and *indomethacin*, sometimes in combination with a *tricyclic antidepressant.* A brief course of cortisone treatment is often effective. The chronic form responds to lithium.

Tension-type Headache

This is probably the most common type of headache. It was previously known as "vasomotor headache." Its clinical features resemble those of postconcussive headache.

Painful Syndromes

13

Table 13.**6**   **Some rare types of primary headache**

Type	Clinical features	Remarks
Hemicrania continua	persistent unilateral headache	responds to indomethacin and perhaps to ASA
"Ice-cream headache"	acute headache, usually temporal, lasting 20–30 seconds, precipitated by a cold stimulus on the palate (such as ice cream)	
Cough headache	precipitated by coughing, abdominal straining, or bending over; an intense, diffuse headache lasting a few seconds	usually innocuous, but sometimes due to a pathological process in the posterior cranial fossa
Coital headache	sudden onset, lasts minutes or hours, sometimes accompanied by vomiting	no meningismus (differential diagnosis: subarachnoid hemorrhage!)

Etiology. The cause of tension-type headache is unknown. It is no longer thought to be due to muscle tension. A current hypothesis attributes it to *abnormal sensitivity to pain in the trigeminal nuclear complex*. This complex, in turn, receives input from other structures in the brain, including the limbic system.

Clinical manifestations. Patients complain of a pressing, aching pain in the head, which is usually *diffuse*, i. e., there is no particular location at which it is most intense. It is of no more than *intermediate severity* and does not worsen with physical activity. It is not associated with nausea, photophobia, or phonophobia, and usually does not keep patients from going about their everyday activities.

There are **episodic and chronic forms** of tension-type headache. Patients with the episodic form suffer from headache on fewer than 15 days per month (180 days per year). The individual episodes of headache may last from 30 minutes to several days. Patients with the chronic form suffer from headache on more than 15 days per month (180 days per year).

Diagnostic evaluation. The *history* is crucial, as the neurological examination and ancillary tests do not reveal any abnormalities.

Treatment. Life-style readjustment is the recommended first line of therapy: removal of headache-producing substances such as alcohol and nicotine, regular physical exercise, regular sleep, stress reduction, and, if necessary, other changes in the patient's living situation and mode of living. If medications are needed, tricyclic antidepressants are the agents of choice, followed by beta-blockers or tizanidine.

Rare Varieties of Primary headache

Table 13.**6** provides an overview of rarer types of primary headache other than migraine, cluster headache, and tension-type headache.

Symptomatic Headache

Symptomatic headache is due to a **structural lesion, infection, or inflammation of intra- and/or extracranial tissue.** Its direct cause is often a *pathological alteration of intracranial pressure*, which excites nociceptive nerve endings in the meninges. The ICP may be either too high (particularly because of space-occupying lesions such as

hematomas, tumors, and hydrocephalus) or too low (e. g., in the intracranial hypotension syndrome after a lumbar puncture).

Symptomatic headache, however, is not necessarily due to neurological disease. **Pathological conditions of the ears, nose, throat, eyes, teeth, or jaw** can also cause head and/or facial pain, which may be quite severe. Even **diseases of the cervical spine** can, rarely, produce headache (*spondylogenic headache*).

Table 13.**7** provides an overview of the major causes of symptomatic headache. We will describe a few of the causative neurological illnesses and spondylogenic headache, in detail in the following paragraphs.

Occlusions and Dissections of Cranial Vessels

Arterial occlusion only rarely causes headache, but, if it does, the site of the headache may be a clue to the identity of the occluded vessel: occlusion of the internal carotid a. produces temporal headache, while occlusion of the basilar a. produces headache in a ringlike distribution around the head. Very intense pain on one side of the neck and face accompanies acute **dissection** of the internal carotid a. Vertebral artery dissection produces pain in the ipsilateral occiput and nuchal region. Dissections can arise spontaneously or after trauma to the head or neck.

Intracranial Hemorrhage

Subarachnoid hemorrhage (SAH) due to a ruptured saccular aneurysm at the base of the brain produces an extremely intense, diffuse headache of lightning-like onset ("*the worst headache of my life*"), possibly accompanied by meningismus and an impairment of consciousness. If the patient is comatose, of course, the headache and meningismus may be masked or absent. **Intracerebral hemorrhage** (e. g., spontaneous hemorrhage due to hydrocephalus, into a tumor, or from a ruptured arteriovenous malformation) causes rapidly progressive headache in addition to hemiparesis and progressive impairment of consciousness. A more slowly progressive headache, perhaps accompanied by a fluctuating level of consciousness, is typical of **chronic subdural hematoma**. Neurological deficits in these patients are surprisingly rare (p. 91).

Cranial Arteritis

Cranial (also called temporal) arteritis is an autoimmune disease of blood vessels that almost exclusively

Table 13.**7** **Important types of symptomatic headache**

Type	Cause	Features	Remarks
Headache of subarachnoid hemorrhage	usually rupture of a saccular aneurysm at the base of the brain	sudden, extremely severe headache, usually diffuse, accompanied by vomiting, drowsiness, and meningism	see p. 108
Headache due to intracranial mass	brain tumor, chronic subdural hematoma, brain abscess	permanent headache of increasing severity; nausea, bradycardia, papilledema, focal neurological deficits	neuroimaging is essential; see p. 94
Headache due to occlusive hydrocephalus	aqueductal stenosis, intraventricular mass, mass in posterior cranial fossa	manifestations like those of a brain tumor	neuroimaging is essential; see p. 84
Headache due to malresorptive hydrocephalus	prior subarachnoid hemorrhage or meningitis, venous sinus thrombosis	diffuse, increasingly severe headache, gait ataxia, incontinence	isotope cisternography or MRI may be useful
Intracranial hypotension	prior lumbar puncture, (rarely) spontaneous	orthostatic headache that improves or resolves when the patient lies down; normal neurological examination, CSF not obtainable by lumbar puncture (or only with aspiration); elevated CSF protein concentration	
Pseudotumor cerebri	often seen in overweight young women; may be secondary to prior head trauma, anovulatory drugs, steroid withdrawal, tetracycline, etc.	chronic headache without any other detectable cause; often papilledema; CT or MRI reveals slit ventricles; elevated pressure on LP	
Headache in meningitis	bacterial or viral meningitis	hyperacute in purulent meningitis; very severe headache, meningism, drowsiness, vomiting	
Headache in carcinomatous or leukemic meningitis	primary tumors of various types, e. g., breast carcinoma	chronic, diffuse headache, cranial nerve deficits or spinal radicular deficits; LP and CSF cytology are essential	can often be diagnosed by MRI
Postinfectious headache	after recovery from a (viral) infection	diffuse, often intractable headache without other neurological abnormalities, resembling tension headache; mild elevation of CSF cell count	
Headache in ENT disease	chronic sinusitis, neoplasia in the pharyngeal cavity	headache or facial pain depending on the site of the disease process; no neurological deficit	
Headache in eye disease	e. g., heterophorias, acute glaucoma, iritis, infectious/inflammatory processes in the orbit	usually frontal and temporal headache	
Headache due to dental conditions	pulpitis, periodontitis, retained teeth, and myofascial pain syndrome due to malocclusion	severe, acute facial pain or chronic facial pain, depending on cause	

affects persons over age 60. Its most prominent, though by no means only, clinical manifestations are in the large and middle-sized extracranial arteries.

Clinical manifestations. The leading symptom is an atypical headache that rapidly worsens over a few days or weeks and then becomes *constant, often in the temporal region.* The affected arteries (particularly the superficial temporal a.) are tender, tortuous, and swollen (Fig. 13.**5**). They may occlude by thrombosis, in which case they cease to pulsate. The headache is often accompanied by further manifestations: pain in the shoulder and pelvic girdle muscles, fatigue, subfebrile temperature, weight loss, and nocturnal diaphoresis—a systemic syndrome known as *polymyalgia rheumatica.* The *complication* to be most feared is involvement of the ophthalmic a. causing occlusion of the central retinal a. and sudden blindness (Fig. 13.**6**).

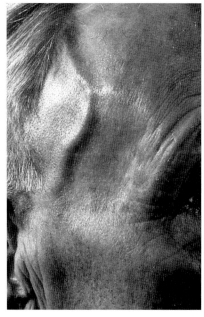

Fig. 13.**5 Temporal arteritis** in a 65-year-old man. Note the thickened, painful, no longer pulsating superficial temporal a.

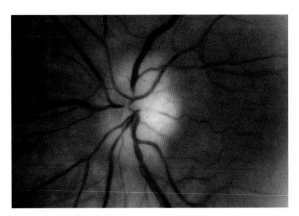

Fig. 13.**6 Atrophic optic disc in a 79-year-old woman with temporal arteritis.** Note the abnormal disc pallor; the patient is blind in this eye.

Table 13.**8 Diagnostic criteria for spondylogenic headache**

Characteristics of pain
- radiating from occipital to frontal
- usually unilateral
- coming in attacks, or
- permanent pain of variable intensity
- not throbbing
- moderately severe

Cervical spine
- prior history of trauma to the head or cervical spine
- or prior whiplash injury
- or episodes of torticollis (wry neck),
- perhaps accompanied by arm pain
- clinical or radiological evidence of cervical spine pathology

Precipitating and alleviating factors
- pain induced by movement (or manipulation) of the cervical spine
- or by keeping the head in a particular position for a longer than usual time
- or by local pressure on the nape of the neck or the occiput
- pain temporarily alleviated by infiltration of the greater occipital n. or the C2 nerve root with local anaesthetic

Accompanying symptoms
- dizziness
- nausea
- blurred vision
- phono- and photophobia
- dysphagia

Diagnostic evaluation. The erythrocyte sedimentation rate is nearly always markedly elevated. The diagnosis is confirmed by *temporal artery biopsy*: histopathological examination reveals giant cell arteritis. A biopsy should be performed in all suspected cases, because there is no other way to establish the diagnosis with the certainty required before starting long-term treatment with corticosteroids. These often need to be given continuously for a year or more.

Spondylogenic Headache ("Migraine Cervicale")

Our experience suggests that this condition is overdiagnosed. The appropriate diagnostic criteria to be used are summarized in Table 13.**8**.

Dangerous Types of Headache

All patients who consult a physician because of headache are in pain and therefore deserve our full attention and respect. More than 90% of them, however, will turn out not to have a serious medical problem. One of the important tasks facing the physician is to be on guard for those few, unusual cases of headache that are, in fact, due to a dangerous underlying condition. The main alarm signals are the following:
- headache of an unusual nature in a patient who never had headaches before;
- headache arising at an advanced age;
- headache of sudden (lightning-like) onset;
- headache that always occurs in precisely the same location (except cluster headache or trigeminal neuralgia, both of which, by definition, always occur in the same place);
- progressively severe headache (crescendo headache);
- continuous headache;
- headache accompanied by:
  - personality change,
  - impairment of consciousness,
  - epileptic seizures;
- neurological deficits revealed on physical examination.

If any of the above applies, further investigation is needed, usually with an imaging study.

Painful Syndromes of the Face

Facial pain is often due to a **lesion of a sensory nerve in the face**, most commonly the trigeminal n. It typically presents with **very brief, but very intense attacks of pain** ("classic" or "genuine" neuralgia in the face). There are also a variety of other kinds of facial pain with other pathogenetic mechanisms, e. g., a structural anomaly of the jaw. The pain may resemble neuralgia in these other conditions as well; thus, patients with any kind of facial pain always require careful evaluation to establish the differential diagnosis.

"Genuine" Neuralgias in the Face

Typical manifestations of "genuine" neuralgia in the face are the following:
- **pain** is located in the face or the mucous membranes of the head,
- usually comes in brief attacks lasting a few seconds to a few minutes at most,
- is usually very intense;
- is described as electrical, knifelike, cutting, stabbing, or lightninglike;
- arises either spontaneously or on provocation by touch or other mechanical or thermal stimuli;

- is always on the same side of the face (in most patients);
- and is always in the same location.
- In addition, the **attacks** are very frequent, up to several times a day,
- with no pain in between attacks, except, possibly, for a dull background pain.
- Finally, there are **no objective neurological abnormalities**, except in the rare forms of symptomatic neuralgia.

The most common "genuine" neuralgias in the face are described in the following paragraphs. The localization and radiation of pain in the various types of neuralgia are depicted in Fig. 13.**7**.

Trigeminal Neuralgia

Idiopathic trigeminal neuralgia, which is far more common than the **symptomatic** type, only affects individuals over age 50.

Pathogenesis. Idiopathic trigeminal neuralgia appears to have more than one possible cause. In many patients, neuroimaging studies reveal a looping blood vessel that makes contact with the trigeminal n. at its zone of entry into the pons. In other patients, defective myelin sheaths are found in the Gasserian ganglion (naturally only at postmortem examination). In symptomatic trigeminal neuralgia, on the other hand, the pain is due to an underlying neurological disease, e. g., multiple sclerosis.

Clinical manifestations. The painful attacks of idiopathic trigeminal neuralgia are usually located in the distribution of the *second trigeminal division* (the maxillary n.), less commonly in that of the first or third divisions. The pain is nearly always unilateral; it is felt on both sides simultaneously, or in alternation, in only 3 % of patients. The individual attacks last only a few seconds and cause a reflexive grimace or pulling of the face ("*tic douloureux*," not to be confused with a tic in the

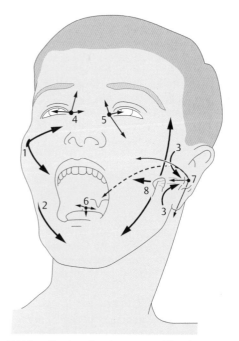

Fig. 13.**7 Localization of various types of facial pain and neuralgia. 1** Trigeminal neuralgia in the distribution of the maxillary nerve (V_2). **2** Trigeminal neuralgia in the distribution of the mandibular nerve (V_3). **3** Auriculotemporal neuralgia. **4** Nasociliary neuralgia. **5** Sluder's neuralgia. **6** Glossopharyngeal neuralgia. **7** Neuralgia of the geniculate ganglion. **8** Temporomandibular joint "neuralgia" (myofacial pain syndrome).

usual sense of a primary movement disorder). The pain is *unbearably intense.* The attacks occur spontaneously or on provocation by eating, speaking, tooth brushing, or touch; they may come dozens of times per day. Some patients eat and speak so little to avoid the pain that they lose weight, even to the point of cachexia. Attacks generally do not occur during sleep. The typical clinical manifestations of trigeminal neuralgia are depicted in Fig. 13.**8**. Sometimes, a long period with frequent attacks

Fig. 13.**8 Trigeminal neuralgia:** schematic diagram.

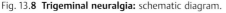

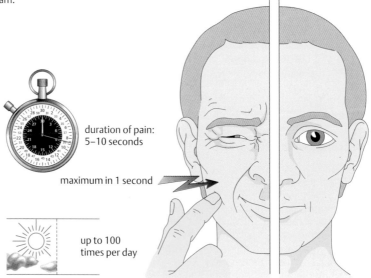

duration of pain:
5–10 seconds

maximum in 1 second

up to 100
times per day

is followed by a pain-free interval that may last for months until the attacks return.

In the rarer **symptomatic** cases of trigeminal neuralgia, the clinical manifestations are slightly different. The attacks are more commonly bilateral (either simultaneously or in alternation) and a neurological deficit may be found, depending on the underlying etiology, e.g., multiple sclerosis or a tumor compressing the trigeminal n.

Diagnostic evaluation. As stated above, the neurological examination generally reveals no abnormality. About one-quarter of patients who have suffered from idiopathic trigeminal neuralgia for a long time have a mild sensory deficit in the affected area of the face.

Treatment. About 80% of patients initially respond to correctly dosed treatment with *carbamazepine* or *gabapentin*. The medication must be taken every day and the dose must be steadily increased until the pain is relieved.

! *The pharmacological treatment of trigeminal neuralgia often fails because of underdosing or irregular consumption of the prescribed drug.*

If pharmacological treatment does not eliminate the pain despite a high dose of medication (in some patients, just below the threshold for intolerable side effects, which varies greatly from one patient to the next), neurosurgical treatment is indicated. The available, effective procedures include open microvascular decompression of the trigeminal n. (requires craniotomy) and percutaneous techniques such as selective radiofrequency coagulation of the Gasserian ganglion, balloon compression of the ganglion, and glycerol injection into Meckel's cave.

Auriculotemporal Neuralgia

In this disorder, the pain is located *in the temple and in front of the ear*. It is usually a sequela of disease of the ipsilateral parotid gland, appearing a few days or months after the parotid condition resolves.

The attacks of pain can be provoked by chewing or by chemical stimuli, particularly sour (acidic) food. The pain is of a burning quality. It is often accompanied by erythema and increased sweating in the preauricular area.

The differential diagnosis of this condition includes temporomandibular joint syndrome.

Nasociliary Neuralgia

The attacks of pain are located *in the nose and on the inner canthus of the eye*. There may be a continuous, background pain in addition to the typical, lightning-like, shooting pain. In this condition, as in the other neuralgias of the face, the pain is provoked by chewing or by touch—here, by touching the eye. The attacks are often accompanied by redness of the eye, swelling of the nasal mucosa, and lacrimation. They can often be aborted by the application of a 5% cocaine solution in-

side the nostril. This condition is sometimes difficult to distinguish from cluster headache (p. 248). On rare occasions, it is also confused with dissection of the internal carotid a., which produces a similar type of pain.

Sluder Neuralgia

This condition is thought to be due to a pathological process affecting the pterygopalatine ganglion. Its clinical manifestations closely resemble those of nasociliary neuralgia (see above). In many patients, the attacks are accompanied by the urge to sneeze. Sluder neuralgia is occasionally associated with sphenoid or ethmoid sinusitis.

Glossopharyngeal Neuralgia

This condition is usually seen in the elderly. Its typical manifestations are lightninglike pain in the *base of the tongue*, the *hypopharynx*, and the *tonsillar fossa*, radiating toward the ear. The pain can be provoked by swallowing (especially of cold liquids), speaking, or sticking out the tongue. The painful attacks are, on rare occasions, accompanied by syncope. The pharmacological treatment of this disorder is like that of trigeminal neuralgia. If surgical treatment is required, resection of the glossopharyngeal n. and the upper root of the vagus n. has a good chance of success.

Rarer Types of Neuralgia

The neuralgias of the geniculate ganglion, the superior laryngeal n., and the auricular branch of the vagus n. are all very rare. The existence of occipital neuralgia is still debated.

Other Diseases Causing

Facial Pain

Temporomandibular Joint Syndrome

This condition has many other names, including myofacial syndrome and Costen syndrome. Our experience suggests that it is overdiagnosed.

Pathogenesis. This condition is thought to be due to abnormal mechanical stress on the jaw joint caused by *malocclusion*, e.g., after tooth extraction, or by local changes in the joint itself. This, in turn, causes the muscles of mastication to be activated in nonphysiological ways, which leads to pain in the muscles, so that their pattern of activation is distorted even further. A vicious circle arises in which pain produces more pain.

Clinical manifestations. Patients typically suffer from more or less continuous *preauricular pain*, which is described as dull or neuralgia-like. The pain can be brought on, or made worse, by chewing.

Diagnostic evaluation. The jaw joint is tender to pressure on one or both sides. CT or MRI occasionally demonstrates an abnormality of the joint.

Treatment. *Optimization of the dental occlusion* (bite) sometimes relieves the pain to some extent. Unfortunately, however, many dental and surgical procedures on the teeth and jaws are performed for this condition to no avail.

Atypical Facial Pain

This term refers to *unilateral, diffuse pain in the face.* The pain is often of a burning or dull character and is maddeningly persistent. The condition generally affects middle-aged women. It may be of spontaneous onset, but, in many patients, the pain first appears (or becomes severe) in the aftermath of a dental procedure. This often leads to a series of further dental procedures, which the dentist or oral surgeon characteristically performs only after being urgently entreated to do so by the patient. Atypical facial pain is difficult to treat; perhaps the most important aspect of treatment is the avoidance of further surgery. Serotonin reuptake inhibitors, flunarizine, or tricyclic antidepressants have been used for this condition.

Glossodynia is a rare type of atypical facial pain consisting of dysesthesia of the tongue, often of a burning character. It usually affects elderly women.

General Differential Diagnosis of Headache and Facial Pain

The location and clinical course of headache and facial pain often provide important clues to its etiology. Important aspects of differential diagnosis are summarized in Table 13.**9**.

Table 13.**9** **Differential diagnosis of headache and facial pain**

Clinical features	Syndrome
Recurrent **attacks** of intense **headache** with pain-free intervals	• migraine (unilateral headache) • cluster headache (unilateral pain in the temporal region, eye, and face) • hypertensive crises (diffuse pain)
Recurrent **attacks** of intense **facial pain** with pain-free intervals	• trigeminal neuralgia (duration, seconds; localization, usually mid-face) • auriculotemporal neuralgia (duration, minutes ; localization, preauricular) • nasociliary neuralgia (duration, minutes to hours; localization, inner canthus) • Sluder neuralgia (duration, minutes; localization, inner canthus) • glossopharyngeal neuralgia (duration, seconds; localization, base of tongue and tonsillar fossa) • geniculate ganglion neuralgia (duration, seconds; localization, external auditory canal and palatal roof)
Continuous facial pain	• atypical facial pain (diffuse, usually unilateral pain) • temporomandibular joint (TMJ) syndrome (preauricular)
Intense **headache** of **sudden onset,** which then persists	• subarachnoid hemorrhage • intracerebral hemorrhage
Diffuse, usually intense **headache** of **subacute onset,** which then persists	• meningitis, encephalitis (accompanied by meningism)
Headache on standing or sitting that improves when the patient lies down	• intracranial hypotension
Chronic, or chronically relapsing, diffuse headache of insidious onset and mild to moderate severity	• tension-type headache • headache due to hypertension • headache due to intracranial mass • posttraumatic headache • headache due to systemic illness (particularly febrile illness); toxic/iatrogenic headache; psychogenic or depressive headache
Chronic, localized headache and facial pain	• spondylogenic headache (pain mainly in the back of the head) • cranial (temporal) arteritis (pain mainly temporal) • eye diseases (pain mainly frontal) • ENT diseases (esp. sinusitis, pain mainly frontal, worse on forward bending of the head) • odontogenic headache (jaw and temporal region)

Painful Syndromes

13

Painful Shoulder–Arm Syndromes (SAS)

Pain in the shoulder and arm is a common complaint. The differential diagnosis includes conditions belonging to widely disparate medical specialties: cervical spine pathology (spondylogenic arm pain); degenerative changes of the joints of the shoulder and upper limb and the adjacent connective tissues (ligaments, tendons, joint capsules); diseases of the cervical nerve roots, brachial plexus, and peripheral nerves (neurogenic arm pain); and vascular diseases. Finally, there remains "arm pain of overuse," a collection of conditions due to nonphysiological stress on the muscles and joints of the upper limb.

An overview of diseases producing pain in the shoulder and arm is provided in Table 13.10. The clinical features of the more common conditions of this type are described in the following paragraphs.

Table 13.10   Overview of shoulder–arm pain

Category	Etiology	Remarks
Spondylogenic pain	• spondylosis	• nuchal pain at first; pain radiation is often diffuse
	• disk herniation	• acute torticollis at first, only later followed by pain radiation in a radicular pattern; demonstrable neurological deficits
Nonspondylogenic nerve root lesion	• tumor	• slowly progressive symptoms
	• dissection of the vertebral a.	• acute, unilateral nuchal or occipital pain
Brachial plexus lesion	• tumor	• e. g., lung apex tumor with lower brachial plexus involvement and Horner syndrome
	• radiation injury	• pain and progressive neurological deficits after a latency period
	• neuralgic shoulder amyotrophy	• intense pain for one or more days, followed by weakness of shoulder girdle or arm muscles
	• thoracic outlet syndrome (TOS)	• overdiagnosed; the diagnosis can be accepted if there is a cervical rib or other anomaly of the thoracic outlet
	• hyperabduction syndrome	• the arm "falls asleep" at night in certain positions
	• posttraumatic brachial plexus dysfunction	• phantom pain, neuroma pain, stump pain
Lesion of an individual peripheral nerve (or branch)	• radial n.	• supinator syndrome
	• median n.	• pronator syndrome, carpal tunnel syndrome (most common cause of nocturnal arm pain)
	• ulnar n.	• sulcus ulnaris syndrome
	• cutaneous sensory branches	• e. g., elbow after paravenous injection
Rheumatologic disorders	• in the shoulder region	• rotator cuff involvement, impingement syndrome
	• in the elbow region	• radial epicondylitis (tennis elbow), ulnar epicondylitis (golfer's elbow)
	• in the distal forearm and hand	• radial styloiditis, metacarpophalangeal joint of the thumb, e. g., in gout
Brachialgia of vascular origin	• arterial	• acute brachial a. occlusion, subclavian steal syndrome
	• venous	• effort thrombosis
Tenomyalgic and pseudoradicular overuse syndromes	• diffuse brachialgia after nonphysiological overuse of an arm, or secondary to weakness of the shoulder muscles	• various professions, e. g., bank teller, or in the wake of trapezius weakness
Rarer causes	• glomus tumor	• a locally painful blue spot is often visible under the fingernail; the pain increases when the arm is dependent

Spondylogenic (Cervicogenic) Shoulder and Arm Pain

Etiology. The cause is usually *degenerative osteochondrosis* producing spondylotic narrowing of the intervertebral foramina; sometimes, cervical disk herniation is also present. These disease processes compress and mechanically irritate the cervical nerve roots.

Clinical manifestations. Conditions of this type always begin with neck pain and/or a painful restriction of head movement. Later on, the pain radiates into the shoulder and usually down the arm (*cervicobrachialgia*). The pain is diffuse in some patients, but often remains mostly within the dermatome of the affected nerve root (i. e., *radicular pain*): thus, C6 lesions cause pain on the lateral aspect of the forearm and the thumb region, C7 lesions cause pain in the middle finger, and C8 lesions cause pain on the ulnar side of the hand and in the fourth and fifth fingers (cf. p. 208). The *objective findings* include painful restriction of head movement and, sometimes, radicular neurological deficits—weakness, loss of reflexes, and diminished sensation in the distribution of the affected nerve root (cf. Table 12.1, p. 208).

Treatment. *Physical therapy* and *analgesic medications* are the mainstays of treatment (cf. p. 211).

Degenerative and Rheumatic Shoulder and Arm Pain

Most cases of pain in the shoulder and arm are probably caused by degenerative changes of the bones, joints, tendons, and other soft tissues.

Degenerative disease of the rotator cuff. This painful syndrome, formerly termed humeroscapular periarthropathy, arises after shoulder trauma (a blow or sprain) or immobilization. The tendons of the short rotators of the shoulder joint undergo degenerative changes, sometimes with calcium deposition, and these changes lead to irritation of the subdeltoid bursa. The highly typical clinical finding is *local shoulder pain on active raising of the arm, particularly with simultaneous internal rotation.* It is painful, for example, for the patient to slip the arm into a sleeve while getting dressed. If the abducted arm is then rested on a surface (table, etc.), the pain disappears. The diseased tendon(s) is (are) tender to palpation, usually ventral to the shoulder joint. Plain radiographs may reveal calcifications. *Rotator cuff tear* produces mechanical weakness of abduction, objectively demonstrable as the so-called "lag sign."

Impingement syndrome is closely related to degenerative disease of the rotator cuff. In this condition, when the arm is abducted, the painful area of the rotator cuff comes into contact with the coracoacromial roof.

Frozen shoulder syndrome sometimes represents the end stage of degenerative disease of the rotator cuff, but more commonly arises as a sequela of hemiparesis or myocardial infarction. It is also rarely caused by phenobarbital use. It is characterized by *very painful restriction of shoulder movement*, with a slowly progressive course.

Regional pain syndrome. This often-intractable condition used to be known as reflex sympathetic dystrophy, algodystrophy, or Sudeck dystrophy. The sympathetic nervous system plays an important role in its pathogenesis, particularly as a cause of the characteristic swelling. Faulty information processing in the neurons of the dorsal horn of the spinal cord is thought to be another contributing factor. Regional pain syndrome can affect any part of the upper or lower limbs, but it is particularly common in the *hand*. It tends to arise after a fracture or other type of trauma, which need not be particularly severe. The clinical findings include *soft tissue swelling, smooth, cool, often cyanotic skin*, and a *very painful restriction of joint mobility*. Plain radiographs reveal patchy osteoporosis of the bones in the affected area.

Epicondylitis is characterized by pain at the origins of the extensor and flexor muscles of the hand and fingers on the humeral epicondyles. The pain can be felt spontaneously, on movement of the affected tendons and muscles, or in response to local pressure. The usual cause is muscle overuse. The commonest type is lateral epicondylitis, so-called *"tennis elbow."* Medial epicondylitis ("golfer's elbow") is rarer and is caused by overuse of the flexor muscles.

Styloiditis. Radial styloiditis is characterized by pain at the tendinous origins of the extensor carpi radialis muscles on the styloid process of the radius; ulnar styloiditis is the analogous condition on the styloid process of the ulna. Both of these conditions are varieties of tendinitis, similar to other varieties occurring elsewhere in the body.

Neurogenic Arm Pain

In these conditions, pain in the arm and shoulder is due to a **lesion affecting sensory nerve fibers**, either in the brachial plexus or in the peripheral nerves. The lesion may be either **mechanical** (common) or **infectious/inflammatory** (less common).

Irritation of the Brachial Plexus

Compression of the brachial plexus at the thoracic outlet can occur at any of several anatomical bottlenecks (the scalene hiatus, the costoclavicular passage, or the subacromial space). This generally occurs, however, only when an additional pathogenic factor is present, such as a cervical rib, fibrous band, anomaly of the scalene attachments, or excessive exogenous pressure. The corresponding clinical syndromes are discussed in Chapter 12 (p. 220).

Brachial plexus tumors sometimes cause progressively worsening arm pain that becomes very severe within a matter of weeks. *Pancoast tumors* of the lung apex are a well-known cause (p. 222).

Painful Syndromes

13

Neuralgic shoulder amyotrophy (p. 222) also causes acute, severe pain.

Peripheral Nerve Conditions

Compressive neuropathies can cause severe, intractable pain in the upper limb. These conditions are described in Chapter 12. The more common types are *sulcus ulnaris syndrome* (p. 232) and *carpal tunnel syndrome* (p. 228), which causes arm pain especially at night (brachialgia paraesthetica nocturna).

Vasogenic Arm Pain

Arterial Diseases

Occlusion or stenosis of the subclavian a. causes diffuse arm pain on movement, forcing the patient to stop using the limb ("*intermittent claudication of the arm*"). If the artery is occluded proximal to the origin of the vertebral a., the arm will be supplied with blood through retrograde flow in the vertebral a. Blood can be "stolen" in this way from the cerebral circulation (**subclavian steal syndrome**): movement of the arm diverts blood flow away from the vertebrobasilar territory in the brain and lightheadedness or sudden falls (*drop attacks*) may result. Arterial insufficiency in the upper limb is demonstrated with the *fist-clenching test*: the patient holds the upper limbs high, then rapidly and repeatedly clenches and reopens both hands. Pain arises within a few minutes on the poorly perfused side and the hand turns pale. When the arms are lowered again, the veins on the dorsum of the hand fill slowly on the affected side. The arterial blood pressure is also always lower when measured in the affected arm.

Venous Thrombosis

Occlusion of the axillary or subclavian v . This condition, also known as *effort syndrome* or *Paget–von Schrötter syndrome*, is seen most commonly in young men, usually on the right side. It is rarely spontaneous; more commonly, it arises after heavy use of the arm, e. g., in sports. The venous occlusion manifests itself as a painful tension in the arm, often accompanied by swelling. The subcutaneous veins in the region of the arm provide an alternative path for venous return and are thus more clearly visible than normal. The thrombosed vein itself can sometimes be palpated in the axilla and is tender. It can often be unequivocally demonstrated with neuroimaging studies and Doppler ultrasonography. The prognosis is usually good; operative thrombectomy is only rarely necessary.

"Arm Pain of Overuse"

The nonphysiological, prolonged, and repeated performance of specific movements of the upper limb(s), particularly at the workplace (e. g., typing, working at a cash register, or long and monotonous use of other kinds of machines), can produce intractable pain in the upper limb extending well beyond the muscles that were used in the repeated movement. Pain of this type leads, in turn, to excessive reliance on other muscle groups, so that these, too, become involved in the pain syndrome. This condition and its pathogenesis are described further under "Pseudoradicular Pain" (below).

Other Types of Arm Pain

Glomus tumors are small, benign growths that originate in the glomus organs of the skin. They are composed of *arteriovenous anastomoses* in close association with autonomic fibers. Clinically, they are characterized by a *dull pain* that worsens when the arm hangs down and, particularly, when the arm swings as the patient walks. Local pressure over the tumor also causes pain. Glomus tumors are often found at the fingertips, where they may be visible as a bluish spot under the fingernail, but they can also arise practically anywhere else, including on the lower limbs.

"Referred pain." Diseases of the internal organs commonly cause referred pain in the shoulder and arm. Pain is felt in the right shoulder in gall bladder disease, for example, and in the left arm in angina pectoris.

Gout. An exacerbation of gout can produce extremely severe, acute pain in a hand (*chiragra*) or foot (*podagra*). Chiragra is sometimes, but not always, restricted to the metacarpophalangeal joint of the thumb.

Pain in the Trunk and Back

The back is by far the most common site of pain in the trunk. It is usually due to **pathological abnormalities of the spine**, which lead, in turn, to abnormal posture and nonphysiological activation of the muscles of the back.

Table 13.**11** provides an overview of these painful syndromes, their localization, and the types of pain they produce. A few of them will be described in detail in the following paragraphs.

Table 13.**11** **Overview of pain in the trunk and back**

Designation	Mechanism	Localization and clinical features	Remarks
Pain in a band-like distribution	uni- or bilateral nerve root lesion	feeling of segmental tightening on one or both sides; continuous pain	e. g., spinal tumor, disk herniation, herpes zoster
Abnormally mobile 10th rib ("slipping rib")	pain on displacement of the free end of the 10th rib	unilateral pain at the costal margin, on bending over or with local pressure; the pain may be continuous	after thoracic trauma, or spontaneous
Tear and hemorrhage in the abdominal wall musculature	lesion (rupture) of the rectus abdominis m., e. g., after strenuous exercise	local pain in the abdominal wall	rarely, compartment syndrome of the rectus abdominis m.
Spiegel hernia	herniation next to the rectus sheath, covered by the abdominal oblique m. and difficult to identify	pain at a paramedian location on the abdominal wall, local tenderness	the pain disappears after the application of local anesthetic
Rectus abdominis syndrome	entrapment neuropathy; a medial cutaneous branch of one of the intercostal nerves is caught in a gap in the fascia	abdominal wall pain on movement; sometimes there is a coin-sized zone of cutaneous anesthesia	differential diagnosis: inguinal hernia, testicular torsion
Ilioinguinal nerve syndrome	compression of the ilioinguinal n., or constriction by scar	groin, external genitalia; dull, continuous pain, worse on hip extension, better on flexion; objective sensory deficit in the distribution of the nerve	
"Referred pain" (zones of Head)	pain from internal organs projected to the surface of the trunk	pain localization depends on the affected organ; e. g., chest pain in diseases of the heart and lungs, abdominal pain in GI diseases, lumbar pain in diseases of the retroperitoneal organs; typically a dull, piercing, or acute tearing pain	
Thoracoabdominal neuropathy	usually diabetic mononeuropathy	continuous pain and paresthesiae of the thoracic or abdominal wall; diminished sensation, or unilateral weakness of abdominal wall muscles	
Ankylosing spondylitis (Bekhterev disease)	in 90 % of cases, associated with the HLA-B27 histocompatibility antigen	the pain usually begins in the low lumbosacral region, usually at night; progressive thoracic kyphosis and diminishing mobility of the spine; rarely, pain in the chest and heels; typical radiologic findings	usually affects younger men
Spondylolisthesis and spondylolysis	prolongation of the pars interarticularis and ventral displacement of the cranial vertebra, ranging to spondyloptosis	lower lumbar pain, worse on exertion and after prolonged standing; palpable "step" in the back; typical radiologic findings	congenital anomaly; spondylolisthesis can be induced by mechanical stress or can occur spontaneously (in the latter case, usually as a symptom of an underlying condition); differential diagnosis: pseudospondylolisthesis in degenerative osteochondrosis
Sacroiliac strain	tension on the ligamentous apparatus of the sacroiliac joint	low back pain, sometimes pseudoradicular radiation into the lower limbs; worse when the patient stands on one leg, or with the Mennell maneuver	relieved by wearing a trochanteric belt
Notalgia paresthetica	entrapment of the terminal sensory branch of the dorsal ramus of a spinal nerve in a fascial gap in the back	local, unilateral pain in the back; objective local tenderness and a coin-sized area of paravertebral cutaneous anesthesia	the pain disappears after the application of local anesthetic

Painful Syndromes

13

Thoracic and Abdominal Wall Pain

Diseases of the internal organs are the most common cause of pain in the thoracic and abdominal wall (see "*referred pain*," above). *Chest pain* is often due to diseases of the heart and lungs. *Band-like pain* suggests a (possibly intraspinal) process irritating one of the spinal nerve roots or segmental nerves. *Abdominal wall pain* often arises from the internal organs, but may also be due, for example, to *compression of the ventral rami of the spinal nerve roots* (e. g., compression of the caudal thoracic nerves in the *rectus abdominis syndrome*). The rare *Spiegel hernia* (cf. Table 13.**11**) is another possibility, as is an *abnormally mobile tenth rib*.

Back Pain

Back pain is a very common problem that often profoundly affects the sufferer's everyday life at work and at home. The pain cannot always be fully explained based on objectively demonstrable skeletal changes. The extent of the visible structural changes is often not commensurate with the intensity of the pain. The major causes of back pain are:

Structural changes of the spine cause the vast majority of cases of back pain. *Osteochondrosis* leads to reactive spondylotic changes and, therefore, increased stress on the intervertebral joints. This, in turn, causes faulty posture, reflex functional disturbances of the musculature, and, therefore, pain. A *herniated intervertebral disk* can compress a nerve root, producing acute pain radiating into the periphery (p. 210). *Abnormal postures of the spine*, as in ankylosing spondylitis or scoliosis, often cause intractable back pain because of the associated nonphysiological stress on the muscles of the trunk and back. *Spondylolisthesis*, the sliding of one vertebral body on another (with or without *spondylolysis*, i. e., a defect of the pars interarticularis of the vertebral arch), is a congenital anomaly that usually remains clinically silent until later in life. It sometimes becomes symptomatic after an accident.

Pathological changes of the sacroiliac joint typically produce pain that worsens when the patient stands on one leg or hyperextends the leg on the affected side (*Mennell maneuver*).

Entrapment neuropathies are responsible for some cases of back pain of nonskeletal origin. *Notalgia paresthetica*, for example, is a rare entrapment neuropathy of the sensory dorsal rami of the thoracic spinal nerves as they pass through small apertures in the fascia (see p. 232).

Coccygodynia , i. e., intractable *pain in the region of the coccyx*, can arise after local trauma (a fall on the buttocks) or spontaneously. In the latter case, the diagnostic evaluation should include a search for tumors or infectious/inflammatory changes in the pelvis, as well as cysts of the lumbosacral nerve root sleeves (= Tarlov cysts).

Groin Pain

Pain in the groin can be caused not only by bladder conditions, gynecologic diseases, and inguinal hernias, but also by *peripheral nerve lesions*. The *ilioinguinal nerve syndrome*, a type of entrapment neuropathy, is described in Table 13.**11**. The pain of *spermatic neuralgia* is felt in the scrotum. In general, when the cause of groin pain is unclear, a pathological process should be sought in the pelvis.

▬ Leg Pain

Pain in the leg, like pain in the arm, has many causes. Common causes are degenerative and traumatic **joint and soft tissue processes**, **lumbar disk herniation**, and **pathology in the lumbar spinal canal**. Others include **polyneuropathies**, **entrapment neuropathies**, and **restless legs syndrome**. **Vascular diseases**, too, play an important role, particularly arterial occlusive disease.

Pain in the hip is usually due to diseases of the hip joint, most often degenerative arthritis (*coxarthrosis*). A diagnosis that is often missed is *periarthropathy of the hip*: in this condition, the joint itself is not diseased, but the soft tissues around it give rise to intractable pain, which frequently lasts for months. In *algodystrophy of the hip*, local pain is followed, some time afterward, by the development of osteopenia of the femoral head. Both the pain and the osteopenia usually resolve spontaneously.

Thigh pain may be due to a local process such as a *sarcoma*. An upper lumbar disk herniation or other lesion causing *nerve root irritation* can produce referred pain in the thigh. *Meralgia paresthetica*, a type of entrapment neuropathy causing pain in the thigh, is described on p. 234. Acute thigh pain and femoral nerve palsy can be caused either by *diabetic neuropathy* or by a *hematoma in the psoas sheath*.

Knee pain is usually of orthopedic, rheumatological, or traumatic origin. A proximal lesion of the obturator n. produces referred pain in the popliteal fossa in *Howship–Romberg syndrome* (p. 236). Spontaneous or mechanically induced lesions of the *infrapatellar branch of the saphenous n.* are a further cause of pain in the knee.

Pain in the lower leg that is present **only when the patient walks** is typical of *vasogenic intermittent claudication*, a syndrome whose cause usually lies in the arteries, less commonly in the veins. *Neurogenic intermit-*

tent claudication is caused by compression of the cauda equina in *lumbar spinal stenosis* (p. 213). Vasogenic intermittent claudication is worse when the patient walks uphill, while the neurogenic type is worse when the patient walks downhill. In the *anterior tibial artery syndrome*, pain develops **acutely** on the anterior aspect of the lower leg, particularly with exercise (p. 239). The *saphenous n.* can be caught in a fascial gap on the medial side of the lower leg, or, alternatively, in Hunter's canal in the thigh; pain ensues in the cutaneous zone innervated by this nerve (*entrapment neuropathy*).

Pain in the foot is a common complaint. It is usually **unilateral** and caused by an orthopedic condition, or by trauma. *Tarsal tunnel syndrome*, which typically arises after an ankle sprain, causes pain in the sole of the foot when the patient walks; it is described on p. 241. *Morton's metatarsalgia* is described in the same section. **Bilateral**, burning pain in the feet characterizes *erythromelalgia of vasomotor origin*, otherwise known as *burning feet syndrome*. Similar symptoms may arise in *polyneuropathy*, but are then usually accompanied by objective neurological findings (loss of Achilles reflexes, distal sensory deficit). In "*restless legs syndrome*," the restlessness, which is perceived as painful, forces the sufferer to stand up, walk around, and move the legs time and again, particularly at night or after prolonged sitting in a soft chair. This syndrome usually responds to small doses of L-DOPA, as well as to dopamine agonists.

Pseudoradicular Pain

This term denotes an etiologically heterogeneous collection of painful syndromes caused by a **faulty synergy of the muscles and joints**. The faulty synergy arises either from structural joint changes or from nonphysiological movements putting excessive stress on the musculoskeletal system.

Pathophysiology. The joints of the body have a continuous, dynamic relationship with the muscles that move them. Afferent nerve impulses arising in the joints are fed back to the muscles to regulate and coordinate the timing and strength of muscle contraction. Thus, *pathological impulses* arising from *mechanically damaged or otherwise dysfunctional joints* lead to nonphysiologic patterns of muscle activation. In addition, *movements that are repeated monotonously or that put the joints in an unfavorable position* ("nonergonomic" movements) cause pain of the participating anatomic structures through overuse. Different names are used for the resulting pain syndromes, depending on the specialty and school of thought of the physician or other expert consulted: tendomyalgia, tendomyosis, pseudoradicular pain, myofascial syndrome, muscular rheumatism, and so forth.

Clinical manifestations. Pseudoradicular pain can arise in many different regions of the body but is particularly common in the *upper limb*. The pain is chronic and difficult to treat, because it is constantly reactivated by the daily (over)use of the involved joints and muscles.

The general features of pseudoradicular pain are as follows:
- the pain is of greater or lesser intensity,
- usually radiates into a single limb,
- is exacerbated by the use of this limb,
- and causes an antalgic restriction of movement;
- there are painful trigger points and painful tendon attachments;
- there is no objectifiable sensory deficit, paresis, or reflex abnormality;
- nonphysiologic, antalgic movement leads to the perpetuation, extension, and chronification of the pain.

Treatment and prognosis. This condition is difficult to treat. The most useful approach consists of good occupational hygiene (use of the affected muscles only up to the pain threshold), changing the illness-producing behavior (switch to a different task at work), and passive measures such as trigger-point therapy. Much patience is demanded of both doctor and patient.

Painful Syndromes

13

14 Diseases of Muscle (Myopathies)

Structure and Function of Muscle

Microscopic anatomy of muscle. The most important structural components of striated skeletal muscle are the muscle fibers (Fig. 14.1). These cells contain *contractile elements* called myofibrils, which, in turn, are composed of interlacing *actin* and *myosin molecules*, which take the shape of filaments. The periodically repeating pattern of molecular structures in skeletal muscle accounts for its characteristic, striped ("striated") microscopic appearance (Fig. 14.1). The actin and myosin filaments are connected to each other by intermolecular "bridges."

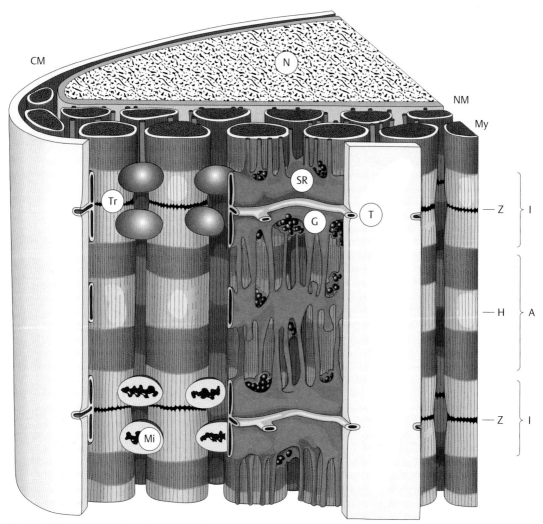

Fig. 14.**1 Microstructure of skeletal muscle fibers** (diagram of a frog preparation). **CM,** cell membrane. **G,** glycogen granule. **Mi,** mitochondrion. **My,** myofibrils. **N,** nucleus. **NM,** nuclear membrane. **SR,** sarcoplasmic reticulum. **T,** tubular system. (After Mumenthaler, M.: Muskelkrankheiten, in Hornbostel H., Kaufmann W., Siegenthaler W.: *Innere Medizin in Praxis und Klinik*, vol. II, 4th edn, Thieme, Stuttgart 1992.)

Physiology of muscle contraction. When a skeletal muscle contracts, the actin filaments pull the myosin filaments toward themselves. The myosin filaments slide over each other by a progressive ratcheting mechanism of the intermolecular bridges, resulting in a net shortening (contraction) of the muscle fiber. The energy for this process is derived from phosphate compounds, mainly adenosine triphosphate (ATP), but also creatine phosphate when the muscle is under acute stress. The regeneration of creatine phosphate after muscle contraction is catalyzed by the muscle-specific enzyme creatine phosphokinase (CK).

When a muscle is first set in contraction, glycogen within the muscle is anaerobically metabolized and lactic acid accumulates in the muscle for five to 10 minutes. After that, if the muscle continues to be contracted, a switch to aerobic metabolism occurs, with increasing consumption of fatty acids and lactic acid. Enzyme defects that interfere with these energy-liberating processes during muscle contraction can cause clinically apparent abnormalities of muscle function. Much of the aerobic energy metabolism in muscle tissue takes place in mitochondria (Fig. 14.1); thus, mitochondrial diseases, too, can impair muscle function.

Impulse transmission at the motor end plate and impulse conduction in the muscle fiber. Skeletal muscle is set in contraction by a nerve impulse arriving at the so-called *motor end plate* (Fig. 14.2) or neuromuscular junction. This "relay station" at the point where a nerve fiber and a muscle fiber meet consists of the *presynaptic membrane*, a specialized component of the terminal segment of the motor neuron; the *synaptic cleft*; and the *postsynaptic membrane*, a specialized component of the cell membrane (sarcolemma) of the muscle fiber.

An action potential arriving at the motor end plate induces the secretion of acetylcholine from the presynaptic membrane. The acetylcholine molecules then diffuse across the synaptic cleft and bind to specific receptors on the postsynaptic membrane. This, in turn, leads to depolarization of the sarcolemma. Having accomplished their task, the acetylcholine molecules are now rapidly broken down within the synaptic cleft into acetate and choline, a step catalyzed by the enzyme acetylcholinesterase. Meanwhile, the sarcolemmal excitation is carried into the interior of the muscle fiber by way of numerous transverse invaginations of the cell mem-

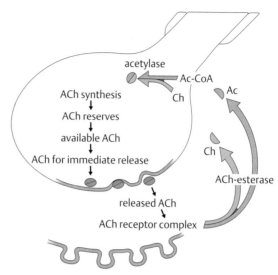

Fig. 14.**2 Impulse transmission at the motor end plate.** Acetylcholine (ACh), the acetic acid ester of the aminoalcohol choline, is released into the synaptic cleft in response to a depolarizing stimulus and then binds to specific receptors on the postsynaptic membrane. Acetylcholine is inactivated by breakdown into its two components, choline (Ch) and acetate (Ac); this step is catalyzed by the enzyme acetylcholinesterase. Choline is taken back up into the presynaptic nerve terminal with the aid of specific transporters and then reacts again with the activated form of acetic acid (Ac-CoA) to form new acetylcholine molecules.

brane (the tubular system or T-system) and is then transmitted to the longitudinal system, a branched network of cisterns of the endoplasmic (sarcoplasmic) reticulum, which surrounds the individual myofibrils (Fig. 14.1). When the depolarizing stimulus arrives here, it induces the secretion of calcium ions from terminal cisterns and the intracellular calcium concentration accordingly rises. This, in turn, activates actomyosin ATPase, which is the final step in the initiation of muscle contraction.

Functional disturbances of these complex processes and structural changes of one or more elements of muscle or of the motor end plate cause various types of myopathy, which will be discussed from the clinical point of view in the remainder of this chapter.

General Symptomatology, Evaluation, and Classification of Muscle Diseases

Muscle weakness can be either **neurogenic** or **myogenic**. The causes and clinical features of neurogenic muscle weakness were already discussed in earlier chapters. The present chapter concerns diseases involving a **structural or functional defect of the muscle tissue itself**, which are called **myopathies**. These, in turn, can be classified as either **primary** or **symptomatic**. Symptomatic myopathies are manifestations of muscle involvement by some other underlying disease or condition— e. g., **endocrine** or **toxic** myopathy. Primary myopathies, in contrast, are due to a pathological process in the muscle itself. Most primary myopathies are genetically determined, e. g., the group of **muscular dystrophies** and the **channelopathies** (functional disorders of the individual ion channels of the muscle fiber membrane), which express themselves clinically either as a myotonic syn-

Table 14.**1** **Characteristics of myopathies**

Criterion	Characteristic findings
Onset and progression	usually progresses slowly (years); exceptions include myasthenia and polymyositis
Appearance of muscles	usually atrophic, sometimes pseudohypertrophic (e. g., calf muscles)
Strength	decreased
Localization of atrophy and weakness	usually symmetrical; exceptions include myasthenia and, sometimes, polymyositis; the weakness is usually proximal; exception, myasthenia (sometimes)
Reflexes	diminished or absent
Sensation	intact
Contractures	usually develop over the course of time (years)
Ancillary testing	pathological EMG, normal nerve conduction velocity, elevated serum creatine kinase concentration, typical biopsy findings
Differential diagnosis	most importantly, spinal muscular atrophy; muscle weakness of metabolic origin; functional pseudoparesis

Table 14.**2** **Classification of muscle diseases**

Muscular dystrophies
Spinal muscular atrophy and other motor neuron diseases, cf. p. 154
Myotonias and periodic paralyses ("channelopathies")
Metabolic myopathies
Mitochondrial myopathies and encephalomyopathies
Congenital myopathies
Infectious/inflammatory myopathies
Myopathy due to endocrine disorders
Muscle involvement by electrolyte disturbances
Toxic and iatrogenic myopathies
Disorders of neuromuscular transmission
Tumors
Trauma

drome or as episodic paralysis. Most of the diseases caused by **enzyme defects** are also genetically determined (including, among others, the mitochondrial encephalomyopathies). There are also numerous types of **autoimmune** myopathy. Prominent among them are **polymyositis** and **dermatomyositis**, as well as **myasthenia gravis**, a disease of the motor end plate.

General clinical manifestations. Myopathies are traditionally considered part of the subject matter of neurology because their most prominent sign is motor weakness. The typical manifestations that are common to all myopathies as a class are summarized in Table 14.**1**.

General diagnostic considerations. The evaluation of myopathy comprises the following steps:
- *a complete and precise case history*, including the family history;

- *physical examination*, with particular attention to:
  - muscle weakness that is already present at rest, or that worsens or is exclusively present on exercise; the examiner should also specifically look for
  - muscle atrophy,
  - fasciculations,
  - diminished or absent reflexes,
  - myotonic reactions (p. 270) to a tap on a muscle, or on muscle contraction, and
  - shortened muscles;
- *electromyography* and *electroneurography* (p. 58);
- *blood tests*, particularly the serum concentration of creatine phosphokinase (CK);
- and, as needed depending on the particular clinical situation, further special tests:
  - *muscle biopsy* with conventional light-microscopic histopathological examination;
  - special stains for the demonstration of abnormal lipid deposition, dystrophin, mitochondrial anomalies, enzyme defects, etc.;
  - electron microscopy;
  - quantitative biochemical analysis of biopsy specimens;
  - stress testing, e. g., measurement of the rise in lactate concentration after anaerobic muscle contraction;
  - genetic analyses.

Classification of muscle diseases. Myopathies can be classified by their etiology and pathophysiology, by their clinical phenomenology, or, as is now increasingly common, by their underlying genetic defects (Table 14.**2**). The genetically oriented classification of the myopathies is currently changing so rapidly that our listings in Tables 14.**3**, 14.**4** must be regarded as provisional.

Muscular Dystrophies

The muscular dystrophies are **genetically determined**. They typically present with **symmetric muscle weakness**, which is at first either mainly proximal or mainly distal, and which slowly worsens over the years. The chronically progressive weakness is not accompanied by pain or by any sensory deficit. The muscles usually become **atrophic**, though this is masked, in some patients, by intramuscular deposition of fatty tissue (**pseudohypertrophy**). Connective tissue deposition can lead to **muscle shortening and contractures**. The reflexes are diminished or lost. Weakness produces characteristic **postural abnormalities** and **deformities**, e. g., to lumbar hyperlordosis (a common finding), Duchenne or Trendelenburg gait (p. 15), winging of the scapula, or scoliosis.

Table 14.**3** provides an overview of the various types of muscular dystrophy. The major types are described in detail in the following paragraphs.

Table 14.**3**   **The muscular dystrophies**

Type	Inheritance pattern	Chromosomal or genomic defect	Missing or abnormal gene product	Incidence (i. e., frequency with respect to live births)	Age of onset	Clinical features	Prognosis
Duchenne	X-linked, 30 % sporadic	Xp21.2	dystrophin absent	20–30/ 100 000 boys	2nd–3rd year	onset in pelvic girdle, pseudo-hypertrophy of calves	rapidly progressive, most patients die by age 25
Becker	X-linked	Xp21.2	dystrophin abnormal	3/100 000 boys	1st(–4th) decade	same as in Duchenne muscular dystrophy, but milder; sometimes cardiomyopathy	ambulatory till age 15 or later, death in 4th or 5th decade or later
Emery–Dreifuss	X-linked, rarely autosomal dominant	Xp28	emerin	1/100 000	childhood, adolescence	scapuloperoneal dystrophy, contractures, and cardiopathy may be prominent	ambulatory till 3rd decade or for entire life; cardiac arrhythmia a frequent cause of death
Facioscapulo-humeral dystrophy (Duchenne–Landouzy–Dejerine)	autosomal dominant	4q35	homeobox gene	5/100 000	childhood to young adulthood	weakness of facial, shoulder girdle, and calf muscles	practically normal life expectancy
Scapulo-peroneal dystrophy	autosomal dominant, autosomal recessive, or sporadic	unknown	unknown	rare	childhood to adulthood	weakness of shoulder girdle and dorsiflexors of the feet and toes	usually normal life expectancy
Limb girdle dystrophy	autosomal recessive, autosomal dominant, or sporadic	5q, 13q, 15q	unknown	rare	childhood to adulthood	mainly proximal weakness of pelvic or shoulder girdle	depending on type, premature death or only minor disability into old age
Distal myopathies (Welander type, Markesbery–Griggs, Finnish variant)	autosomal dominant	unknown	unknown	rare	middle age	mainly distal atrophy and weakness	only minor disability into old age
Distal myopathies (Nonaka and Miyoshi types)	autosomal recessive	Miyoshi: 2p12–14 Nonaka: unknown	unknown	rare	adolescence to young adulthood	mainly distal weakness	progression to inability to walk

Diseases of Muscle

14

Continued →

Table 14.**3** **The muscular dystrophies** (Continued)

Type	Inheritance pattern	Chromosomal or genomic defect	Missing or abnormal gene product	Incidence (i. e., frequency with respect to live births)	Age of onset	Clinical features	Prognosis
Oculopharyngeal dystrophies	autosomal dominant	unknown	unknown	rare	middle age	oculofaciobulbar paresis	often premature death due to dysphagia and aspiration pneumonia
Congenital dystrophies (for variants, see text)	autosomal recessive	unknown	unknown	rare	at birth	depending on type: involvement of muscles, eyes, and brain; contractures, arthrogryposis multiplex	ranging from mild disability to severe mental retardation
Steinert myotonic dystrophy	autosomal dominant	19q13.3	protein kinase	13.5/100 000, prevalence 5/100 000	young adulthood, rarely congenital, earlier age of onset in each successive generation ("anticipation")	mainly distal weakness, faciobulbar paresis, myotonia, cataracts	age of significant disability depends on age of onset, usually middle age; premature death
Proximal myotonic myopathy (PROMM)	autosomal dominant	unknown	unknown	0.5/100 000	3rd and 4th decades, sometimes earlier	mainly proximal weakness, myotonia, and cataracts	disability in old age

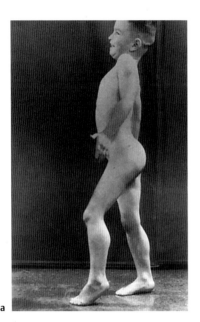
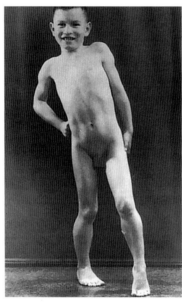

a   b

Fig. 14.**3** **Duchenne muscular dystrophy** in a 10-year-old boy. **a** Lateral view: note the lumbar lordosis and pseudohypertrophic calves. **b** When the child walks, the trunk inclines to the side of the stationary leg (Duchenne limp). (From: Mumenthaler M.: *Didaktischer Atlas der klinischen Neurologie.* 2nd edn, Springer, Heidelberg 1986.)

Hereditary Muscular Dystrophies of X-chromosomal Inheritance– Dystrophinopathies

The diseases in this group are caused by a genetic defect on chromosome Xp21.2. They are, therefore, almost exclusively seen in boys whose mothers are (healthy) carriers. Dystrophin, a structural protein of the muscle fiber membrane that is also expressed in the brain, is present in reduced amounts or completely absent.

Duchenne Muscular Dystrophy

Clinical manifestations. Boys develop the first signs of the disease in the first decade of life, usually in the preschool years. The conspicuous abnormalities at first are *difficulty climbing stairs, hyperlordosis of the lumbar spine,* and *waddling gait* (Fig. 14.**3**). Over the next few years, weakness becomes progressively severe in the proximal muscles of the lower limbs and then of the upper limbs as well. The affected boys can stand up from a squatting position only by climbing up their own legs with their hands and arms (*Gowers sign,* Fig. 14.**4**). Fat deposition leads to *pseudohypertrophy of the calves.* The waddling gait is due to bilateral hip adductor weakness (*Duchenne* or *Trendelenburg gait*, p. 15).

Diagnostic evaluation. The *CK* is markedly elevated in the initial stages of the disease. The absence of dystrophin can be demonstrated by *muscle biopsy* with special tissue staining (Fig. 14.**5**).

Prognosis. The disease progresses relatively rapidly, rendering the affected boys unable to walk in the second decade of life. The scoliosis worsens and causes respiratory difficulty. The cardiac muscle is also affected, though usually not to any clinically evident extent. As dystrophin is expressed in the brain, most of the affected boys are mentally retarded. They usually die of respiratory insufficiency or secondary complications between the ages of 18 and 25.

Becker Muscular Dystrophy

This type of muscular dystrophy is about one-tenth as common as the Duchenne type. Dystrophin is not wholly absent, but is expressed in reduced amounts (Fig. 14.**5**). The affected boys show the first signs of the disease in the first or second decade; the progression is much slower than in the Duchenne type. Many patients are still able to walk after age 30, but most die in their fourth or fifth decade of life. The EMG and laboratory findings are similar to those of Duchenne muscular dystrophy.

Autosomal Muscular Dystrophies

The genetic localization of the autosomal muscular dystrophies is known in most patients, though the gene products are not. We will only describe the more common forms here.

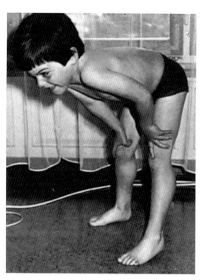

Fig. 14.**4 Gowers sign** in Duchenne muscular dystrophy. This 7-year-old boy stands up by climbing up his own thighs. (From: Mumenthaler M.: *Didaktischer Atlas der klinischen Neurologie.* 2nd edn, Springer, Heidelberg 1986.)

Facio-Scapulo-Humeral Type

This is a disease of autosomal dominant inheritance due to a genetic defect in the 4q35 region of chromosome 4, near the telomere. It begins in the second or third decade of life with *weakness of the facial and shoulder girdle musculature* (eye closure, whistling; raising the arms) (Fig. 14.**6**). Sensorineural deafness is often present as well. The muscles of the pelvic girdle and the distal muscles of the limbs are not affected until later decades. The life expectancy is normal.

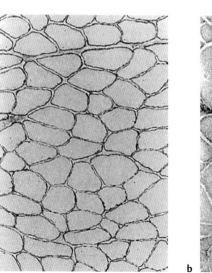
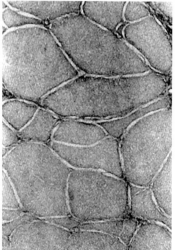
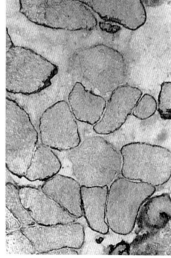
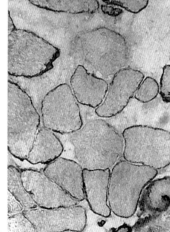

a b c

Fig. 14.**5 Dystrophin stain. a** Normal skeletal muscle. Regular, homogeneous distribution of dystrophin on the inner surface of the sarcolemma of each muscle fiber (black contours). **b** Duchenne dystrophy. Dystrophin is absent. **c** Becker dystrophy. Dystrophin is expressed to a varying extent on the individual muscle fibers, in diminished quantity and abnormal distribution; in some fibers, it is not expressed at all. The presence of dystrophin—albeit in subnormal amounts—distinguishes Becker from Duchenne dystrophy.

Diseases of Muscle

14

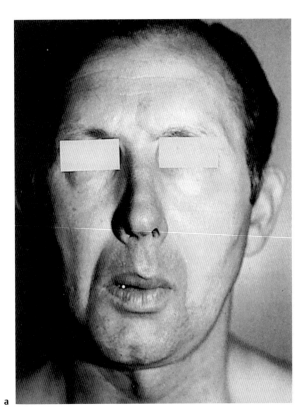

a

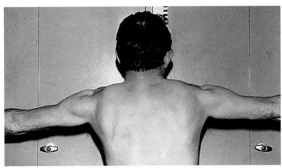

b

Fig. 14.**6 Facio-scapulo-humeral muscular dystrophy** in a 37-year-old man. A photograph of the face **(a)**,reveals weakness of the orbicularis oris m., because of which the patient cannot whistle. A rear view of the upper body **(b)**, shows the protruding scapulae. The patient cannot raise his arms laterally above a horizontal line. (From Mumenthaler, M., in Hornbostel H., Kaufmann W., Siegenthaler W.: *Innere Medizin in Praxis und Klinik*, vol. II, 4th edn, Thieme, Stuttgart 1992, cf. Fig. 14.**1**)

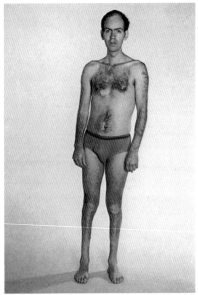

Fig. 14.**7 Steinert myotonic dystrophy** in a 28-year-old man. Note the flaccid facial features and sunken temples (myopathic facies) and the predominantly distal muscle atrophy in the limbs, particularly the lower limbs. (From: Mumenthaler M.: *Didaktischer Atlas der klinischen Neurologie*. 2nd edn, Springer, Heidelberg 1986.)

Limb Girdle Types of Muscular Dystrophy

This is a genetically heterogeneous group of diseases: the inheritance pattern is autosomal dominant for some, autosomal recessive for others. Causative genetic defects have been found on chromosomes 5q, 13q, and 15q. The onset of disease can be in childhood or in adulthood. The first sign is always *mainly proximal weakness of the muscles of either the shoulder girdle or the pelvic girdle*; over time, the other limb girdle is affected as well (*ascending vs. descending type*). The prognosis is highly variable: some patients experience rapid progression of the disease within one or two decades, while others live on into old age with hardly any impairment.

Myotonic Dystrophy of Curschmann–Steinert Type

Epidemiology. This is the most common myopathy of adulthood (see also Table 14.**3**).

Etiology. This is a disease of autosomal dominant inheritance due to an unstable CTG trinucleotide sequence expansion in a gene on chromosome 19q13.3. Clinical manifestations arise when the sequence contains more than the usual five to 30 trinucleotide repeats. The expansion lengthens from generation to generation when transmitted in the maternal line; this explains the onset of the disease at an earlier age in each successive generation (*anticipation*).

Clinical manifestations. *Muscle involvement* is the most prominent sign. *Weakness of the facial and distal limb muscles* usually becomes apparent in young adulthood. The face develops a typical "tired" appearance with sunken temples, mild ptosis, and loose folds around the often slightly open mouth (*myopathic facies*, cf. Fig. 14.**7**). Weakness and atrophy of the dorsiflexors of the feet produce a steppage gait. *Myotonia* is a striking phenomenon that may appear in a very early stage of the disease: after the patient firmly grips an object, he or she has difficulty letting it go. Delayed muscle relaxation can also be demonstrated after a sharp blow to a muscle (e. g., tongue, ball of the thumb). *Other organs*, too, are affected: early cataracts, dysphagia, sluggish bowel function, cardiomyopathy, pulmonary involvement, diabetes, testicular atrophy, and infertility are all possible manifestations of the disease.

Diagnosis. The diagnosis can be made tentatively based on the typical clinical features and the demonstration of myotonic discharges in the EMG. It is confirmed by genetic testing.

Prognosis. The life expectancy is markedly lowered; most patients die around age 50.

Congenital Myotonic Dystrophy

This disease is due to a genetic defect involving a very large trinucleotide expansion (more than 2000 copies). It is usually passed on from mothers to their children, particularly when the mother already possesses a long expansion. The affected individuals suffer from birth onward from dysphagia and weakness of drinking, flaccid facial muscles, a high palate, mental retardation, and other signs like those of Curschmann–Steinert myotonic dystrophy.

Rarer Types of Muscular Dystrophy

Congenital muscular dystrophies are a heterogeneous group of diseases characterized by dystrophic changes in muscle fibers that are present at birth and then either remain constant or slowly progress. Muscular dystrophy that has already exerted its effects in prenatal life presents in the newborn with *arthrogryposis multiplex*, i. e., fixed, abnormal positions of the joints.

Oculopharyngeal dystrophy is a disease of autosomal dominant inheritance that first becomes evident in middle age. The initial signs are progressively severe ptosis and restriction of eye movements, without diplopia. Later, dysphagia develops, which may be life threatening. Other muscle groups are sometimes paretic as well. This condition requires diagnostic differentiation from myasthenia gravis (p. 275) and Kearns–Sayre syndrome (p. 273).

Myotonic Syndromes and Periodic Paralysis Syndromes

These inherited muscle diseases belong to the group of so-called **channelopathies**: they involve abnormalities of the chloride, sodium, or calcium channels in the muscle fiber membrane. They are caused by a variety of different genetic defects and manifest themselves clinically either with **myotonia** (delayed relaxation of muscle after active contraction) or with **episodic paralysis**.

Table 14.**4** provides an overview of the major types of channelopathy. A selection of these will be discussed in the following paragraphs.

Table 14.**4** Myotonias and periodic paralyses ("channelopathies," channel diseases)

Type	Inheritance pattern	Chromosomal or genomic defect	Missing or abnormal gene product	Incidence (i. e., frequency with respect to live births)	Age of onset	Clinical features	Prognosis
Myotonia congenita, Thomsen type	autosomal dominant	7q35	abnormal chloride channels	1/23 000	early in 1st decade	generalized myotonia	stable, nonprogressive
Myotonia congenita, Becker type	autosomal recessive	7q35	abnormal chloride channels	1/23 000–1/50 000	end of 1st decade	generalized myotonia	stable, nonprogressive
Myotonia fluctuans, myotonia permanens, acetazolamide-sensitive myotonia	autosomal dominant	17q23–25	abnormal sodium channels	very rare	1st decade; myotonia fluctuans in adolescence	generalized, myotonia fluctuans only episodic, other types severe, potassium loading worsens myotonia, acetazolamide-sensitive myotonia is painful	nonprogressive

Diseases of Muscle

14

Continued →

Tabelle 14.**4** **Myotonias and periodic paralyses ("channelopathies," channel diseases)** (Continued)

Type	Inheritance pattern	Chromosomal or genomic defect	Missing or abnormal gene product	Incidence (i. e., frequency with respect to live births)	Age of onset	Clinical features	Prognosis
Paramyotonia congenita of Eulenburg	autosomal dominant	17q23–25	abnormal sodium channels	very rare	1st decade	generalized myotonia induced by cold and worsened by exertion, occasionally combined with paramyotonic and hyperkalemic paralyses	persistent, tendency to improve over time
Hyperkalemic periodic paralysis	autosomal dominant	17q23–25	abnormal sodium channels	very rare	1st decade	paralysis occurring on fasting, or rest after physical activity	persistent, often improves over time. Permanent myopathy and weakness are less severe than in hypokalemic paralysis
Hypokalemic periodic paralysis	autosomal dominant	1q31–32	abnormal calcium channels	very rare	age 5–30, usually in 2nd decade	paralysis occurring after carbohydrate consumption or physical activity	persistent, often slowly developing permanent myopathy and weakness

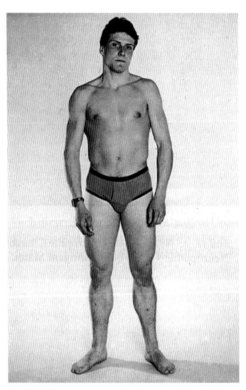

Fig. 14.**8 Thomsen congenital myotonia** in a 20-year-old man. The patient is of athletic build and has normal muscle strength, but active muscle contraction during the physical examination is followed by marked myotonia. (From: Mumenthaler M.: *Didaktischer Atlas der klinischen Neurologie.* 2nd edn, Springer, Heidelberg 1986.)

Diseases Mainly Causing Myotonia

Congenital Myotonia

Congenital myotonia has both dominant (**Thomsen**) and recessive (**Becker**) forms. Both are due to a genetic defect on chromosome 7q35 that impairs the transporting ability of chloride channels.

Clinical manifestations. The most prominent manifestation is *myotonia*, i. e., markedly slowed muscle relaxation after active contraction. A tightly grasped object can be let go again only after a delay. The patient cannot make any sudden movements, but the movements do become more fluid after a few attempts (the *warming-up phenomenon*). Raw muscle strength may be transiently diminished after a powerful contraction (= *myotonic paralysis*) but is otherwise normal. There is no atrophy; on the contrary, patients often have a markedly athletic habitus (Fig. 14.**8**). In the Becker form, the myotonic manifestations are more severe and mild distal atrophy may be present in the late stage of the disease.

Diagnostic evaluation. Tonic muscle relaxation and transient indentations of muscle, the key features of myotonia, can be seen after a contraction induced by a tap or electrical stimulation of the muscle (Fig. 14.**9**). The diagnosis is confirmed by the typical electromyographic findings (Fig. 14.**10**).

Treatment. Antiarrhythmic drugs such as procainamide and mexitil, antiepileptic drugs such as phenytoin, or acetazolamide can be used.

Prognosis. The prognosis is favorable, in that the severity of disease manifestations tends to lessen over the years and the life expectancy is normal.

Other Diseases with Myotonic Manifestations

Other diseases with myotonic manifestations are listed in Table 14.**4**. Curschmann–Steinert myotonic dystrophy is described above on p. 268; a few more rare diseases are described in the following paragraphs.

Proximal myotonic myopathy (PROMM). In this disease, *mainly proximal muscle atrophy* (particularly of the thigh muscles) is accompanied by *mild myotonia*. Cardiac arrhythmias and cataracts may also be present. The progression of the disease, and the impairment that it causes, are mild. The responsible gene is located on chromosome 3q.

Neuromyotonia is also known as the syndrome of continuous muscle fiber activity and as Isaacs syndrome. Its characteristic feature is *continuous stiffness of the musculature, with myokymia.* The patient's movements are correspondingly viscous. The EMG reveals continuous spontaneous muscle activity. This disease can arise at any age and is thought to be due to an autoimmune process. Antiepileptic drugs are an effective form of treatment, as is plasmapheresis in some patients.

"Stiff man" syndrome is also characterized by *continuous muscle fiber activity*, as revealed by EMG. The muscles are stiff and subject to *painful spasms*, which worsen in response to external stimuli and emotional stress. The disease manifestations progress slowly over months or years. Here, too, the pathogenesis is thought to be autoimmune. Effective treatments include diazepam, antiepileptic drugs, baclofen, and immunoglobulins.

Diseases Causing Periodic Paralysis

The genetically determined periodic paralyses are characterized by suddenly arising abnormalities of the serum potassium concentration leading to transient inexcitability of the muscle fiber membrane and therefore to muscle dysfunction. They share the following clinical features:

- *episodes of paralysis of sudden onset*, of varying severity and duration, which may last for hours to days;
- usually, sparing of the facial and respiratory muscles;
- in some patients, permanent muscle weakness later on in the course of the disease.

There are **normokalemic, hyperkalemic,** and **hypokalemic types** (Fig. 14.**4**). We will describe only the last-named type here as a paradigmatic example.

Hypokalemic Periodic Paralysis

Pathogenesis. This is a disease of autosomal dominant inheritance caused by dysfunction of the dihydropyridine-sensitive calcium channels in the transverse tubular system of muscle fibers. These channels are encoded by a gene on chromosome 1q31–32. The disease has higher penetrance in men.

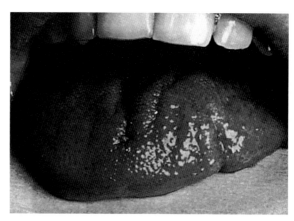

Fig. 14.**9 Myotonic reaction of the tongue musculature** in Steinert myotonic dystrophy. Repeated tapping of the edge of the tongue (here, the left edge) produces a lasting indentation. (From: Mumenthaler M.: *Didaktischer Atlas der klinischen Neurologie.* 2nd edn, Springer, Heidelberg 1986.)

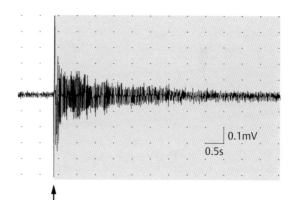

muscle percussion

Fig. 14.**10 Electromyogram in a 29-year-old woman with Steinert myotonic dystrophy.** Tapping on the thenar muscles evokes long-lasting high-frequency electrical activity, whose amplitude dies down slowly.

Clinical manifestations. The initial *paralytic attacks* occur between the ages of five and 30, usually in the second decade of life. Their frequency is highly variable, ranging from daily attacks in some patients to a few attacks per year in others. Each attack lasts from a few hours to an entire day.

Diagnostic evaluation. The CK is usually normal. The EMG during an attack reveals only a few low-voltage potentials, or none at all. There are flat T and U waves in the ECG. Rare symptomatic (nonfamiliar) cases have been described in persons with hypothyroidism.

Treatment. The prognosis of each individual attack is good. The frequency of attacks can be reduced by a low-salt and low-carbohydrate diet, as well as by potassium supplementation. Intravenous administration of potassium shortens the duration of an attack.

Diseases of Muscle

14

Metabolic Myopathies

Normal muscle function depends on an adequate supply and continuous regeneration of the energetic molecule ATP. ATP can be derived from a number of different sources; glycogen and lipid metabolism, and normal mitochondrial function, play a central role in these processes. Insufficient availability of energy to muscle tissue results in **exercise-induced muscle weakness**, **myalgias**, and, in the later course of disease, **contractures**. The underlying metabolic disorder is usually due to an **inherited enzyme defect**. The major clinical entities of this type are the **glycogenoses, carnitine deficiency**, and the group of **mitochondrial (encephalo-)myopathies** (with dysfunction either of the tricarbonic acid cycle, or of the respiratory chain and oxidative phosphorylation).

These metabolic diseases often do not become apparent until adolescence or young adulthood. The following findings suggest the presence of one of these conditions:

- *Muscle exercise* is followed by *muscle weakness, myalgias, and/or contractures*. Rhabdomyolysis sometimes occurs, causing myoglobinuria and an elevated CK concentration.
- *Permanent muscle atrophy and weakness* may develop over time.
- *The serum CK concentration is often elevated and* sometimes the lactate concentration as well (particularly in mitochondrial diseases).
- The EMG is usually normal; only in rare cases is there any evidence of myopathy.
- Muscle exercise under ischemic conditions normally leads to a fourfold rise of the lactate concentration. This rise does not occur in persons suffering from one of the glycogenoses. If, on the other hand, an exaggerated rise is found after only mild exertion, a mitochondrial disease is probably present.

The individual types of metabolic myopathy are summarized in Table 14.5. In the following paragraphs, we will discuss only rhabdomyolysis and the mitochondrial encephalomyopathies in detail.

Acute Rhabdomyolysis

Rhabdomyolysis is the **acute destruction of skeletal muscle tissue**, resulting in the passage of myoglobin into the bloodstream and a marked rise of the serum CK concentration. There are both *idiopathic* forms, with an *autosomal dominant* inheritance pattern, and *symptomatic* forms of rhabdomyolysis, caused either by toxic influences—e. g., the consumption of alcohol, heroin, or certain medications, such as statins—or by a disease of muscle metabolism, e. g., one of the glycogenoses. Rhabdomyolysis can thus be the symptomatic expression of a wide variety of pathological processes.

Clinical manifestations. The patient develops *rapidly worsening muscle pain and weakness*. Examination reveals loss of reflexes and often muscle swelling; urinalysis reveals myoglobinuria. There is no sensory deficit. The most feared complication is acute renal failure.

Treatment. If the patient has myoglobinuria, optimal hydration is given to prevent renal failure. If renal failure nevertheless occurs, dialysis is necessary.

Mitochondrial Encephalomyopathies

Mitochondrial function. Mitochondria are present in every cell of the body; they are the sites of pyruvate, fatty acid, and amino acid metabolism. These processes result in the production of ATP, an essential energy carrier for cellular metabolism and muscle contraction.

Table 14.**5**   **Metabolic myopathies with exercise-induced manifestations**

Group of diseases	Enzyme defect	Clinical manifestations	Diagnostic evaluation
Glycogen metabolism	phosphorylase phosphorylase kinase phosphofructokinase phosphoglycerate kinase	exercise-induced weakness, myalgias, contractures, and sometimes myoglobinuria, even after brief exertion	lactate ischemia test electromyography muscle biopsy with histochemistry biochemical study of muscle DNA analysis
Lipid metabolism	carnitine deficiency carnitine palmitoyl transferase deficiency	exercise-induced weakness, myalgias, and sometimes myoglobinuria, with prolonged muscle activity	muscle biopsy with histochemistry and perhaps biochemical analysis; in carnitine deficiency, the serum carnitine concentration is low
Mitochondrial myopathies	decoupling of oxidative phosphorylation defects of the tricarbonic acid cycle defects of the respiratory chain	muscle involvement almost always includes progressive external ophthalmoplegia; the brain is usually involved as well	serum lactate concentration, muscle biopsy with electron microscopy and biochemical analysis, DNA analysis
Purine nucleotide cycle	myoadenylate deaminase	rarely clinically relevant, exercise intolerance	absence of rise in ammonia concentration with exercise

The mitochondrial genome. Mitochondria have two copies of the nuclear DNA (nDNA) at their disposal, but also multiple copies of their own mitochondrial DNA (mtDNA). Mitochondrial DNA is transmitted from generation to generation through the oocyte, independently of the nuclear genome. Thus, mitochondrial diseases caused by mtDNA defects are inherited in a maternal pattern.

General clinical manifestations of mitochondrial disease. Disturbances of mitochondrial metabolism impair the function of nearly all cells in the body. Muscle and brain cells are particularly strongly affected because of their high-energy requirements. Thus, mitochondrial diseases often express themselves clinically as an *encephalomyopathy*. The typical clinical features are summarized in Table 14.**6**.

Examples of Mitochondrial Myopathies

Progressive external ophthalmoplegia usually has its onset in adulthood and progresses very slowly. Its typical features are *progressive ptosis and restriction of ocular motility*, so that, in the end, all movements of the eyes are impossible. Skeletal muscle biopsy with Gomori trichrome staining reveals accumulations of mitochondria in so-called "*ragged red fibers.*" The condition can appear as a familial disease of maternal inheritance or as a component of Kearns–Sayre syndrome (see below).

Kearns–Sayre syndrome (KSS) is characterized by *progressive external ophthalmoplegia* combined with retinal pigment degeneration and an intracardiac conduction defect. There may be further clinical manifestations as well (cf. Table 14.**6**). KSS is usually familial and is due to a point mutation in the mitochondrial DNA.

MELAS syndrome consists of mitochondrial **m**yopathy, **e**ncephalopathy, **la**ctic acidosis, and "**s**trokelike epi-

Table 14.**6**   Clinical manifestations of mitochondrial diseases

Organ	Manifestation
Muscle	myopathy with ragged red fibers progressive external ophthalmoplegia exercise intolerance
Nervous system	myoclonus and generalized seizures stroke in younger individuals ataxia dementia polyneuropathy deafness optic neuropathy migraine basal ganglionic calcification (Fahr syndrome) dystonia elevated CSF protein concentration
Eye	retinitis pigmentosa cataract
Heart	cardiomyopathy conduction abnormalities
Gastrointestinal system	intestinal pseudoobstruction diarrhea
Endocrine system	short stature diabetes goiter hypogonadism
Skin	multiple lipomas ichthyosis

sodes." It presents in childhood with transient cerebral ischemia, episodic vomiting, and often, later, dementia. The serum lactic acid concentration is elevated.

MERRF syndrome (**m**yoclonus **e**pilepsy with **r**agged **r**ed **f**ibers) is a rare syndrome characterized by myoclonus, generalized epileptic seizures, myopathy, and dementia.

Myositis

Myositis is an **infectious or inflammatory disease of muscle**. The various types of myositis include:
- **autoimmune diseases affecting muscle**, either as the major disease manifestation (as in polymyositis, which sometimes affects the skin as well = dermatomyositis) or as an accompanying manifestation in a larger syndrome;
- muscle involvement by a **primary, systemic, noninfectious, chronic inflammatory disease;**
- **direct infection of muscle** (infectious myositis).

The most important types of myositis are listed in Table 14.**7**.

General clinical manifestations. The common features of infectious and inflammatory myopathies are:
- usually symmetrical muscle involvement;
- usually very rapid progression, within a few months;
- sometimes, local pain;
- lack of a sensory deficit;
- sometimes, very high serum CK concentration;
- lack of a family history.

In this chapter, we will restrict ourselves to a description of polymyositis and dermatomyositis.

Polymyositis and Dermatomyositis

Epidemiology. The incidence of these conditions is low: they strike only five to 10 per 100 000 individuals per year. Women are more commonly affected. The disease usually appears either before puberty or around age 40.

Diseases of Muscle

14

Table 14.**7** **Infectious and inflammatory myopathies (myositides)**

Autoimmune inflammatory disorders mainly affecting muscle	dermatomyositis and polymyositis in adults dermatomyositis and polymyositis in children dermatomyositis and polymyositis accompanying malignancy inclusion body myositis myofasciitis with macrophages
Autoimmune inflammatory disorders affecting muscle as well as other organ systems	scleroderma Sjögren syndrome systemic lupus erythematosus rheumatoid arthritis mixed collagenosis (mixed connective tissue disease, Sharp syndrome) periarteritis nodosa Behçet disease
Other noninfectious myositides	giant cell myositis diffuse fasciitis with eosinophilia eosinophilic polymyositis polymyalgia rheumatica sarcoidosis myositis in Crohn disease myositis ossificans myosclerosis
Infectious myositides	viral (e. g., influenza virus) bacterial borrelial fungal protozoal helminthic

Pathogenesis. Humoral factors play a role in dermatomyositis, while cellular immune mechanisms are involved in pure polymyositis.

Clinical manifestations. The illness often begins with *constitutional symptoms* such as fatigue, myalgias, joint pain, and sometimes even fever. Thereafter, a *usually symmetrical, mainly proximal muscle weakness* develops. Patients have difficulty rising from a squatting position, getting up from a chair, or raising the arms above the horizontal position. The muscles are often *tender to pressure.* The symptoms and signs progress rapidly over a few weeks or months. About one-third of patients suffer from *dysphagia*, which may result in *aspiration pneumonia.* If the skin is involved as well (**dermatomyositis**), it is discolored to a reddish-purple hue. The discoloration may involve the face in "butterfly" fashion (nose and both cheeks), or it may be visible on the chest, on the dorsum of the hand, or around the fingernails. Subcutaneous calcinosis, joint pain, joint effusions (rare), and Raynaud-like phenomena may also be present. The heart may be involved (extrasystole, heart failure). When polymyositis appears as a component of a collagenosis (Table 14.**7**) ("*overlap syndrome*"), other organs are affected as well. The only other disease affecting both the muscles and the skin is scleroderma.

Diagnostic evaluation. Ancillary testing is usually necessary. The *serum CK concentration* is elevated to 10 times the normal value or more, at least initially. The *EMG* reveals markedly shortened, low, polyphasic potentials, to a highly variable degree in different portions of the same muscle. Pathological spontaneous activity and denervation potentials are also present. Muscle biopsy typically reveals diffusely distributed muscle necrosis and inflammatory infiltrates.

Treatment. Children tend to respond well to treatment with *corticosteroids.* Adults often require treatment with other immunosuppressive drugs, usually *azathioprine. Immunoglobulins* are beneficial in the initial stage of treatment but must always be supplemented with corticosteroids or immune suppressants over the course of time.

Other Diseases Affecting Muscle

Myopathies Due to Systemic Disease

A variety of general medical conditions cause muscle weakness, among them certain **endocrinopathies** (hypo- and hyperthyroidism, hyper- and hypoparathyroidism, Cushing disease, Addison disease). **Paraneoplastic syndromes** causing muscle weakness include paraneoplastic poly- and dermatomyositis, as well as Lambert–Eaton syndrome, in which neuromuscular transmission is impaired (p. 277). Among the **electrolyte disorders**, hyper- and hypokalemia (not of genetic origin) can cause muscle weakness, as can medications such as colchicine, chloroquine, fluorocortisone, and antilipemic agents. **Toxic substances** such as gasoline vapor and toluene can produce rhabdomyolysis (be aware of recreational sniffing as a possible cause!), while alcohol can produce an acute alcoholic myopathy. **Malnutrition**, e. g., in prison camps, can lead to myastheniform disturbances, and **vitamin E deficiency** can lead to severe myopathy.

Congenital Myopathies

A number of types of congenital myopathy have been described and the genetic basis of some of them is now known. Their common features are:
- markedly reduced muscle tone from infancy onward;
- delayed motor development;
- later, mainly proximal muscle weakness;
- often, generally diminished muscle bulk;

- often, a narrow head with a raised, "Gothic" palate and possibly other skeletal deformities;
- slow progression, or none;
- sometimes, cardiomyopathy and/or dementia.

Table 14.**8** contains a list of congenital myopathies classified by the histopathological findings of muscle biopsy.

Table 14.**8** Congenital myopathies
Central core myopathy
Nemaline (rod) myopathy
Centronuclear myopathy
Multicore myopathy
Fingerprint body myopathy
Sarcotubular myopathy
Hyaline body myopathy (= myopathy with disintegration of myofibrils in type I fibers)

Disturbances of Neuromuscular Transmission–Myasthenic Syndromes

> The myasthenic syndromes are characterized by **abnormal fatigability of muscle.** The weakness may affect individual muscle groups in more or less isolated fashion, or, alternatively, all of the muscles of the body. Pathophysiologically speaking, these conditions are due to a **disturbance of impulse transmission at the motor end plate**, usually because of an underlying **autoimmune disorder.** For example, the most common myasthenic syndrome, **myasthenia gravis**, is due to the destruction of acetylcholine receptors on the postsynaptic membrane by cross-reacting autoantibodies.

The cellular processes involved in impulse transmission at the motor end plate are discussed on p. 263 and shown pictorially in Fig. 14.**2**. Theoretically speaking, these processes were impaired in a number of different ways:

- inadequate synthesis of acetylcholine, or defective storage of acetylcholine in axon terminals;
- inadequate release of acetylcholine from axon terminals;
- impaired transport of acetylcholine in the synaptic cleft;
- impaired binding of acetylcholine to its specific receptors on the postsynaptic membrane.

The last-named mechanism is at work in the commonest and clinically most important type of myasthenia, namely, myasthenia gravis. In Lambert–Eaton syndrome (p. 277), on the other hand, the underlying problem is inadequate release of acetylcholine from the presynaptic membrane.

Myasthenia Gravis

Epidemiology. The incidence of this disorder is one to four per 100 000 individuals per year; its prevalence in the general population is 140 per million. Women are more commonly affected, in a female-to-male ratio of 3:2. The onset of the disease is usually in the second through fourth decade of life in women, but in the sixth decade in men. In principle, however, myasthenia gravis can appear at any age.

It is not uncommon for myasthenia gravis to be accompanied by certain other diseases: thymoma occurs in about 15% of patients with the disease, hyperthyroidism in 5%, hypothyroidism likewise in 5%, and polyarthritis in 4%.

Pathophysiology. Three-quarters of all patients with myasthenia gravis have hyperplasia of the thymus and 15% harbor a thymoma. Antibodies are generated against the myoid cells of the thymus; owing to a misdirection of the immune response, these antibodies also attack the acetylcholine receptors of the motor end plate. **Acetylcholine receptor antibodies** are present in the serum in elevated concentration in a large majority of patients with generalized myasthenia. If the serum of an affected patient is injected into an experimental animal, the animal develops a myasthenic syndrome. The antibodies can be transmitted across the placenta from a myasthenic mother to her child (see below). They are highly heterogeneous and bind to the acetylcholine receptor at a number of different locations.

Clinical manifestations. The clinical features of myasthenia are summarized in Table 14.**9**. The most prominent manifestation is **abnormal fatigability of muscle**. Initially, the muscles most obviously affected are those that carry out very fine movements and that accordingly contain unusually small motor units. These are the muscles that react most strongly to a decline in acetylcholine receptor density, i. e., the extraocular muscles, the levator palpebrae m., and the muscles of mastication and deglutition. Thus, the early manifestations of myasthenia gravis often include *diplopia, ptosis, dysphagia* with frequent aspiration, and *difficulty chewing food.* Nevertheless, practically any other muscle group can be involved, even at the onset of the disease. The disease manifestations worsen over the course of the day and are worst in the evening. Repeated activation of an affected muscle group leads to rapidly worsening weakness. This phenomenon forms the basis of a number of clinical diagnostic tests.

Diagnostic evaluation. Myasthenic ptosis worsens visibly over the course of a single minute if the patient rapidly and repeatedly closes and opens the eyes, or looks upward for a prolonged period (the **Simpson test**, Fig. 14.**11**).

Diseases of Muscle

14

Table 14.**9**   **Clinical features of myasthenia**

- Progressive weakness of individual muscles
- The weakness increases on rapid, repeated contraction of the affected muscles
- Recovery within minutes, or a fraction of an hour, at rest
- The weakness usually worsens toward evening
- The eye muscles are often affected first (ptosis, diplopia), or else the pharyngeal muscles (dysphagia, nasal speech)
- Variably severe weakness of muscles belonging to different motor units
- Occasionally, crises with sudden deterioration of muscle strength
- No atrophy or fasciculations
- More or less complete resolution of disease manifestations after the administration of a cholinesterase inhibitor, e. g., test injection of edrophonium chloride I.V. (Tensilon test)
- Usually, elevated serum titer of antibodies against the acetylcholine receptor (though this is a rare finding in ocular myasthenia)

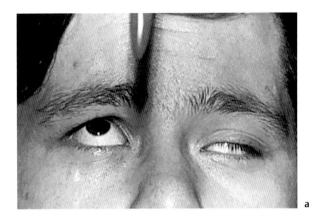

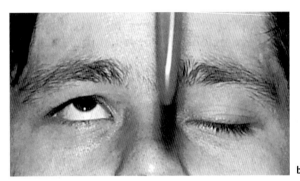

Fig. 14.**11   Myasthenia of the extraocular muscles and a Simpson test** in a 23-year-old man. The left ptosis **(a)**, becomes increasingly evident on looking up repeatedly in rapid succession—this is a maneuver that activates the levator palpebrae muscle **(b)**. (From: Mumenthaler M.: *Didaktischer Atlas der klinischen Neurologie*. 2nd edn, Springer, Heidelberg 1986.)

Further diagnostic tests serve to confirm the clinical diagnosis. In the **Tensilon test**, 10 mg of the acetylcholinesterase inhibitor edrophonium chloride are injected intravenously over 10 seconds. This drug inhibits the breakdown of acetylcholine in the synaptic cleft, so that acetylcholine is available to its receptors on the muscle cell membrane for a longer time and the deleterious effect of diminished receptor density is counteracted. An improvement is seen within 30 seconds and lasts for about three minutes. A marked ptosis, for example, can transiently disappear.

When a motor nerve is repeatedly stimulated, the **electromyogram** recorded from the corresponding muscle through a surface electrode reveals a progressive fall-off (*decrement*) in the amplitude of the muscle potential (Fig. 14.**12**).

Antibodies against the acetylcholine receptor are demonstrable in the serum of 85 % of patients with myasthenia gravis. They are not found, however, in 50 % of patients with the purely ocular form, as well as in about

15 % of patients with generalized myasthenia (see below). A *chest CT or MRI* must be performed to disclose or rule out a thymoma. *Other diseases* that can mimic or accompany myasthenia must be sought and excluded as well (see below).

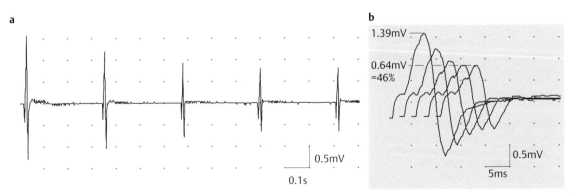

Fig. 14.**12 Electromyogram of a 59-year-old man with ocular myasthenia.** Electrical activity is recorded from the nasalis m. on repetitive stimulation of the facial n. in the stylomastoid fossa (frequency of stimulation, 3 Hz). The EMG tracing is shown in **a**. In **b**, the same curve is shown on an expanded time scale, and the responses to successive stimuli are superimposed. The summed muscle potential diminishes from one stimulus to the next; the response to the fifth stimulus is 54 % smaller than the initial response. Normally there should be no more than a 10 % diminution in amplitude.

Classification. Myasthenia can be subdivided into a number of stages depending on the extent and severity of muscle involvement. Ossermann classification has four main stages and is reproduced in Table 14.**10**.

Spontaneous course. The severity of the disease manifestations fluctuates markedly without treatment, even over longer periods. Spontaneous remissions may be long lasting, but true spontaneous cures are rare. The eyes are initially affected in 50% of patients and are eventually affected at some point in 90%. Myasthenic manifestations remain confined to the eyes in 16% (ocular myasthenia). Generalization of manifestations from the eyes to the rest of the body, if it occurs, usually occurs within three years of onset. Transient neonatal myasthenia, caused by placental transmission of antibodies from a myasthenic mother to her child, rarely lasts longer than two weeks.

Treatment. Cholinesterase inhibitors improve the disease manifestations by delaying the breakdown of acetylcholine and thereby prolonging its effect on the remaining functional acetylcholine receptors of the muscle fiber membrane. *Pyridostigmine* is given several times a day in individual doses of 10 to 60 mg.

Immune therapies with short-lasting effect are used to treat acute exacerbations of myasthenia gravis with impending respiratory failure (myasthenic crises). These include *plasmapheresis* and *intravenous immunoglobulins*. *Corticosteroids* and other im*mune suppressants*, e. g., azathioprine, are given chronically to influence the disease process in the long term. Most patients with myasthenia gravis need these drugs. Steroid treatment can transiently worsen the manifestations of disease and should therefore be initiated very slowly or during an in-patient hospitalization. It usually takes two to four weeks for the positive effect to appear.

Thymectomy should be considered for every patient with myasthenia: the operation brings cures, or at least substantially improves, of myasthenia in 80% of operated patients, after a latency period of several months or years. There is little controversy regarding the indication for thymectomy in patients below age 60, except for those with the mild ocular form of the disease. Good results have also been obtained in older patients. A *thymoma*, if present, must be surgically removed whatever the age of the patient. Adjuvant radiotherapy must be given if the resection is subtotal, because 25% of these tumors undergo malignant degeneration. The operative approach should be chosen to allow the surgeon to inspect the mediastinum thoroughly, so that the thymus or thymoma can be completely resected.

Complications. Patients in the midst of a myasthenic crisis may require such high doses of cholinesterase inhibitors that they develop toxic manifestations such as nausea, diaphoresis, abdominal cramps, excessive tracheobronchial secretions, agitation, and anxiety. This syndrome is referred to, somewhat simplistically, as a **cholinergic crisis**. Long-term immunosuppressive therapy can also cause complications, including leukopenia, increased susceptibility to infections, etc.

Table 14.**10** **Ossermann classification of myasthenia**

I	Ocular myasthenia, i. e., limited to the eye muscles
IIa	Mild generalized myasthenia
IIb	Moderately severe generalized myasthenia, not involving muscles of respiration
III	Acute, rapidly progressive myasthenia, beginning abruptly and progressing to involve the muscles of respiration within 6 months of onset
IV	Chronic, severe myasthenia; may develop from previous Class I or Class II disease after two years of a relatively stable course
	Patients in Classes III and IV are subject to higher mortality and suffer more frequently from thymoma

Seronegative myasthenia gravis and anti-MuSK antibodies. About 70% of "seronegative" myasthenia gravis patients have antibodies to muscle-specific receptor typrosine kinase (MuSK). These patients are typically women under age 40 at disease onset in whom the cranial and bulbar muscles are severely affected. They often suffer from respiratory crises. Anticholinesterase drugs often yield no useful benefit and may even worsen the manifestations of disease. Thymectomy is also of no benefit. Immunosuppressive therapy, however, is usually effective, just as it is in seropositive myasthenia gravis.

Lambert–Eaton Syndrome

Etiology and pathogenesis. The clinical manifestations of this disease are caused by antibodies against voltage-sensitive calcium channels in the motor nerve terminals at the motor end plate. Inactivation of these channels lessens the calcium influx induced by an incoming action potential and therefore results in the release of inadequate amounts of acetylcholine from the nerve terminal. The *impairment of neuromuscular transmission* in Lambert–Eaton syndrome is therefore *located in the presynaptic cell* (unlike myasthenia gravis). The underlying etiology in two-thirds of patients is a small-cell carcinoma of the lung: voltage-sensitive calcium channels on the cell membranes of the carcinoma cells initiate a misdirected autoimmune response. In cases of nonneoplastic origin, Lambert–Eaton syndrome is often seen in combination with other autoimmune conditions, such as pernicious anemia, hypo- or hyperthyroidism, myasthenia gravis, Sjögren syndrome, and others. The thymus is not enlarged.

Clinical manifestations. The hallmark of this condition is *weakness* and, above all, *abnormal fatigability of the muscles*, predominantly in the pelvic girdle and lower limbs. The extraocular muscles and the levator palpebrae m. are sometimes mildly affected. Muscular strength transiently *increases*, at first, with exercise. The intrinsic muscle reflexes are often absent and many patients complain of dry mouth or other autonomic manifestations (orthostatic hypotension, impotence).

Diseases of Muscle

14

Diagnostic evaluation. In the electromyogram, the first few muscle action potentials on repeated stimulation are low, and the subsequent ones are larger. This is particularly evident with high-frequency stimulation.

Treatment. The weakness and fatigability of muscle respond to *immunoglobulins* and *plasmapheresis*, and, in the long term, to corticosteroids and azathioprine. Cholinesterase inhibitors are not very effective.

Rare Myasthenia-like Syndromes

Hereditary myasthenic syndromes are usually of autosomal recessive inheritance. These genetic diseases may be due to either pre- or postsynaptic disturbances of neuromuscular transmission. Clinically, they are characterized by *ocular manifestations* and *generalized muscle weakness*. Cholinesterase inhibitors are therapeutically effective, as is 3,4-diaminopyridine in rare cases. *Congenital myasthenia gravis* and *familial infantile myasthenia* are hereditary syndromes whose manifestations are present over the patient's entire lifetime. The last-named disease can cause potentially lethal episodes of respiratory insufficiency in affected children, but its severity tends to lessen in later life.

"Slow channel" syndrome is of autosomal dominant inheritance. It usually becomes clinically evident in young adulthood. The underlying abnormality of neuromuscular transmission is that the cation channels of the acetylcholine receptors open too slowly. In addition to exercise-dependent muscle weakness, patients suffer from muscle atrophy. The usual treatments for myasthenia are ineffective in this disease.

Myasthenic weakness can be produced by a number of different substances, including organophosphates and penicillamine. Other substances can worsen myasthenia that is already present, such as aminoglycosides, quinine, antiarrhythmic drugs, and anticonvulsants.

15 Diseases of the Autonomic Nervous System

Anatomy

The autonomic nervous system is responsible for the neural control of all of the organs and tissues of the body whose function is involuntary. It thus innervates the internal organs of the throat, thorax, and abdomen, the blood vessels, and the lacrimal, salivary, and sweat glands (among other organs). It can be divided on structural and functional grounds into a **sympathetic** and a **parasympathetic** nervous system. These two systems largely exert mutually antagonistic effects on their target organs. The fundamental structural unit of each system is a two-neuron chain, in which the first neuron has its cell body within the central nervous system, i.e., in the brainstem or spinal cord (the **preganglionic neuron**) and the second neuron has its cell body in an autonomic ganglion or plexus (the **postganglionic neuron**). The hypothalamus is the "command center" of the autonomic nervous system: it exerts a major degree of control on both sympathetic and parasympathetic activity. **Diseases of the autonomic nervous system** very often manifest themselves in the form of disturbances of sweating, impairment of bladder, bowel, and sexual function, orthostatic hypotension, and Horner syndrome.

Sympathetic nervous system. The cell bodies of the preganglionic neurons lie in the lateral horns of the spinal cord at levels T1 to L2/3 (the *intermediolateral nucleus*; the entire system is thus sometimes called the **thoracolumbar system**). These cell bodies receive neural input from the hypothalamus, whose efferent projection (the central sympathetic pathway) descends through the brainstem and down the spinal cord to the sympathetic nuclei within the cord. The axons of the preganglionic neurons exit the spinal cord in the *anterior roots* and then travel by way of the *rami communicantes* into the *sympathetic chain*, which lies lateral to

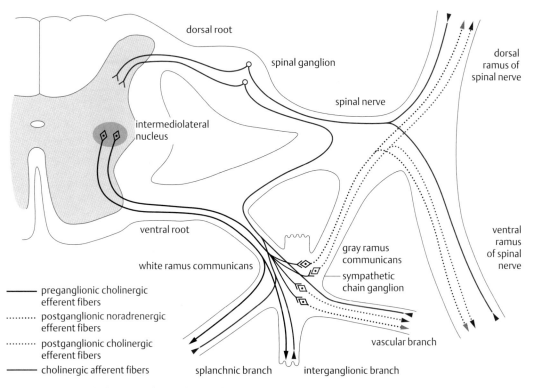

- preganglionic cholinergic efferent fibers
- postganglionic noradrenergic efferent fibers
- postganglionic cholinergic efferent fibers
- cholinergic afferent fibers

dorsal root
spinal ganglion
spinal nerve
dorsal ramus of spinal nerve
intermediolateral nucleus
ventral root
ventral ramus of spinal nerve
white ramus communicans
gray ramus communicans
sympathetic chain ganglion
vascular branch
splanchnic branch
interganglionic branch

Fig. 15.**1 Anatomy of the sympathetic efferent fibers leaving the spinal cord.** The sudomotor fibers accompany the spinal nerves (dorsal and ventral rami) to their areas of cutaneous distribution, while the autonomic fibers to the blood vessels and internal organs follow their own paths to their respective targets (vascular ramus, splanchnic ramus).

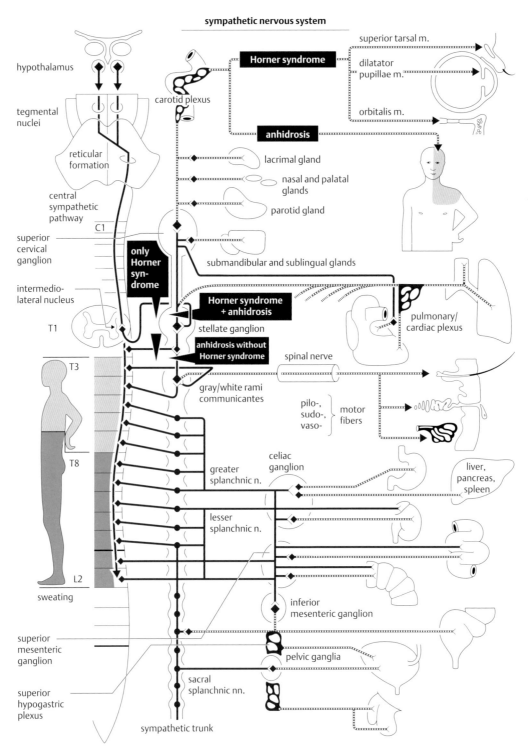

sympathetic nervous system

hypothalamus

tegmental nuclei

reticular formation

central sympathetic pathway

C1

superior cervical ganglion

intermedio-lateral nucleus

T1

T3

T8

L2

sweating

superior mesenteric ganglion

superior hypogastric plexus

sympathetic trunk

carotid plexus

Horner syndrome

only Horner syn-drome

Horner syndrome + anhidrosis

stellate ganglion

anhidrosis without Horner syndrome

spinal nerve

gray/white rami communicantes

greater splanchnic n.

lesser splanchnic n.

sacral splanchnic nn.

anhidrosis

superior tarsal m.

dilatator pupillae m.

orbitalis m.

lacrimal gland

nasal and palatal glands

parotid gland

submandibular and sublingual glands

pulmonary/cardiac plexus

pilo-, sudo-, vaso- motor fibers

celiac ganglion

liver, pancreas, spleen

inferior mesenteric ganglion

pelvic ganglia

Fig. 15.**2 Anatomy of the sympathetic nervous system.**

the spinal cord and consists of a chainlike arrangement of ganglia and the fibrous connections between them (interganglionic branches). Some of the fibers form a synapse with a postganglionic neuron inside the sympathetic chain, while others ascend the entire sympathetic chain without a synapse, not meeting their corresponding postganglionic neuron till they have arrived in the

vicinity of the target organ (either in an *autonomic plexus* or in an *intramural ganglion,* i. e., a ganglion located within the wall of the organ in question). The postganglionic neurons project efferent fibers to the target tissue, e. g., the smooth muscle of the internal organs and blood vessels, and various glands. The relationship of the sympathetic fibers exiting the spinal cord to the

parasympathetic nervous system

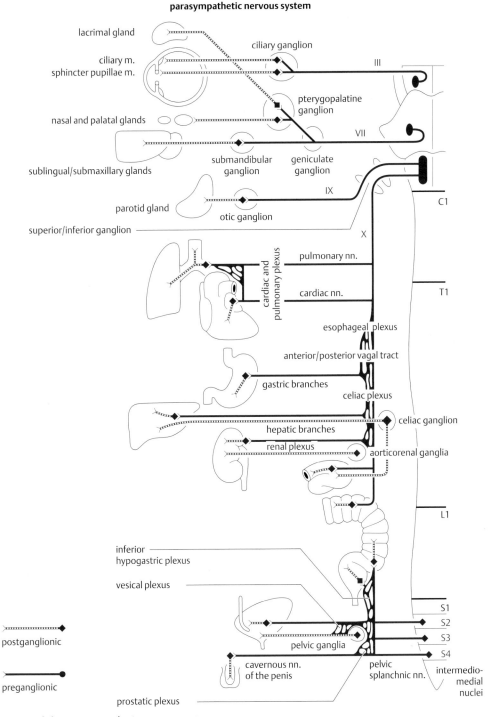

Fig. 15.**3 Anatomy of the parasympathetic nervous system.**

nerve roots, sympathetic chain, and peripheral nerves is depicted in Fig. 15.**1**, while Fig. 15.**2** provides an overview of the anatomy of the sympathetic nervous system.

Parasympathetic nervous system. The preganglionic neurons of the parasympathetic nervous system, unlike those of the sympathetic nervous system, are located in two parts of the central nervous system that lie at a con-

siderable distance from each other. Some of the preganglionic neurons lie in the visceral motor and visceral sensory *brainstem nuclei*, the remainder in the *lateral horns of spinal cord segments S2–S4* (the **craniosacral system**). The axons of the cranial preganglionic neurons exit the brainstem in *cranial nerves III, VII, IX, and X* and then travel onward to *parasympathetic ganglia* in the periphery, some of which are intramural, i. e., already located in the wall of the target organ; inside the parasympathetic ganglia, the preganglionic fibers form synapses onto the postganglionic neurons. The parasympathetic fibers of cranial nerves III, VII, and IX innervate the smooth musculature and glands of the head, while those of the vagus n. descend in an extensively branched fiber system to innervate the viscera of the throat, thorax, and abdomen, all the way down to the level of the left colic flexure. Beyond this point (the so-called point of Cannon and Böhm), the abdominal and pelvic viscera are innervated by the sacral portion of the parasympathetic nervous system. The axons of the preganglionic neurons whose cell bodies lie in the lateral horns of the sacral spinal cord reach the periphery by way of the *anterior roots* or the *pelvic nerves.* They form synapses onto the postganglionic neurons in the *pelvic plexus* (= inferior hypogastric plexus) and in the *intramural ganglia* of the abdominal and pelvic viscera. The anatomy of the parasympathetic nervous system is shown in Fig. 15.**3**.

Normal and Pathological Function of the Autonomic Nervous System

The sympathetic and parasympathetic nervous systems regulate the functions of the internal organs and are the substrate for all of the autonomic reflexes of the body. The neurotransmitter used at the synapses of the parasympathetic nervous system is *acetylcholine*, while the sympathetic nervous system uses *acetylcholine* at the synapse onto the preganglionic neuron, *norepinephrine* at the synapse onto the postganglionic neuron, and *epinephrine* in the adrenal cortex (whence the name, epinephrine). An overview of the major functions of the two halves of the autonomic nervous system is provided in Table 15.**1**.

In the following paragraphs, we will describe just a few, clinically relevant functional disturbances and diseases of the autonomic nervous system.

Sweating

The autonomic fibers innervating the sweat glands are exclusively sympathetic. They run in the peripheral nerves in close association with the somatosensory fibers innervating the same area of skin. A lesion of a peripheral nerve, therefore, always impairs sweating in the sensory distribution of the nerve. The impairment of sweating can be demonstrated with various tests, such as the *ninhydrin test* (Fig. 15.**4**).

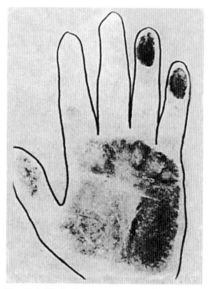

Fig. 15.**4 Ninhydrin test in a right median nerve lesion.** The patient lays his hand on a piece of paper that is subsequently "developed" with several applications of a 1% ninhydrin solution, followed by drying in a hot air chamber. Sweating is diminished or absent in the cutaneous sensory distribution of the median n.

Table 15.**1 Functions of the sympathetic and parasympathetic nervous systems**

Effect of the sympathetic nervous system	Organ	Effect of the parasympathetic nervous system
+ pupillary dilation	eye: ● dilator pupillae m. ● sphincter pupillae m.	+ pupillary constriction
+ vasoconstriction in certain areas of the body, e. g., the skin	vascular smooth muscle	− vasodilatation in certain areas of the body, e. g., gastrointestinal tract
− diminished secretion	salivary glands	+ increased secretion
+ increased secretion	sweat glands lacrimal glands glands of the GI tract	+ increased secretion + increased secretion
− diminished motility and peristalsis	smooth muscle of the GI tract	+ increased motility and peristalsis
− bronchodilation	bronchial smooth muscle	+ bronchoconstriction
+ increased heart rate	heart	− decreased heart rate
− urinary retention	smooth muscle of the vesical wall	+ micturition
+ urinary retention	sphincters	− micturition

Fig. 15.**5 Spastic neurogenic bladder.** The bladder is cut off from the influence of the CNS above the level of the lesion, but the spinal reflex arc controlling micturition is intact. It is automatically activated whenever the bladder is filled to a certain volume.

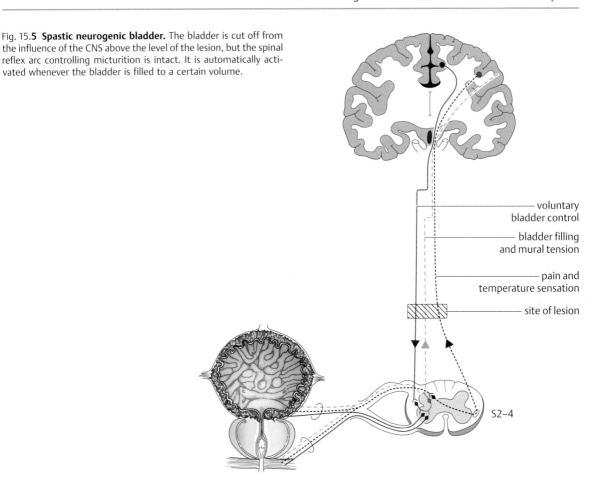

voluntary
bladder control

bladder filling
and mural tension

pain and
temperature sensation

site of lesion

S2–4

Bladder, Bowel, and Sexual Function

Anatomy. The neural elements controlling bladder, bowel, and sexual function are the following:

- **Sympathetic fibers from spinal cord segments T12–L2** and **parasympathetic fibers from spinal cord segments S2–S4** innervate the smooth muscle of the urinary bladder, rectum, and internal genitalia, including the corpora cavernosa. The sympathetic fibers travel to their target organs after a synaptic relay in the superior hypogastric plexus, while the parasympathetic fibers do so after a synaptic relay in the inferior hypogastric plexus. There are ganglion cells and synapses not just in the plexuses, but also within the walls of the target organs. Visceral sensory (afferent) fibers return to the spinal cord from the urinary bladder, genitalia, and rectum.
- The spinal center for micturition and defecation receives **supranuclear input from multiple higher cortical areas** (paracentral lobule → voluntary initiation of micturition and defecation) through a number of different pathways in the spinal cord, and it also conveys afferent information back upward to the brain (→ conscious perception of bladder filling and of noxious and thermal stimuli). These mechanisms are the basis of the voluntary control of micturition and defecation.
- The striated skeletal muscle of the pelvic floor and of the external sphincters of the bladder and rectum,

which are under voluntary control, is innervated by the **pudendal n.**, whose fibers are derived from spinal cord segments S2–S4. This nerve also conveys afferent impulses arising in the urethra, prostate gland, anal canal, and external genitalia.

Disturbances of bladder, bowel, and sexual function. The clinical manifestations depend on the site of the lesion (peripheral/central, unilateral/bilateral):

- Spinal cord transection above the sacral level cuts off the bladder and bowel from the supraspinally derived (cortical) impulses subserving the voluntary control of micturition and defecation, but all of the afferent and efferent nerve pathways of the bladder remain intact, including the spinal reflex arc for bladder emptying. The result is a **spastic (automatic) neurogenic bladder**, which empties itself reflexively whenever it is filled to a certain volume (Fig. 15.**5**). Penile erection remains possible, though there may be retrograde ejaculation into the bladder.

Lesions of the conus medullaris, cauda equina, sacral plexus, and pelvic plexus. Lesions of these structures inactivate the sacral centers for micturition and defecation. The result is **atony of the bladder and bowel musculature**, leading to severe impairment of emptying. Bladder filling can no longer be perceived, either consciously or unconsciously. Tone is preserved in the sympathetically elevated vesical sphincter; the bladder,

15

Diseases of the Autonomic Nervous System

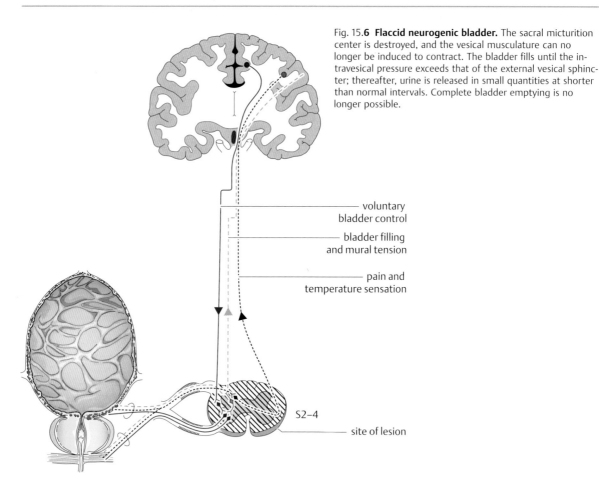

Fig. 15.**6 Flaccid neurogenic bladder.** The sacral micturition center is destroyed, and the vesical musculature can no longer be induced to contract. The bladder fills until the intravesical pressure exceeds that of the external vesical sphincter; thereafter, urine is released in small quantities at shorter than normal intervals. Complete bladder emptying is no longer possible.

voluntary
bladder control

bladder filling
and mural tension

pain and
temperature sensation

S2–4

site of lesion

therefore, continues to fill until the passive intravesical pressure overcomes the closing force of the sphincter. The continually overfilled bladder lets out small amounts of urine at short intervals (**overflow incontinence**, Fig. 15.**6**). Defecation, meanwhile, occurs passively and in uncontrolled fashion through a *patulous anal sphincter*. In the male, lesions of these structures cause **erectile impotence**. Psychosexually mediated arousal remains possible in rare cases because of the preserved sympathetic efferent innervation through the hypogastric plexus. Thus, a small number of affected men are still able to have an emission of semen, but without ejaculation, and without rhythmic contraction of the pelvic floor muscles.

Lesions of the pudendal n. An isolated lesion of the pudendal n., which contains parasympathetic fibers from segments S2–S4, causes **erectile dysfunction**: the sacral erection center can no longer be activated because its somatosensory afferent input has been interrupted. Moreover, because the somatic efferent impulses to the bulbocavernosus and ischiocavernosus mm. no longer reach their targets, the maximal tumescence of the corpora cavernosa mediated by these muscles also fails to occur.

Impairment of the sympathetic innervation of the pelvic organs can be caused, for example, by tumor infiltration or by surgical procedures. Bilateral lesions of the

sympathetic chain and lesions of the superior hypogastric plexus abolish seminal emission into the proximal urethra; if ejaculation does occur, then the semen goes into the bladder, in retrograde fashion. As long as the parasympathetic innervation of the genital organs by the pelvic plexus and their somatic sensory and motor innervation by the pudendal n. remain intact, the affected men are still able to have erections, and affected persons of both sexes can still experience pelvic floor contractions and orgasm. This constellation of symptoms (preserved ability to experience orgasm, in the absence of seminal emission) is seen in about half of all men who have undergone bilateral sympathectomy. It does not occur after unilateral lumbar sympathectomy.

The Cervical Sympathetic Pathway and Horner Syndrome

Anatomy. As already discussed at the beginning of this chapter, the spinal cord nuclei in which sympathetic impulses originate are present only from the T2 level downward. Thus, the sympathetic fibers innervating the head must ascend from the thoracic spinal cord and the thoracic segments of the sympathetic chain, by way of the interganglionic branches, to the **cervical sympathetic chain**, where they make a synaptic relay onto the second neuron in one of the three **cervical ganglia** (including the **stellate ganglion**). From these ganglia, the sympathetic fibers continue upward in **periarterial nerve plexuses** until they reach their destinations. Sympathetic fibers in the head innervate the walls of the blood vessels, the sweat glands, and the salivary, lacrimal, nasal, and palatal glands, as well as the smooth muscle of the dilator pupillae m. See also Fig. 15.**2**, p. 280.

Lesions of the cervical sympathetic pathway. Destruction of the stellate ganglion or of the cervical sympathetic chain causes **Horner syndrome**: the pupil is (unilaterally) narrow and, when the patient looks slightly downward, ptosis is evident (p. 192). Horner syndrome is usually seen in conjunction with loss of sweating on the ipsilateral upper quadrant of the body, particularly on the neck and face. Depending on the level of the lesion, the arm, hand, and axilla may be affected as well. If the sympathetic chain is interrupted immediately below the stellate ganglion, anhidrosis of the upper quadrant of the body results, but without Horner syndrome. On the other hand, isolated Horner syndrome without anhidrosis can occur as the result of a lesion of the C8–T2 nerve roots between the spinal cord and the sympathetic chain.

Generalized Autonomic Dysfunction

Polyneuropathy. Damage to autonomic fibers is often a component of polyneuropathy. Affected persons suffer from impaired regulation of blood pressure and sweat-

ing, as well as from diarrhea, urinary disturbances, and erectile dysfunction. Autonomic manifestations of these kinds are particularly common in *diabetic polyneuropathy.*

Acute pandysautonomia. This condition is due to a neuropathy affecting either preganglionic or postganglionic autonomic nerve fibers. Patients suffer from orthostatic hypotension, an invariant heart rate, a lack of sweating and lacrimation, nonreactive midsized pupils, impotence, and an atonic bladder. The etiology of this condition is not known; it gradually resolves spontaneously over the course of a few months.

Familial dysautonomia (Riley). This autosomal recessive disease is probably due to a disturbance of norepinephrine synthesis. Its manifestations, which are already evident in infancy, include dysphagia, lack of tears when the infant cries, abnormally intense sweating, diminished sensitivity to pain, and impaired temperature regulation. The prognosis is poor.

Other generalized autonomic disturbances. A number of degenerative conditions of the basal ganglia can impair autonomic function; further diseases that can affect the autonomic nervous system include *orthostatic hypotension of Shy–Drager type, botulinus intoxication,* and *congenital sensory neuropathy with anhidrosis.*

Diseases of the Autonomic Nervous System

15

Index

Entries in italics indicate figures